LABELS ON NEXT PAGE

ESSENTIALS OF COMMUNICABLE DISEASE

Essentials of communicable disease

MARY ELIZABETH McINNES
R.N., B.Sc.N., M.Sc. (Ed.)

Co-ordinator, Learning Resources Centers
for Health Sciences, Department
of Nursing, Mohawk College of Applied Arts and
Technology, Hamilton, Ontario, Canada

WITH 34 ILLUSTRATIONS

SECOND EDITION

The C. V. Mosby Company

SAINT LOUIS 1975

SECOND EDITION

Printed in the United States of America

Distributed in Great Britain by Henry Kimpton, London

Library of Congress Cataloging in Publication Data

McInnes, Mary Elizabeth, 1931-
Essentials of communicable disease.

Bibliography: p.
1. Communicable diseases. I. Title.
[DNLM: 1. Communicable diseases–Nursing. WY153 M152e]
RC111.M24 1975 616.9 74-28353
ISBN 0-8016-2545-9

VH/VH/VH 9 8 7 6 5 4 3 2 1

PREFACE

The second edition of *Essentials of Communicable Disease* maintains the original author's format; however, the information has been updated and revised into a more concise form so that the text may be used as a quick reference. Emphasis is placed on presenting basic information on the communicable diseases still surrounding us in the world today.

As this book is not an exhaustive coverage of all aspects of communicable diseases, it is suggested that it be used in conjunction with related references on microbiology, pharmacology, nursing, and nutrition when extensive detail is required.

Six basic and interlocking purposes are inherent in the development of this text. They are as follows:

1. To show that the scientific age has given us the means by which some communicable diseases may be prevented and ultimately eradicated.
2. To show that all people do not have equal opportunities to receive the help of research and scientific achievement.
3. To show how some of the unresolved problems of society affect the incidence and dissemination of communicable diseases.
4. To present nursing care that the nurse may be required to use in daily patient care for specific communicable diseases both in the hospital setting and the community.
5. To present specific information on the diseases themselves: etiology, epidemiology, incubation period, communicability period, clinical manifestations, diagnosis, treatment, prevention, and control.
6. To show how far we have come and how far we must still go to achieve prevention, control, and eventually global eradication of communicable diseases.

The overall changes in this edition include updating of all statistics, with particular emphasis on the statistics of the United States and Canada. World statistics are reported where available. New sections have been added on jet-borne communicable diseases, rashes, the common cold, roseola infantum, congenital rubella, sociological factors influencing the spread of venereal diseases, and the new role of the nurse in caring for patients with venereal diseases. Several new tables have been added and many of the old illustrations deleted to make the text a more concise, quick reference. Information has been updated on each specific disease on the topics of treatment, diagnosis, nursing care, prevention, and control.

Of particular interest to the nurse is Section One, which provides a quick overview of the role communicable diseases have played in the history of mankind. This section also deals with the past and the present scope of control over infectious diseases and the role played by public health departments, voluntary health agencies, and foundations. The science of immunology is discussed in relation to its role as a defense against infectious diseases. An attempt is made to elucidate some of the factors in our society that contribute to the incidence of communicable diseases and what such diseases mean to the psychic constitution and economic status at all levels of society. The nurse's role in caring for patients suffering from infectious diseases is discussed not only in relation to clinical manifestations and immediate patient care but also in relation to the role played in controlling the spread of diseases throughout the world.

It would be unreasonable to expect that every new case of a notifiable disease will actually be recorded. The likelihood that a particular case will be counted in official statistics depends on a variety of circumstances—the severity of the illness, the availability and accessibility of a medical practitioner, the correctness of diagnosis, and so forth. Even if every provider of health care in the country reported every observed case of a notifiable disease, the data would in many instances still not reflect the total cases occurring. Many cases of infectious diseases are never seen by a provider of health care. Subclinical cases of infectious diseases are seldom detected except in the course of special studies. Therefore a fair summary would be that the degree of reporting is influenced by (1) the nature of the disease, (2) the diagnostic and control measures available, (3) the interest and activity of health officials responsible for disease control and surveillance, and (4) monetary support.

Many persons have contributed to this revision, and special thanks and appreciation are extended to them. Acknowledgement is given to Mrs. Helen Stewart, nurse-librarian at St. Joseph's Campus, Department of Nursing, Mohawk College of Applied Arts and Technology, Hamilton, Ontario, who gave valuable assistance in locating and researching current literature.

I am indebted to the McMaster University Medical Center, Hamilton, Ontario, and to St. Joseph's Hospital, Hamilton, Ontario for the use of their libraries.

I also wish to acknowledge the contribution made by Statistics Canada, Ottawa, Ontario, and the United States Department of Health, Education, and Welfare, Center for Disease Control, Atlanta, Georgia, for the contribution of recent statistics.

Appreciation is also extended to my secretary, Miss Yoka Koelewijn, for patiently typing the manuscript.

BETTY MCINNES

CONTENTS

SECTION THREE
Viral diseases

SECTION FOUR
Arthropod-borne diseases

SECTION FIVE

Diseases caused by fungi

SECTION SIX

Helminth infections

ESSENTIALS OF COMMUNICABLE DISEASE

SECTION ONE

Introductory material

1

HISTORICAL EVENTS

Archeologists have examined the material remains of prehistoric animals and found evidence that many diseases probably existed millions of years before the earth was inhabited by man.

Prehistoric man led a nomadic way of life with almost no contact outside his own tribe. With the progress of civilization human beings began to live together in some form of organized society. Since the beginning of group life, man has waged an endless battle against the destructive forces of disease. Throughout centuries history reveals the suffering and sorrow of physical affliction.

Determination of the cause of infectious diseases was based on the prevailing theory and philosophy of the period. All civilizations throughout history had some form of religion and belief in a Supreme Being. Therefore, the cause of disease and deliverance from its scourge permeated most theories of early periods. Although the prevailing belief held that infectious disease was divine punishment for sin, emphasis was also placed on environmental causes. During some periods, the disease was attributed to celestial bodies in the heavens such as the moon, stars, and sun. The direction of the wind, rain, and floods was considered a causal factor. At other periods the miasmas, poisonous vapors arising from decaying animal and vegetable matter, were considered the cause of infectious disease. Thus man has taken the long arduous road from the world of spirits, superstition, and fallacious reasoning to that of scientific investigation and systematic inquiry. Along the way millions have perished, and noble men have sacrificed their lives in the pursuit of knowledge.

The tragedy of epidemic disease has been well documented by eminent historians. Although there is evidence that epidemics of infectious disease existed centuries before Christ, there is limited information concerning them. From the fourteenth to the twentieth centuries there were regular, relentless, and destructive visitations of great epidemics and pandemics of infectious disease. The peoples of Asia, Europe, the British Isles, and the United States lived with the constant fear of disease and death. The sciences of bacteriology and epidemiology were unknown, and Jenner, Pasteur, Lister, and Koch were unborn; therefore, the causes and the methods of the spread of infectious diseases remained a mystery.

The great epidemics and pandemics of earlier periods have passed into oblivion; however, in many parts of the world infectious disease continues to flourish and take its toll of human lives. The modern means of transportation have closed the distance between countries, and a catastrophic epidemic of infectious disease is a constant threat. No country is safe until all are safe. Efforts are being made by the United States, assisted by other countries, to eradicate poverty, unsanitary conditions, and ignorance in countries where infectious diseases are prevalent.

Many historians have focused attention upon the great epidemics resulting in wanton destruction of human life. Frequently, less attention has been given to the concomitant effects suffered by society. The entire social order was affected by the great epidemics of the period. Death may have been a welcome relief from disease and suffering, but thousands were left incapacitated and unable to pursue their normal activities. The fields lay untended and crops unharvested, shops and businesses were closed, commerce and trade were restricted, education was interrupted, and the orderly procedure of courts and justice became disorganized. Lawlessness and crime increased, titles to property were lost, and the master frequently lost control over the serf.

When disease became epidemic, thousands fled to other towns and the country, which often only served to spread the disease. Many towns would not permit persons to enter if they came from areas where epidemic disease existed. As a rule only the most affluent were able to leave. The poor were left to the ravages of the scourge or to death from starvation. Fear was so great that men would offer no help to neighbors lest they contract the disease, and friends lay dying in the street while others passed by at great distance. During the great epidemics of plague, entire families perished and their property was seized by others. Politicians frequently sought to conceal the existence of disease, but when this was no longer possible, they also fled from the scene of death and destruction.

Regardless of the lack of knowledge concerning the cause of disease, the foundations for public health were being laid. Many efforts failed because of lack of knowledge, but the rudiments of isolation, quarantine, sanitation, disinfection, and vaccination for smallpox had their origin during the great epidemics of past centuries. Scientific knowledge and understanding concerning infectious disease have greatly modified many of these early efforts; however, some of the early procedures have been modified within the past thirty years.

It is impossible to explore in detail all of the epidemics of the past. The following pages provide a synopsis of some of the most important ones. Additional information will be found in chapters dealing with specific diseases. For those who wish to do more intensive study, the references at the end of the chapter will provide interesting and stimulating reading.

THE GREAT EPIDEMICS AND PANDEMICS

Plague (black death)

Plague is caused by *Pasteurella pestis,* or plague bacillus. Several forms of the disease are recognized, including bubonic plague, pneumonic plague, septicemic form, and sylvatic plague. Sylvatic plague occurs in wild rodents and continues to be a reservoir of infection in many areas of the world, including the western part of the United States. (See Chapter 45.)

Historic evidence indicates that epidemics of plague occurred as early as 1100 B.C. Since the cause of infectious disease was unknown, it is difficult to trace the history of any specific disease. It seems possible that other infectious diseases as well as plague probably existed hundreds of years before Christ. Probably the earliest authenticated record of plague was that of an epidemic occurring during the reign of Justinian (A.D. 527-565), emperor of the Byzantine Empire. The disease became widespread throughout the known world and has been documented as "the plague of Justinian." Although the disease was not considered to be contagious, Justinian imposed a quarantine of forty days on all infected or exposed persons.

From the thirteenth to the seventeenth centuries plague was epidemic over all of Asia, Europe, the islands of the Mediterranean, and the British Isles. The exact number of persons who succumbed to the disease is unknown, since accurate mortality records were not maintained. It is believed that deaths far exceeded those indicated in the records. Various estimates placed the number of deaths from one fourth to three fourths of the entire population. It has been reported that some towns had a 90% mortality rate and that some small villages were completely wiped out. Defoe reports that during the 1665 epidemic in London there may have been as many as 10,000 deaths a week.[3]

In 1333 an epidemic of plague began in China, spreading to India and Persia. By 1345 it invaded Italy, and every town and hamlet in its wake suffered from its devastating effects. The number of deaths had reached millions, and about one third of the population had succumbed to the disease.

During 1630 and 1631 half of the population in many Polish towns died. The disease continued to spread eastward to France, Russia, and the British Isles. Plague continued to exist for hundreds of years, decreasing only to increase again to epidemic proportions. In 1418 there were 16,000 deaths in Florence and 50,000 in Paris. In 1477 and 1478 Venice had 30,000 deaths. In 1650 it was estimated that 412,000 persons in Ireland had died from plague. In 1711 two thirds of the population of Italy, Spain, and Constantinople had died, and 300,000 in Austria. In 1769 Moscow lost 80,000 people, mostly young healthy individuals.

Plague does not seem to have been a serious problem in the United States. Records indicate that an epidemic occurred among the Indians in New England about 1618 and 1619. This is probably the first recorded epidemic of infectious disease in the United States.[9] Small outbreaks occurred in 1919 and 1924 in California.[1]

The history of plague in England spans more than a thousand years. In A.D. 558 and 664 England suffered visitations of plague in a mild form. From that time until 1665 the country was not free of the disease for periods of more than five years at a time. Of particular interest are the four great epidemics occurring in 1602, 1625, 1636, and 1665. The epidemic of 1665 has been referred to as the "Black Death" and was by far the most devastating. The disease disappeared from England after this epidemic; the reason remains unknown.

In 1602 the epidemic began in some of the small towns, finally reaching London, a city of about 225,000 population. During this epidemic 34,000 of the inhabitants of London succumbed to the disease. Between 1606 and 1610 there was an average of 7400 to 9600 deaths annually from plague.

The epidemic of 1625 claimed 35,417 persons in London and the suburban areas about the city. The plague continued with about 2000 deaths a year until 1636, when two fifths of all the deaths in London were caused by plague. During the last visitation in 1665 the number of persons who died from the disease was estimated to be 100,000. The smaller towns suffered as severely as London.

During these serious epidemics the country was in a state of chaos. Thousands fled to the country, including members of the Royal family. Many persons already exposed to the disease died along the way, and their bodies lay unburied. The heaviest toll occurred among the poor in the slums.

Many theories existed concerning the cause of the epidemics, among which were that the south wind opened the pores and that swarming flies, air infected by dirty streets and gutters, standing water, and shallow burials caused infection. Many sanitary regulations were passed with emphasis on the environmental factors. Quarantine was imposed, with proctors (guards) stationed at the door to prevent persons from leaving or entering houses where the disease existed. Public gatherings, feasts, fairs, and public baths were forbidden. Walls of houses were to be scraped and whitewashed and the house fumigated with sulfur. Domestic animals were to be penned up. During one period, destruction of cats and dogs was ordered, and an estimated 40,000 dogs and about 200,000 cats were exterminated. Cleaning of streets and gutters was ordered, and throwing any kind of refuse into ditches or into the river was prohibited. Regulations concerning the depth of burials were established and enforced. There was an effort to quarantine exposed persons as indicated in the following:

> If any nurse keeper shall remove herself out of any infected house before twenty-eight days after the decease of any person dying of the infection, the house to which the said nurse keeper doth so remove herself shall be shut up until the said twenty-eight days shall be expired.*

The medical practice and treatment of plague varied widely among the physicians. The disease was not considered contagious, and a fatalistic at-

---

*Defoe, Daniel: History of plague in London, New York, 1894, American Book Co.

titude toward prognosis prevailed. By 1818 the question of contagiousness and noncontagiousness had received extensive review in the literature. The Royal College of Physicians in London assumed the attitude that no one had proved that the disease was noncontagious or that quarantine was of no value. However, they did agree that some modification could be made in the rigid quarantine procedure.

Nursing had entered what has generally been referred to as the "dark period" of nursing. Many nurses were of questionable character and had little interest in nursing or in the patient. This decline in nursing was destined to continue for a long time. Throughout the history of plague in England most persons received no nursing care. From the literature it would appear that the available nurses did little to relieve the suffering of their patients. The following excerpts show the nursing situation of the period:

> . . . the searchers and nurses were usually "dirty, ugly, unwholesome hags." All too often nurses abused or strangled their patients, stole their effects, and reputedly infected the well to insure future employment.*
>
> We had at this time a great many frightful stories told us of nurses and watchmen who looked after the dying people, that is to say, hired nurses, who attended infected people, using them barbarously, starving them, smothering them, or by other wicked means hastening their end, that is to say, murdering them.†

Many women employed as servants were turned out when employers left the city. Large numbers of these women posed as nurses to tend the sick and were responsible for much of the stealing of clothing, linens, jewelry, and money. One such nurse admitted thievery while on her deathbed. The situation became so critical that the local parish officers recommended nurses and maintained records of who was sent so that they could be held accountable if patients or homes were abused.

Although some physicians refused to care for patients with plague, many did care for rich and poor alike. However, in general, there was little concern among the physicians about the kind of nursing care given.

Many theories about the cause of plague had existed for centuries, but the first significant research occurred in Hong Kong in 1894. The reports of the research by Alexander Yersin stimulated interest in further work toward establishing the specific organism responsible for plague. Many individuals and persons in the United States Public Health Service and in Russia contributed toward the work. The final work in 1906 completed identification of the specific vector and the bacillus organism. Thus the cause and method of transmission of a disease that had cost millions of lives had finally been established on a scientific basis.

---

*Mullett, Charles F.: The bubonic plague and England, Lexington, Ky., 1956, University of Kentucky Press.

†Defoe, Daniel: History of plague in London, New York, 1894, American Book Co.

Leprosy

Leprosy (Hansen's disease) is a chronic infectious disease caused by *Mycobacterium leprae* (Hansen's bacillus). There are two recognized types of the disease, lepromatous and tuberculoid; also, a combination of the two types may occur in the same individual. (See Chapter 9.)

The origin of leprosy is controversial. It is believed that it probably existed several thousand years before Christ. These are numerous references in the Bible, particularly in the book of Leviticus, which was written 1400 years before Christ. The translations from the Hebrew have been questioned, since other skin diseases may have existed at the same time. Whether the biblical references actually refer to leprosy or to some other skin disease, the contagiousness of the diseases was recognized.

Hippocrates (460-377 B.C.) did not refer to or describe leprosy. However, Aristotle (384-322 B.C.), a Greek philosopher, did describe the disease. Records indicate that the disease was known to the Greeks in 500 B.C. and that it was epidemic along the Greek coast and Asia Minor in 200 B.C. In A.D. 180 the disease was discovered in Germany, and Claudius Galen, a Greek physician, wrote about it.

The disease may have originated in central Africa, from where it gradually spread over all of Europe and the British Isles, Scotland, and Wales. During the twelfth and thirteenth centuries the disease became widespread. Laws were passed in England in 1346 requiring persons with leprosy to leave the city within fifteen days after contracting the disease. During the great epidemics of plague in England it is believed that many persons with leprosy succumbed to plague. Leprosy remained prevalent over all of Europe for more than a thousand years.

The first known case of leprosy in the United States was discovered in Louisiana in 1758, although there is evidence that it may have been brought to the United States by way of Spain and Portugal as early as 1543. By the end of the nineteenth century the disease had spread to islands of the Pacific Ocean and to South America.

The disease has shown a significant decline in the temperate zones of Europe but continues to be a problem in Asia, Africa, South America, and some islands of the Pacific Ocean. Complete data concerning the incidence of the disease are not available. Estimates of the number of cases of leprosy vary widely and have been placed as low as 3 million and as high as 10 million cases in the world. The disease is endemic in Florida, Louisiana, and Texas, and cases have been reported from New York and California.

Until the latter part of the nineteenth century the disease was considered to be contagious. During the Middle Ages severe regulations were enforced to prevent the spread of the disease. Among some of the precautions taken were the granting of a divorce from an infected spouse, the removal of an infant from an infected mother, and the compulsory segregation of lepers for life.

During the sixth and seventh centuries leper houses (lazarettos) were established in many parts of Europe and England in an effort to isolate leprous persons. In 1894 a leper home was opened in the United States at Carville, Louisiana. During its first six years of operation forty patients were admitted. In 1909 the state of Louisiana provided funds, and the home was rebuilt and enlarged. In 1922 the United States government took over the home and established the National Leprosarium. The institution is under the supervision of the Division of Hospitals of the United States Public Health Service and is considered the finest institution of its kind in the world.

In 1942 Nigeria established a colony system to care for lepers. Oji River Leprosarium is staffed with missionary doctors and receives its support from the Nigerian government and philanthropy. The institution provides care for 1000 resident patients and 13,000 outpatients. There is also a colony at Uzuakoli that provides care for 15,166 resident patients and, in addition, provides dispensary service to fifty-four outlying areas. In 1934 Sudan, operating a colony system, cared for 7075 cases of leprosy.

In 1848 a controversy arose concerning the contagiousness of leprosy. One theory stated that the disease was hereditary and another stated that it was a blood dyscrasia. The controversy of contagiousness or noncontagiousness continued for some time. The Royal College of Physicians in London supported the noncontagious theory and in 1865 suspended all isolation procedures and closed its lazarettos. In 1871 Hansen discovered the bacillus of leprosy, but the method of transmission remained unknown. However, since 1897 the disease has been considered contagious.

Smallpox (variola)

Smallpox is caused by a virus known as *poxvirus variolae.* Two forms of the disease are recognized, variola major (classical smallpox) and variola minor (alastrim). (See Chapter 34.)

Most historians consider bubonic plague the most devastating disease of all time; according to mortality and morbidity reports, smallpox was a close second in its destruction of human life. As with many epidemic and endemic diseases, the origin of smallpox is unknown. The disease may have existed centuries before Christ; however, the early history of the disease remains obscure. It is generally believed that the disease had its origin in China, India, and Africa and was carried to other parts of the world by military conquest and explorers.

Among the early records concerning the disease we find that in A.D. 625 Bishop Gregory of Tours, France, described a disease "yellow plague" that is believed to have been smallpox. Very accurate descriptions of the disease were given in A.D. 850 by a Persian scholar and in A.D. 900 by an Arabian physician.

The disease first appeared in England during the sixteenth century and was first reported in the United States around 1630. Between 1600 and 1775 the disease was prevalent over all of Europe and America. In 1519 a Negro slave is believed to have brought the disease to Mexico, where it was communicated to the Aztec population. During the Spanish conquest of Mexico it was estimated that one half of the Aztec population died from smallpox. The disease spread to the West Indies, and in 1520 approximately 3 million persons in Central and South America succumbed to the disease. Between 1731 and 1765, smallpox accounted for about 2000 deaths annually in this area.

During the early colonization of America the ravages of smallpox nearly annihilated the population. Although other diseases plagued the early settlers, smallpox was responsible for the most devastating epidemics in the early colonial period. The exact date of the first outbreak is unknown, but it appears to have occurred after 1630. Boston suffered severely as the result of four visitations of the disease. In 1722 there were 844 deaths among 5980 cases, with more than one half of the population of Boston infected with the disease. In 1742 there were 6000 cases among which one in seven persons died. In 1752 there were 5545 cases, with 539 deaths. In the same year London experienced the worst epidemic in its history, with 3538 deaths from smallpox.

The Indians in New England provided a fertile field for smallpox, and during epidemics entire tribes were wiped out. It has been estimated that in 1738 one twentieth of the Cherokee tribe succumbed to the disease. All of the New England towns suffered outbreaks of smallpox, and ships arriving at ports brought the disease with them. In 1675 Charleston suffered a severe outbreak after the arrival of a ship at that port.

Throughout the seventeenth and eighteenth centuries ships arriving from countries where smallpox existed were a constant threat to the colonies. The problem was so serious that in 1647 laws were passed in Boston to prevent ships from entering the harbor if they carried sick persons.

Prior to the beginning of formal quarantine for smallpox, Boston required that a red flag be displayed on all homes where smallpox existed. The first efforts to quarantine smallpox occurred in Virginia in 1667. In 1699 Massachusetts passed a similar law and in 1717 appropriated money to construct a quarantine hospital. In 1718 the hospital was built on Rainsford Island. Soon after, other states including New Hampshire, Rhode Island, and South Carolina built quarantine hospitals.[4]

Throughout the history of epidemic smallpox there has been variation in the age groups attacked. In the sixteenth and seventeenth centuries the disease was primarily one of adults. In the eighteenth century children under 10 years of age were the victims. In England more than 90% of the cases occurred in children under 10 years of age. In the nineteenth century adults were attacked more frequently than children; however, during the severe epidemic in Boston all age groups were affected.

During the nineteenth century smallpox began to decline, but there are countries where it remains endemic. In 1950, 157,322 cases with 41,092 deaths occurred in India, 18,373 deaths in Pakistan, and 1354 deaths in Nigeria.[6] In 1947 an outbreak occurred in New York City, which had been imported from Mexico. During the outbreak twelve cases occurred with two deaths.

Sir William Jenner (1815-1898) is credited with the discovery of a vaccine against smallpox. The forerunner of vaccination was a procedure called "inoculation" or "variolation." The process was one of deliberately infecting a person with active smallpox virus. The importance of the procedure in the psychologic preparation of people for vaccination was recognized by Jenner. Inoculated individuals developed smallpox usually in a mild form; the disease was contagious, and some cases were severe enough to result in the death of the individual.

The origin of inoculation is uncertain, but evidence seems to indicate that it had been practiced in various places, including Africa, Persia, China, Constantinople, and Greece. Information concerning the practice was brought to the colonies by a Negro slave who was familiar with the custom.

The first inoculation was performed in England in 1721, and during the same year three persons in Boston, including the son of a physician and two Negro slaves, were inoculated. The results of all three proved successful.

The new procedure was not readily accepted, and so much criticism and controversy arose that in 1722 the town officials in Boston forbade its practice without their permission. The practice in England was not popular. The Royal College of Physicians of London did not approve the procedure. Clergymen preached against it, saying it was interfering with the will of God and that it was of the Devil. After several deaths, believed to be caused by inoculation, the practice fell into disuse but was later revived. Finally in 1840 the English parliament suppressed the procedure.

In 1738 Charleston suffered from a very severe epidemic of smallpox with a very high mortality. A physician in Charleston inoculated about 800 persons with only eight deaths. The success of inoculation in Charleston revived the practice in England. The Royal family and the Royal Society of London supported inoculation, and several members of the Royal family submitted to the procedure. Experience had shown that the death rate from inoculated smallpox was far less than that for naturally acquired smallpox. In 1743 inoculation was made mandatory for all children in the Children's Foundling Hospital in London, and the procedure was continued until the introduction of vaccination. By 1750 many of the prominent clergymen supported inoculation and took an active part in promoting it.

In 1776, during the colonial period, Cotton Mather (1663-1728), an American clergyman, learned about the procedure from Negro slaves. Smallpox was epidemic in England at the time, and Mather wrote to a member of the Royal Society of London asking why the procedure was not being used in England. Mather also stated that when another epidemic of smallpox occurred in Boston, he intended to persuade the physicians to adopt the practice of inoculation.

Wealthy persons were able to pay for inoculation, but the poor were unable to afford it; thus, while smallpox attacked rich and poor alike, it was the poor who suffered most. In 1746 a county hospital was established at Middlesex, England, to care for the poor who acquired smallpox.

The hospital was later moved to Bath-field, where it had a capacity of 130 beds. The hospital provided a separate area where inoculations were done and where such patients were cared for.

It was customary to establish hospitals outside the town; however, the fear of smallpox was so great that people refused to pass by the hospital. In 1773 a hospital near Marblehead, Massachusetts, was attacked and destroyed by fire.

Cholera (Asiatic cholera)

Cholera is an acute infectious disease caused by Vibrio *cholerae (Vibrio comma).* The organism was first identified by Robert Koch in 1883; however, the disease was described as early as 1769 during an epidemic in India. (See Chapter 19.)

The disease probably existed for centuries, but early in the nineteenth century it became worldwide. The source of the disease is believed to have been the delta of the Ganges, from where it was spread by pilgrims and along trade routes. Between 1817 and 1896 five great pandemics occurred, including one in the United States. In 1826 an epidemic occurred along the Ganges and spread over all of India, finally reaching Russia and countries of the Near East in 1830. By 1831 cholera had spread to England and from there to Ireland. In 1832 Irish immigrants arriving in Montreal and Quebec were infected with the disease. In about the middle of the same year the first cases appeared in Canada, and during the epidemic there were as many as 100 deaths a day. Before the end of 1832 the disease had reached the United States, where New York City suffered 400 deaths. There were 900 deaths in Philadelphia, 800 in Baltimore, and 400 in Norfolk. Plantations were especially hard hit by the infection, and one plantation reported that every one of its 100 slaves had succumbed to the disease. During the same epidemic Tampico, Mexico, reported 900 deaths in less than three weeks.

In 1833 cholera invaded New Orleans, where 1008 persons died within three weeks, and during the same period more than 1000 died in Wheeling, West Virginia. In 1854 and 1855 there were 1936 cases in Pittsburgh, with 865 deaths. In 1840 a very severe epidemic of virulent cholera developed in Calcutta, India, spreading over China, Serbia, and Russia and finally reaching Asia and Europe.

It has been estimated that in 1847 and 1848 more than 1 million persons died from cholera. France had 150,000 deaths. By 1849 the disease invaded New York City and appeared again in New Orleans. In the same year one fifth of the population of Matamoras, Mexico, died from cholera. There were 2000 deaths in the Rio Grande valley. The heaviest loss of any city in the United States occurred in St. Louis, Missouri, where a mortality of one death in every ten cases occurred. Approximately 4500 to 6000 deaths resulted from the epidemic. At the same time Chicago lost 1000 persons with the disease.

The third great epidemic occurred in 1866, when ships bringing immigrants arrived in New York. One ship arrived with sixty cases of cholera aboard, and fifteen dead from the disease. An unreliable report estimated that in fifty-three cities and in the army of the Civil War there had been 10,805 deaths from cholera.

The fourth great pandemic occurred in 1873. There has been no epidemic in the United States since that time. However, during the pandemic of 1873, Hungary had 500,000 cases, while Russia had 500,000 deaths. Migration in the United States was westward, and many smaller towns suffered severely from the disease.

While the United States had escaped the scourge, other parts of the world were not so fortunate. In 1883 the disease continued to cause epidemics in the East and in Europe. France and Italy had 50,000 cases and Russia 800,000. In 1892 there were 17,000 cases in Hamburg, Germany, with 50% mortality.[2] Egypt suffered a severe epidemic in 1902, when there were 34,000 deaths among 40,000 cases.

While the disease has been disappearing from many parts of the world, largely because of vaccination and improvement in living conditions, it continues to remain endemic in India and China. During the period from 1946 to 1955 there were 783,793 deaths from cholera in India. The number of cases in China is unknown but is believed to be greater than that in India.[5]

As long as the disease remains endemic in various parts of the world, it must be regarded as a constant threat to all of the world.

Yellow fever (jungle yellow fever or sylvatic form)

During the nineteenth century yellow fever was frequently referred to as "black vomit" because of old blood contained in the vomitus, giving it a black appearance. Two forms of the disease are recognized, both of which are caused by the same virus. Yellow fever in humans is transmitted by a vector, the *Aedes aegypti* mosquito. The vector feeds on persons ill with the disease during the first three days of illness. After a twelve-day incubation period in the mosquito the disease is then transmitted to humans. The second form of the disease is transmitted by a strain of the *A. aegypti* and is found to exist in the rhesus monkey. The disease exists in jungle and forest areas where there is limited human habitation, and the rhesus monkey is believed to be the reservoir of infection.

Like other endemic and epidemic diseases, yellow fever has taken its toll in human life. The disease is now almost nonexistent in North America. However, in 1966 the *A. aegypti* mosquito was discovered in the southern United States. During the eighteenth and nineteenth centuries the disease was prevalent. Probably the most severe outbreak in the United States occurred in Philadelphia in 1793. The epidemic caused the death of one fifth of the population, or about 5000 persons.

In 1820 the city of Savannah, Georgia, reported that the number of deaths from yellow fever during each fourteen-year period was equal to the entire population of the city. During a period of thirty-seven years there were about 3000 deaths. Analysis of death records indicated that very few deaths occurred among the native population but were found to be among foreigners, including immigrants and migrants.

Over a period of 500 years Havana, Cuba, had about 750 deaths annually from yellow fever. Charleston was constantly menaced by ships arriving from infected ports, carrying persons ill with yellow fever and other infectious diseases.

During 1878 an epidemic of yellow fever spread to eight states, and Memphis, Tennessee, had 17,500 cases with 5150 deaths. The city of New Orleans, Louisiana, experienced at least thirty-seven severe outbreaks after 1803.

Until the twentieth century, when the specific vector was identified and the method of transmission confirmed, the prevailing theory was miasma. Reports of city officials in Savannah, Georgia, and Charleston, South Carolina, provide extensive information concerning the miasma theory of that time.

In 1819 persons in Savannah placed emphasis upon the atmosphere. A mild winter and early spring accompanied by unusual heat and prevailing easterly winds increased the prevalence of yellow fever. Among other conditions believed to be the cause was unusual shade (because of a failure to prune shade trees), dilapidated frame houses, and the ruins from fires that left open cellars. The surrounding marshlands and the increase in a population that was unaccustomed to the climate were also cited as possible causes.

A difference of opinion existed in Charleston in 1859. Some persons believed that rigid quarantine would prevent epidemics, while others believed that it was a question of sanitation. All infected persons arriving on ships and those in the homes of the town were sent to the lazaretto. Houses of the sick were cleaned, whitewashed, and fumigated, after which they remained unoccupied for one month.

The city officials admitted that the cause of yellow fever was unknown but that its devastating effect was well known. Sanitary conditions in the town were described as filthy. Yards were crowded with horses, cows, goats, hogs, and dogs, while the houses were crowded with human beings. There were 800 privies existing in the town and their contents emptied into pits on the same lot. Other environmental factors believed to contribute to the disease included the location of burial grounds within the city limits, sewers and drains that overflowed, and the manure and filth that was placed into the streets for the scavenger's cart to remove.

In 1881 there had been some suspicion that yellow fever was transmitted by a mosquito. In 1900 a commission of army surgeons with Walter Reed as chairman was sent to Cuba to study the disease. After intensive investigation and research they were able to identify the virus and the *A. aegypti* mosquito as the vector. Subsequently W. C. Gorgus was sent to Panama to clear the area so that work on the Panama Canal could proceed.

Through the combined efforts of the Rockefeller Foundation, the West

African Yellow Fever Commission, and the Yellow Fever Research Institute in Uganda, progress has been made toward eradication of yellow fever. International regulations have been established to prevent spread of the disease from infected countries. Mass immunization programs in countries where the *A. aegypti* mosquito exists has gradually reduced the incidence of the disease.

Influenza

Influenza is caused by influenza virus A, identified in 1933, and by influenza virus B, identified in 1940. Influenza virus C was identified in 1949 and influenza virus D in 1953. Influenza virus C and D rarely cause disease in humans. Since the original discovery of influenza virus D, it has been reclassified as para-influenza 1. As research continued concerning influenza viruses, two new strains of influenza virus A were isolated. One has been designated as A-prime, discovered during an epidemic in 1946 and 1947, and the other as an Asian strain A_2, isolated during 1957. Both of these strains have resulted in widespread epidemics.[6]

The earliest recorded evidence of influenza appeared when Hippocrates described its symptoms. The armies of Marcus Claudius Marcellus, a Roman general, suffered an outbreak of influenza in A.D. 212. Symptoms of the disease were described as a sudden onset of chills, cough, sweating, and a dry throat and mouth, accompanied by difficulty in swallowing and expectoration, and wasting. A similar epidemic occurred in the fifth century.

A disease known as "sweating sickness" appeared in England in 1485, lasting about five weeks. The disease attacked all economic levels, causing a very high mortality. From England the disease spread to other countries, where it became generally known as the "English sweat." In subsequent years epidemics occurred, some of which were very virulent, with victims dying within twenty-four hours after the onset of the disease. In 1552 John Cains described the sweating sickness, and it has been rather generally believed that the disease was influenza. In 1743 John Huxham, an English physician, described the disease and was the first to use the name "influenza."

Historic records seem to indicate that epidemics of influenza have occurred at fairly regular intervals in various countries. Epidemics have been overshadowed by the great pandemics. Between 1510 and 1930 about thirty visitations of the disease were sufficiently widespread to be considered pandemics. The greatest pandemic occurred in 1918 and 1919. The cause of the disease was unknown until 1933. During the eighteenth century it was believed to be caused and spread by prevailing winds. However, in 1892 Pfeiffer discovered the *Haemophilus influenzae* organism, and during the epidemic in 1918 and 1919 it was believed that this organism was the cause of the disease.

The origin of the pandemic in 1918 is not entirely clear. The disease was given the name "Spanish influenza," and one theory stated that it originated in Spain and was transported to military camps in the United States. Others believed that it was first encountered in France in 1918 and came to the United States by troops arriving from Europe. Since the disease was widespread, it seems possible that both theories may be correct.

Paul states that more people were attacked by the disease than were attacked by the "black death"; however, the mortality rate for the black death was about 90%, whereas for the Spanish influenza it was about 3%.

The number of persons attacked by the Spanish influenza in 1918 and 1919 has been estimated at 700 million, with total deaths of 22 million. Over 50% of the deaths were in the United States. Two hundred thousand persons died in England and Wales, and about 5 million died in India. In some military camps the death rate was as high as 12%, while the civilian death rate varied from 3% to 4%. Persons living today who experienced the pandemic will never forget it; however, there was no apparent fear or panic throughout the duration of the infection.

The second pandemic of historic significance occurred in 1957 and 1958 and to a much lesser extent into 1959. The origin of the disease known as "Asian influenza" is believed to have originated in China in February, 1957. In two months it had spread to Hong Kong, where 10% of the population was attacked. Prior to the summer it had spread throughout all of Asia and the Pacific islands, and by fall all of Europe and America had been invaded.

The first outbreak in the United States occurred in Rhode Island, where United States Navy personnel became ill with the disease. Within one month an outbreak occurred among civilian persons in California, and the disease then spread rapidly throughout the country. The mortality from Asian influenza was not as great as that during the pandemic of 1918; however, thousands of people died, and many more were ill. The greatest mortality occurred among persons over 50 years of age with chronic diseases such as cancer, cardiovascular disease, and diabetes. There were 750,000 cases and 216 deaths in New York City, where a substantial number of the deaths occurred among pregnant women and persons with rheumatic fever.

Typhoid fever

Typhoid fever is an acute infectious disease caused by the *Salmonella typhosa* organism. The name "typhoid" was first used by Pierre C. A. Lewis of Paris, France, in 1829. The disease had probably existed for centuries before Christ, and it was recognized by Hippocrates who called it "continued fever." Hippocrates recognized the disease as being different from other diseases. (See Chapter 23.)

For centuries confusion existed between typhoid fever and typhus fever. A common theory was that typhoid fever could turn into typhus fever. Although there is some evidence that a French physician differentiated between typhoid fever and typhus fever in 1818, credit is generally given to Gerhardt, an American who made the first differentiation between the two diseases in 1837. The cause of the disease remained unknown until 1880, when Carl Eberth, a German, discovered the typhoid bacillus. In 1859 the disease was not considered contagious; therefore, physicians did not consider it a medical problem. A prevailing theory stated that the disease was caused by some unknown decomposing material that contaminated the air, food, and water. In 1861 about 50,000 cases occurred in England.

During the eighteenth century there was a growing awareness that problems of sanitation, overcrowding, and other environmental factors were related to the cause of typhoid fever. At about 1859 attention was being given to providing a safe water supply. In 1856 William Budd, an Englishman, was convinced that typhoid fever came from excreta of patients ill with the disease. Later, publication of his book intensified the belief that typhoid fever was a waterborne disease.

In 1875 there were 50,000 cases in England, with 9000 deaths. At about the same time a public health act was passed that resulted in the improvement of environmental sanitation. These improvements brought a remarkable decrease in the incidence of typhoid fever in England.

During the early colonial period in America typhoid fever was probably present. Diseases known as "long fevers" and "nervous fevers" were widespread. In 1750 long fever accounted for 150 deaths in Connecticut, and in 1769 there were 425 deaths from "bloody flux" in Boston.[4] Typhoid fever has often been considered a disease of wars, and it was prevalent during the Civil War and World War I. Because of immunization for typhoid fever the incidence was not significant during World War II. With the exception of the period from 1906 to 1910, typhoid fever rate among United States military personnel has been lower than that for the United States as a whole.

Sporadic outbreaks of typhoid fever have occurred throughout the United States, primarily caused by infected water supplies and carriers. At the present time from 600 to 700 cases occur annually in the United States. The incidence in urban areas has showed a steady decline, with most of the reported cases being in rural areas. Only a small percentage of those recovering from the disease become carriers.

After the discovery of the typhoid bacillus and its isolation by Gaffky in 1880, immunization became possible. The first inoculation for typhoid fever was performed in England in 1896 by Sir Almroth Wright.

Thousands of cases of typhoid fever occur annually throughout the world. The primary reservoir of infection is in countries of the Far and Middle East, Europe, Africa, and Central and South America.

Paratyphoid fever

Paratyphoid fever is caused by *Salmonella paratyphi* and is classified as paratyphoid A, B, and C. The source of most cases in the United States is from type B. Clinically the disease is similar to typhoid fever but is milder and has a lower mortality rate. Two laboratories are maintained where differentiation of the specific pathogens are determined. These laboratories are the National Communicable Disease Center, Atlanta, Georgia, and the International Salmonella Laboratory at Copenhagen, Denmark. Since there is a large number of the *Salmonella* pathogens, extensive laboratory procedure is necessary for diagnosis of paratyphoid fever.

Typhus fever

Typhus fever is an acute infectious disease caused by the *Rickettsia prowazekii* organism and transmitted through a vector. Several forms of the disease are recognized; typhus fever transmitted by the body louse, *Pediculus humanus corporis;* Brill-Zinsser disease, a mild form of typhus fever occurring several years after the initial attack without evidence of louse infestation; murine typhus fever, transmitted to humans by the rat flea *Xenopsylla cheopis,* and caused by the organism *Rickettsia mooseri.* (See Chapter 47.)

Typhus fever has caused millions of deaths throughout the world and has been known for centuries. The first description of the disease was recorded in 1546. During the sixteenth and seventeenth centuries numerous outbreaks of the disease occurred in England. During 1740 and 1741 and again in 1846 and 1847, epidemic typhus fever occurred in England. The disease first appeared in North America in about 1570, when outbreaks occurred in Mexico and Peru. The first cases reported in the United States and Canada were observed early in the nineteenth century, when infected Irish immigrants arrived.

After World War I the disease was epidemic in Russia, where an estimated 3 million deaths occurred. At about the same time several million persons died in Serbia, Poland, and Germany. The last important outbreak of typhus fever in the United States occurred in 1921 on the Navajo Indian Reservation in the Southwest.

Epidemic typhus fever remains prevalent in areas of the Near East, Europe, Egypt, Algeria, South Africa, and South America. It was not until 1909 that the human body louse was identified as the vector in the transmission of epidemic typhus fever, and in 1916 the causative organism was named by da Rocha-Lima.

Brill-Zinsser disease was first observed in 1898 and in 1912 was proved to be caused by typhus organisms. The disease had been recognized in immigrants who migrated to the United States from typhus areas. Persons found to have the disease were not louse infested. The name "murine typhus" was given to the disease until 1928, when Mooser identified murine typhus as another form of typhus fever.

Murine typhus fever is a worldwide problem and exists in the same areas as epidemic typhus fever. In 1935 an increase of the disease was observed, which continued until 1944, after which it began to decline. Between 1931 and 1944 there were 34,000 cases of murine typhus fever in the United States. The incidence has decreased so that at the present time less than 100 cases are reported annually. However, in any area where human beings and rats inhabit the same place, murine typhus fever is a constant threat. The disease is confined largely to rural areas along the gulf and south Atlantic seacoast.

CONCLUSIONS

The reader should not conclude that the foregoing diseases were the only ones causing high mobidity and mortality during past centuries. Measles was prevalent throughout Europe and North America. Paul reports that in 1850, 1000 children out of every million died from measles before the age of 15 years.[8] Epidemics of measles occurred in North America, where the Indians and early colonists suffered heavy mortality. In 1875 about one fourth of the population of the Fiji Islands succumbed to the disease.

Scarlet fever was often confused with measles until about 1553, and it caused many deaths in children under 15 years of age. Diphtheria probably existed for centuries before Christ. During the early days it was referred to as "throat distemper" and was not called diphtheria until 1826. From the eighteenth century the disease was prevalent over parts of Europe, England, and North America, and by the nineteenth century it was worldwide.

Between 1847 and 1849 about 63,000 deaths occurred from pertussis. In 1878 the disease occurred in England and Wales, where about 17,784 persons died. Between 1951 and 1955 there were 2463 deaths in the United States from pertussis.

The history of infectious disease throughout the world is an endless story of high mortality and morbidity. It has frequently been surrounded by poverty, unsanitary environmental conditions, and ignorance. In some parts of the world control measures have been effective in reducing the incidence of infectious diseases, but in other parts of the world they remain a threat to all human beings.

REFERENCES

1. Anderson, Gaylord W., Arnstein, Margaret G., and Lester, Mary R.: Communicable disease control, ed. 4, New York, 1962, The Macmillan Co.
2. Chambers, J. S.: The conquest of cholera, New York, 1938, The Macmillan Co.
3. Defoe, Daniel: History of plague in London, New York, 1894, American Book Co.
4. Duffy, John: Epidemics in Colonial America, Baton Rogue, La., 1953, Louisiana State University Press.
5. Harris, C. H. Stewart: Influenza and other virus infections of the respiratory tract, Baltimore, 1965, The Williams & Wilkins Co.
6. Horsefall, Frank L., and Tamm, Ignor, editors: Viral and rickettsial infections of man, ed. 4, Philadelphia, 1965, The Macmillan Co.
7. Mullett, Charles F.: The bubonic plague and England, Lexington, Ky., 1956, University of Kentucky Press.
8. Paul, Hugh: The control of communicable diseases (social and communicable), Baltimore, 1964, The Williams & Wilkins Co.
9. Winslow, C.-E. A., Smillie, Wilson G., Doull, James, A., Gordon, John E., and Top, Franklin H.: The history of American epidemiology, St. Louis, 1952, The C. V. Mosby Co.

2

SCOPE OF CONTROL

PUBLIC HEALTH DEPARTMENT

The prevention and control of infectious disease is a responsibility of every citizen. However, there are certain responsibilities that have been defined by statute with authority vested in a public health department. Until about the last decade the primary function of public health departments was the control of communicable diseases. Now, however the control of communicable diseases has lessened as a result of scientific research, which has made protection against such diseases possible, and further changes in certain activities of health departments are slowly emerging.

Public health departments were essentially unknown until late in the nineteenth century. Prior to their establishment, boards of health were appointed. Probably the first board of health was established in Venice in 1848, when the city was suffering from a severe epidemic of plague. During early colonial periods the town selectmen were responsible for the health of the people. Their efforts were directed toward sanitary reforms and quarantine measures to prevent epidemic disease. Numerous regulations were related to environmental sanitation and quarantine of ships arriving in ports from countries or states where epidemic disease existed. The health of the community was determined exclusively upon the number of cases of infectious disease and the number of deaths from such diseases. As an epidemic of disease passed, most of the regualtions passed with it and were forgotten until the next epidemic occurred.

For many years physicians did not believe that they had any responsibility in preventing disease; therefore, they assumed no role in helping to control infectious diseases. But by the middle of the eighteenth century there was some evidence of physicians beginning to work with the town selectmen. In 1779 the selectmen in Boston appointed a physician, Joseph Whipple, to act as a quarantine officer. His duties included the care of persons quarantined with infectious disease at the Rainsford Island Hospital. His position was actually that of the town's health officer.

In 1794, after a severe epidemic of yellow fever, the town of Philadelphia appointed a board of health, and in 1793 Baltimore did likewise. In 1799 a board of health was appointed by the General Court of Boston. None of the appointees were physicians, and none had any competence in matters of public health. Almost all of the early boards of health were permissive in nature. Controversy has existed concerning the appointment of the first permanent board of health. However, the American Public Health Association gives credit to Baltimore, which established a permanent board of health in 1793.[4]

Although regulations were passed by boards of health, responsibility for compliance was placed upon the individual. Most persons paid little attention to the regulations, and little was accomplished. In 1823 Boston began to employ men with horses and carts to remove the dirt and filth from the streets. It has been reported that in one month 3000 tons were removed.[1]

Between 1800 and 1850 there was very little progress made in public health. The miasma theory continued to persist, and environmental factors were believed to be responsible for epidemic diseases. Most physicians did not accept the theory of the contagiousness of disease, and, therefore, they did not assist in the prevention and control of infectious diseases. Although the period included some of the most disastrous epidemics of infectious disease, a decline in the incidence of epidemic disease began to occur near the end of the period and before the establishment of health departments.

Between 1850 and 1900 the public health movement was influenced by several men, including Lemuel Shattuck (1793-1883) whose report, *Sanitary Survey,* has been considered a public health classic. General health conditions had deteriorated to a horrible degree, and boards of health were noted for their incompetence. Physicians continued to ignore the infectiousness of disease. However, it was during this period that the discoveries of Louis Pasteur, Joseph Lister, Robert Koch, Walter Reed, William Sedwick, and others provided the basis for the control of communicable diseases. Progress was further delayed because of incompetent public health administrators and political appointments. There were no trained pubilc health personnel, and health officers were frequently physicians who were unable to adjust to their position in society.

In spite of the conditions that existed, the foundations for modern public health were being laid. In 1639 Boston had begun to register births and deaths, but the information was used only to determine the health of the town. Eventually the collection of vital statistics and their scientific use became a part of municipal and state health departments.

The first public health laboratory was opened in New York City in 1892, and about the same time municipal and state health departments were becoming mandatory. The board of health that was established in Baltimore in 1793 became a public health department in 1900. The establishment of health departments began with lay boards of health and worked upward to town and municipal health departments, county health departments, and state health departments. The movement was facilitated by the increase in population and the industrial revolution.

There is no national health department. As early as 1799 the United States Congress authorized federal personnel to assist states with quarantine laws aimed at preventing and controlling the introduction of infectious diseases into their ports. In 1887 the government established the Hygienic Laboratory on Staten Island, which eventually became the National Institute of Health. In 1891 the Hygienic Laboratory was moved to Washington, D. C., where it remained. In 1798 Congress authorized the United States Marine Hospital Service to care for sick and disabled seamen. In 1902 the name was changed to Public Health and Marine Hospital Service, and in 1912 it was changed to United States Public Health Service. Since 1937, when the National Cancer Institute was established, additional institutes have been established to meet the increasing emphasis in medicine and public health. At the present time there are nine institutes known collectively as the National Institutes of Health. In 1946 the Communicable Disease Center was created and is now established in Atlanta, Georgia. The United States Public Health Service is a vast comprehensive organization presently within the United States Department of Health, Education and Welfare. Its services encompass all phases of health and related services that extend beyond the borders of the continental United States.[7]

At the present time, the public health department is a complex structure with its role in health services in a state of flux. Communicable disease control is still an important problem, but its character has changed. In 1900 influenza and pneumonia were leading causes of death, while today these diseases rank sixth. For the first four months of 1968, 7200 cases of infectious syphilis were reported in the United States and its territories, and the number continues to increase up to the present day. Tuberculosis remains a problem, but most patients are no longer confined in a hospital for years. The health department today is concerned with degenerative diseases, heart disease, cancer, diabetes, and problems of the aged. Its activities include air pollution, safe water, fluoridation of water, and rabies control.

The shortage of trained public health personnel has been increasing. In 1955 one state reported having only two trained public health physicians in their county health departments. Some persons believe that in general there is a slow deterioration of health department activities, partly caused by the serious shortage of trained personnel. There is increasing federal control of health services with socialization of health and medical services.[2]

James has stated that today man is responsible for his own illness and death. Chronic disease has become an accepted way of life, environmental factors related to illness and death are man-made, and today health is in competition with economic gain. If the health department is to meet the present needs of society, it must become a center for total comprehensive family care. It must be concerned not only with the patient who visits the center but also with the family members who do not come in.[6]

VOLUNTARY HEALTH AGENCIES AND FOUNDATIONS

The voluntary (nonofficial) health agency had its beginning before 1900. Some organizations had their beginning on the local level and became national in scope, while others originated on the national level and filtered down to state and local levels. The overall objective of the voluntary agency was the promotion of health and the prevention of illness. Many agencies have been devoted to one particular phase of health work. Some have had their beginning as a demonstration project. It was anticipated that on completion of the demonstration the efficacy of the work would be recognized and continued by an official agency such as the health department. Programs of many agencies, past and present, have been incorporated into health department programs. Some activities that began as voluntary programs were established on a national level under the National Institutes of Health of the United States Public Health Service. Chief among these are tuberculosis, cancer, and venereal disease.

Nursing played an important role in the voluntary agency. In 1877 the Women's Branch of the New York City Mission organized a program of visiting nurses to provide home care for the poor. Since that time, many visiting nurse associations have come into existence sponsored by non professional groups of persons. In 1902 Lillian Wald organized a program of school nursing in New York City. The American National Red Cross organized county nursing under local Red Cross chapters, and insurance companies provided home nursing service to certain of their policy holders.

Voluntary health agencies concerned with communicable diseases included the National Tuberculosis Association, the American Social Hygiene Association, and the National Poliomyelitis Foundation.

The National Tuberculosis Association had its beginning in Philadelphia in 1892 as the Antituberculosis Society. In 1904 the society became the National Tuberculosis Association. The tuberculosis Christmas seal originated in Denmark in 1904, and the first seals sold in the United States were in Wilmington, Delaware, in 1907. This effort promoted interest in tuberculosis and the belief that control was possible. In 1908 and 1909 the sale of the Christmas seals was sponsored by the American National Red Cross, and beginning in 1910, it has been the sole responsibility of the National Tuberculosis Association.

The American Social Hygiene Association was organized in 1914, incorporating the activities of the American Federation for Sex Hygiene and the American Vigilance Association. The overall objective of the association was public education concerning the prevention and treatment of venereal disease and control of social factors such as prostitution, which was related to the incidence of venereal disease. At the time the organization was established the term *venereal disease* was spoken only in hushed tones behind a closed door. It was believed that the term *social hygiene* would be a more acceptable term and would help to bring the disease into the open. The association is now known as the American Social Health Association.

At about the same time that voluntary health agencies came into existence, foundations were being established. The foundations, some small and some large, represent the private fortunes of individuals. Many of these foundations were devoted to helping persons with specific diseases. In 1938 the National Foundation for Infantile Paralysis came into existence. Later it was called the National Foundation for Poliomyelitis, and presently it is called the National Foundation. Voluntary contributions are solicited through the annual March of Dimes campaign, which is timed to coincide with the birth date of the late President Franklin Roosevelt, who was a victim of poliomyelitis. Since the development of vaccine for the active immunization for poliomyelitis, activities of the National Foundation have been broadened to include metabolic diseases and birth defects.

Activities of some of the foundations such as the Rockefeller Foundation and the W. K. Kellogg Foundation have been of international scope. They have sponsored programs in the prevention and control of communicable diseases among many of the developing countries of the world.

During a period of about fifty years it was estimated that as many as 20,000 voluntary agencies came into existence, many of which were not enduring. After 1950 there was a gradual decline in the number of such agencies. With the new emphasis on chronic and metabolic diseases a number of new voluntary agencies have appeared, each competing with the other for the health dollar. Although millions of dollars are raised annually, it is necessary to spend a large proportion for promotional activities. In addition there is increasing resistance of the public, particularly for those activities that are being supported by tax funds. Many voluntary agencies have become affiliated with community organizations such as the Community Chest and the United Fund. In some instances employed persons are not only encouraged but are pressured to sign pledges for specified contributions for which a payroll deduction is made over a period of time.

METHODS OF CONTROL

Quarantine and isolation

Quarantine of infectious disease is the oldest method known for controlling disease. Probably the first recorded attempt at quarantine occurred during the plague of Justinian in the sixth century. A quarantine of forty days was imposed on persons with or exposed to bubonic plague. From the fourteenth century England, Europe, and colonial America imposed quarantine restrictions on ships from countries where epidemic disease existed. None of these efforts proved very successful in preventing the spread of communicable diseases.

In 1718 Boston built a quarantine hospital on Rainsford Island. Persons infected with disease were removed from ships arriving in port and taken to the quarantine hospital, where they were detained until they had recovered. Gradually other towns built similar hospitals, and eventually they became known as "pest houses." The pest house became the forerunner of the modern communicable disease hospital.

Quarantine, as a method to prevent the spread of communicable disease, has continued into the twentieth century. In fact, prior to World War II almost all persons with communicable disease were quarantined. The patient and his contacts were restricted to their premises and advised that under penalty of law no person could leave the premises and no person could enter. The wage earner was frequently allowed to leave but was required to live outside the home. The procedure was never completely satisfactory bcause it placed hardship on the family, and a certain amount of going in and out of the home occurred during hours when detection was less likely to occur. Professional nurses accepting duty with communicable disease patients were quarantined with the family. After the termination of their service they were restricted from caring for another patient for at least seven days.

Isolation and quarantine are terms frequently used synonymously. However, there is a rather fine distinction between them, both in meaning and in practice. Originally quarantine meant the detention of ships and/or persons for forty days. Quarantine restricts the movement of persons with or exposed to certain diseases such as smallpox to a given area. Quarantine may be for the incubation period for exposed persons and a given number of days for the patient. Isolation generally refers to the infected person and covers the period of communicability. There may be limited or no restriction of contacts. For example, a person with staphylococcal pneumonia is isolated, but his contacts are not. Patients isolated in the hospital with infectious hepatitis are usually permitted to have visitors.

In preventing the spread of communicable disease, emphasis is placed on isolation of the patient. Several factors operate to affect isolation procedures. In some diseases isolation is dependent on bacteriologic examination of body fluids such as spinal fluid, urine, sputum, or feces as in typhoid fever, or nose and throat cultures in diphtheria. In some cases isolation and its duration are dependent on the use of chemotherapeutic agents. States and municipalities may establish laws concerning the isolation of specific communicable diseases, and there may be considerable variation in communicable disease regulations between states. The interpretation of state regulations may vary among health departments in the same state. Large cities may have a communicable disease hospital, and some general hospitals may have segregated units for communicable diseases. However, hundreds of small general hospitals exist in which patients must be isolated on a regular medical unit. The physician orders the isolation and determines when it is to be terminated.

The effectiveness of quarantine and isolation cannot be easily determined. Frequently a large reservoir of unknown infection exists, and isolation of cases may fail to prevent or control an epidemic. Public education, understanding, and cooperation are always important if results are to be achieved through isolation. The nurse who cares for an isolated patient must have a basic understanding of communicable disease and medical asepsis. (See Chapter 6.)

In colonial America regulations required that a red flag be placed on the house. The practice of placarding houses is outmoded and obsolete and is rarely done at the present time.

Disinfection, fumigation, and sterilization

Concurrent disinfection means the immediate and continuous disinfection of infectious discharges or articles contaminated by infectious material.

A variety of chemical compounds having bactericidal effect are used for this purpose. Spores are not destroyed by chemical disinfection. The nurse should be familiar with the resistance power of the particular organism. Some pathogens may be easily destroyed, while others are highly resistant to most disinfectants. Several factors must also be considered, including the strength of the disinfecting solution, the temperature of the solution, and the extent of contamination. There is no disinfectant that gives immediate action. When disinfectants are used for body excretions such as feces, the disinfectant must reach every particle of the mass. Articles to be disinfected must be completely immersed in the solution.

Terminal disinfection is a procedure in which the room and its contents are thoroughly cleaned after discharge, transfer, or death of the patient. With modern methods of housekeeping and emphasis on concurrent disinfection, routine cleaning and airing is usually all that is necessary. However, regulations may vary among hospitals and health departments.

During the thirteenth and fourteenth centuries houses of plague victims in England were fumigated by burning sulfur. The practice continued in the American colonies, where the homes of smallpox and yellow fever victims were fumigated with sulfur. In Charleston, houses were ordered closed for one month after fumigation, during which they had to remain unoccupied. The practice of fumigation continued well into the twentieth century. After the release from a communicable disease, all bedding, clothing, etc. were exposed, windows and doors were sealed, and sulfur or formaldehyde candles were burned. The dwelling remained closed for eight to twelve hours before it was opened, aired, and the family allowed to return. Health departments frequently employed persons with the sole responsibility of placarding and fumigating. The practice of terminal fumigation became so entrenched in controlling communicable diseases that even today some persons will demand that it be carried out. Fumigation with gaseous agents is used for the destruction of certain rodents, insects, or arthropods. The procedure has no place in present-day control of communicable disease except as just indicated.

Sterilization and disinfection are terms used interchangeably. However, they do not always mean the same thing. Disinfection with chemical agents does not guarantee the destruction of all pathogens, while sterilization by heat assures complete destruction of pathogens including spores, and is generally preferred when possible. Disposable items from the communicable disease unit or in the home should be burned. Most hospitals use steam under pressure (autoclaving) to sterilize many nondisposable items. (See Chapter 6.)

Reporting

Most states and provinces have laws requiring the reporting of communicable diseases to the health department. Regulations specify the diseases and conditions under which they are reportable. Some diseases are reportable only in case of epidemics. Responsibility is placed on the private physician, who may be prosecuted for failure to report a communicable disease, unless a previous report has been made. The rules generally require that the case be reported within twenty-four hours following diagnosis. The report includes the patient's name, address, sex, race, and the disease. Diseases for which a positive diagnosis cannot be immediately established may be reported as suspected.

Reporting begins on the local level, where the disease is reported by telephone or postcard by the physician to the local health department. Almost any person or agency may report a suspected case of communicable disease. Cases of diseases in animals that may be transmitted to humans are also reported to the health department. According to regulations established, the local health department reports communicable diseases occurring within their jurisdiction to the state health department. Finally, states and territories report to the National Communicable Disease Center, where data are assembled for the entire nation.

Relationships have been established among nations of the world and defined according to the International Sanitary Regulations for universal reporting of certain diseases including cholera, smallpox, plague, yellow fever, louse-borne typhus fever, and louse-borne relapsing fever. During severe epidemics or pandemics daily telegraphic reports may be required from all reporting agencies.

Epidemiologic investigation

The methods used to search out the source of an infectious disease and to correlate the findings are known as epidemiologic investigation. Such investigation requires training and experience and an understanding of methods as well as the interrelationships among the data obtained. Not all diseases require such a comprehensive investigation, but some such as typhoid fever, smallpox, diphtheria, and certain kinds of meningitis, encephalitis, and chickenpox in an adult may be investigated.

The investigation is the responsibility of the health officer and should be initiated as soon as the case is reported. It is important that the source of the case be located as soon as possible to prevent spread of the disease. The investigation may include an interview with the patient and family, an examination of household contacts, the location of community contacts for examination, and problems of environmental sanitation such as water, milk, food, and sewage and refuse disposal. In an epidemic, cases may be located on a spot map to determine geographic distribution. During such investigation missed cases, carriers, and unreported cases may be uncovered. It may also result in proper medical and nursing care of the patient or in the institution of a broad program of immunization.

Immunization

Immunization of susceptible persons against preventable diseases is the most potent weapon available for preventing and controlling epidemics of communicable disease. In most instances this is accomplished through public education. A vigorous program must be promoted to keep the need for protection before the people. In spite of the best efforts, there will always be a reservoir of susceptible persons who remain unprotected. Van Avery has illustrated the lag in securing protection again poliomyelitis. Three years after the introduction of the Salk vaccine the city of Detroit experienced one of the worst epidemics of poliomyelitis in its history. The city reported 877 cases with twenty-three deaths. Investigation showed that nearly every patient had not received the vaccine or had not completed the required number of injections.[8] In April, 1966, a daily newspaper reported a 2-year-old child with poliomyelitis. The state epidemiologist noted that the child had been born since the last mass immunization campaign. This indicates that immunization must be a continuing program and not a sporadic campaign. A few years ago three children of a family in Gainesville, Georgia, died from diphtheria. None had been immunized.

A few states or cities have enacted legislation making a certificate of immunization mandatory for every child entering school for the first time. Much of the failure to secure immunization for preventable diseases may be attributed to ignorance, prejudice, and general apathy.

Community facilities

Every community must provide facilities for immunization, diagnosis, and treatment if an effective program of communicable disease control is to be maintained. Ideally the private physician should provide the leadership for immunization programs. In practice, however, this is not always the case. There are thousands of underprivileged families who are financially unable to secure the services of a private physician. Where infants and young children are under regular supervision of the pediatrician, a valuable contribution has been made by the physician in immunizing such children. The public health department is a major factor in promoting immunization and usually maintains clinics where protection may be secured without cost. Many hospitals have outpatient clinics where inoculations are offered at a nominal cost. Occasionally community organizations maintain and support private clinics.

As long as a reservoir of susceptible persons exist, the community will need to provide diagnostic and treatment facilities. Diagnosis is within the field of medical practice, but facilities are the responsibility of the community. Close working relationships among private physicians, health departments, and health care facilities such as hospitals and outpatient clinics will enhance these services. In some diseases the epidemiologic investigation and the public health laboratory may assist the private physician in diagnosis. The public health officer should be available for consultant service with private physicians, while public health nurses play a vital role in home care of communicable diseases by teaching isolation and basic nursing care. School nurses provide supervision of children who may be contacts and interpret to teachers and parents the importance of observing children for symptoms of communicable disease.

International control

International controls affect international travelers, immigrants, goods, animals, and animal products, and their means of transport, as may arise from provisions of International Sanitary Regulations, conventions, intergovernmental agreements or national laws. They also include any controls that may protect populations of one country against the known risk of infection from another country when a disease may be present in endemic or epidemic form. Immunization of persons and animals, deratting, control of arthropods, the quarantine and surveillance of travelers, and international exchange of epidemiological information are included.*

The administration of the sanitary regulations is by the Sanitary Conventions and Quarantine Section of the World Health Organization's secretariat. Among the activities of the World Health Organization is the publication of *Weekly Epidemiological Record* and a monthly *Epidemiological and Vital Statistics Report*. The activities of the World Health Organization in many countries has brought about a remarkable decrease in epidemic disease.

Environmental control

The earliest efforts to prevent and control communicable diseases were directed toward the environment. It took centuries to delineate and differentiate specific environmental factors that contribute to or cause infectious disease. Many of these factors involve various aspects of sanitation, while others are generally placed in the category of nuisances with little if any relationship to communicable disease. Today pure water, safe milk, and proper disposal of excreta are taken for granted by most persons; however, their importance is just as relevant now as it was several hundred years ago (Fig. 1).

Social change has had a profound effect upon certain aspects of environmental sanitation and has increased the need for constant surveillance. Concern is being voiced about the pollution of streams by industrial waste and the overtaxed sewage systems of many large cities. In some places raw (untreated) sewage is being poured into rivers from which cities obtain their water supplies, thus creating a potential health hazard. Harry Heimann states "Data are now available indicating we are running out of safe, clean, usable water, partly because we are dumping so much of our refuse into our main water sources, our streams."† (See Fig. 2.)

The rapid growth of suburban development beyond municipal sewage systems has led to an increased use of septic tanks and oxidizing ponds. Although in most cases these are satisfactory, there is always the possibility of a defect or an overflow of septic tanks leading to contamination of the water supply. More leisure time and the high mobility of an increasing pop-

*Gordon, John E.: Control of communicable diseases in man, ed. 10, New York, 1965, American Public Health Assn. Inc.

†Heimann, Harry: Air pollution and respiratory disease, Public Health Service Bulletin no. 1257, Washington, D. C., 1964, U. S. Government Printing Office.

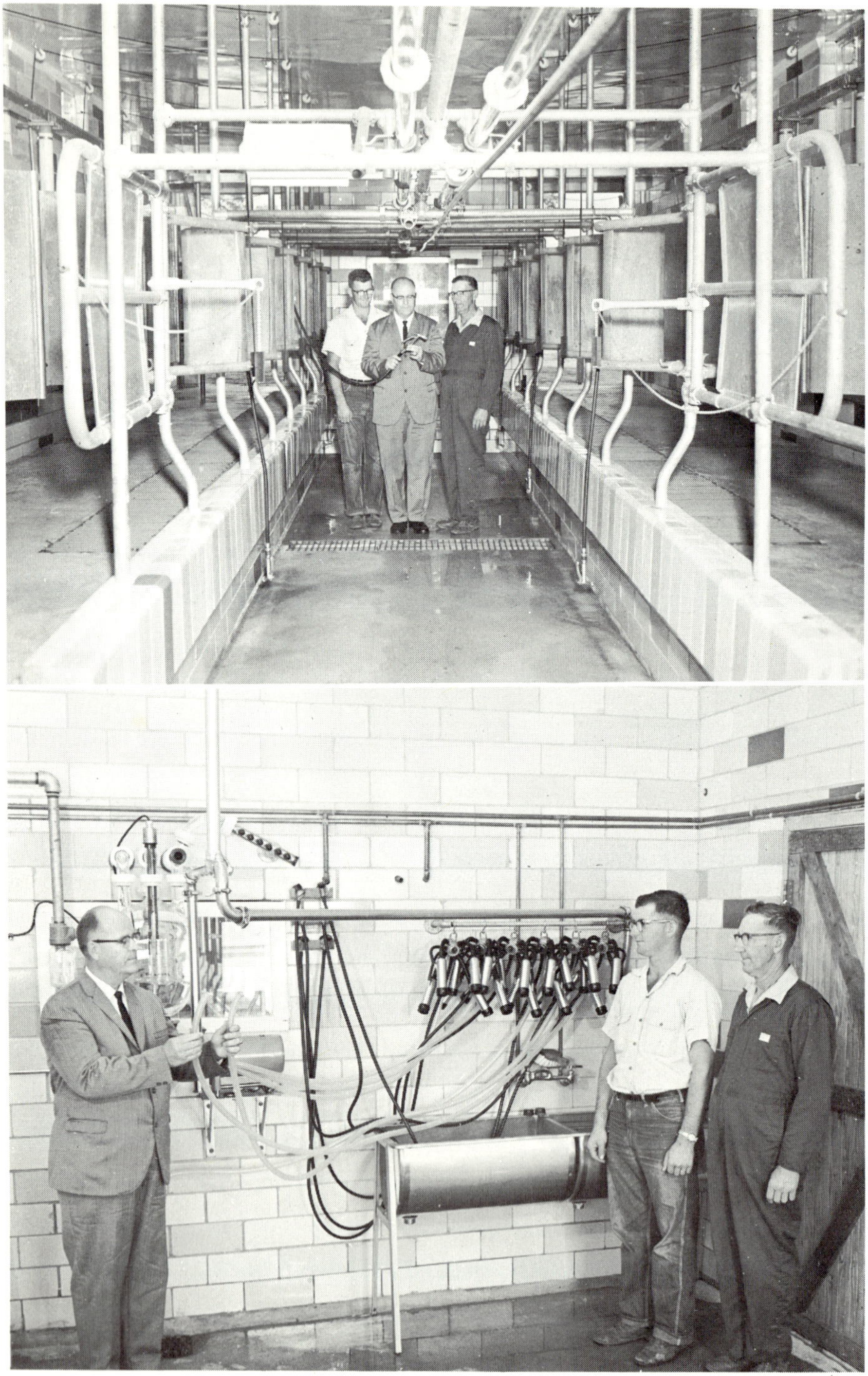

A

B

Fig. 1. For legend see opposite page.

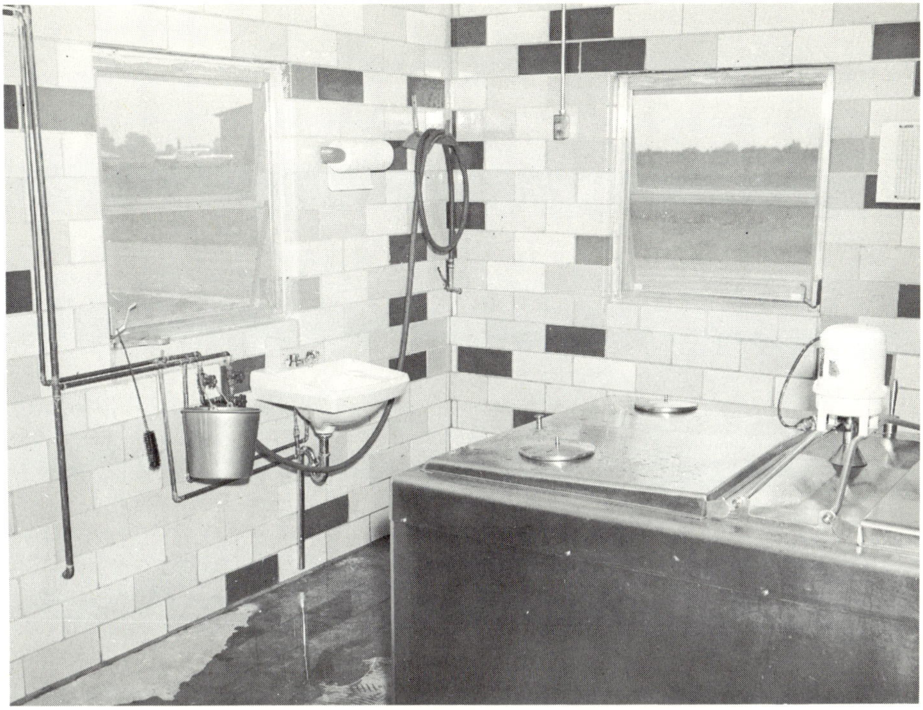

C

Fig. 1. Milk sanitation. **A,** Inspection of animal quarters. **B,** Inspection of milking equipment. **C,** Handwashing facilities where milk is processed. (Courtesy Athens, Clark County Health Department, Athens, Ga.)

ulation who are seeking recreational outlets has increased the number of roadside parks, camping grounds, trailer parks, and resort areas. Overcrowded substandard housing with broken-down sanitary facilities further contributes to the problem of environmental sanitation. The federal governments of the United States and Canada in cooperation with state, provincial, and local governments have provided money for slum clearance and urban redevelopment programs. Housing projects for low-income families are helping to reduce city slums. Large cities are undertaking the inspection of substandard housing and through their building codes require demolition or repair to meet the standards stated in the code, whereas failure to comply may be punishable by law.

Many communities are concerned with the increasing problem of collection of garbage and trash. Where facilities are unable to cope with the problem, it provides an environment for the increase of rodents and insects, which survive and multiply. The increased use of precooked and packaged food has been a major factor in problems of garbage and trash collection.

It has been well established that certain pathogens may be carried by air currents. During certain seasons of the year, pollens from plants, trees, shrubs, and grasses are carried by the air, causing pollinosis in certain sus-

A

B

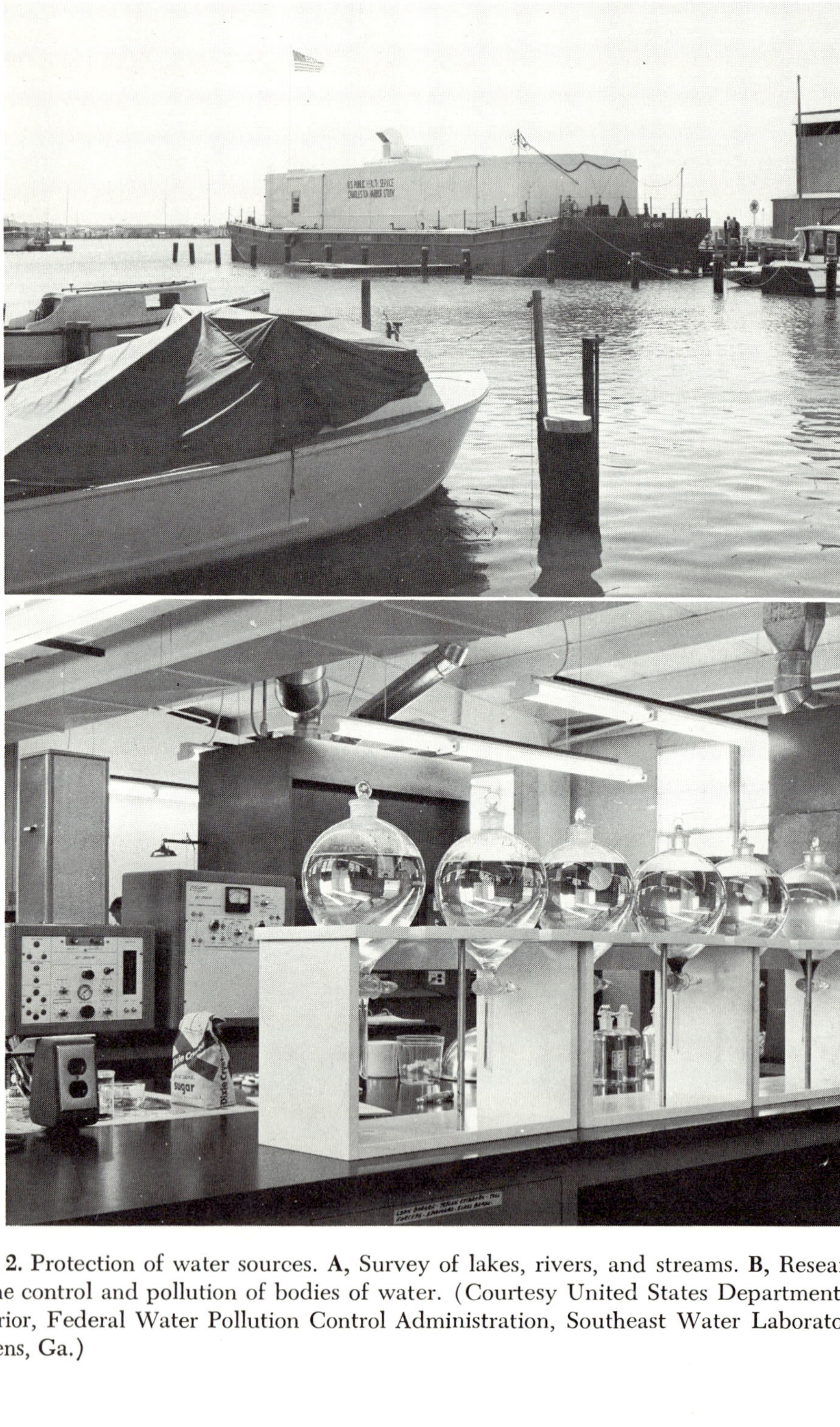

Fig. 2. Protection of water sources. **A,** Survey of lakes, rivers, and streams. **B,** Research in the control and pollution of bodies of water. (Courtesy United States Department of Interior, Federal Water Pollution Control Administration, Southeast Water Laboratory, Athens, Ga.)

ceptible persons. Industrial dusts in the air may be inhaled and contribute to respiratory disease. The pollution of air by man-made pollutants has become serious enough to be regarded as a threat to individual health. In 1963 Congress passed the Clean Air Act, initiating a broad program of control of community air pollution. There is unquestionable evidence that the combustion of fuels and their derivatives discharged into the air has a deleterious effect upon health. Although considerable data have been collected to substantiate the relationship between air pollution and respiratory disease, the extent of the problem has not been fully established. The pollution of air by radioactive materials is another aspect of the problem that is under study.

Arthropod control

Arthropods as vectors in the transmission of disease have been recognized since the beginning of this century. The reservoir of arthropods varies with the season of the year, since some exist for one season only, while others survive from year to year. Frequently organisms transmitted by arthropods are very virulent and cause high mortality in man. About 75 viruses have been identified and are known to be transmitted by arthropods. The principal vectors are mosquitoes, ticks, mites, and flies. Some species of these vectors are uncommon in the United States and Canada, and those that are common may be geographic in distribution. In areas where there is a high reservoir of vectors and a highly susceptible population of hosts, epidemics may occur.

Control measures vary with the specific vector and are based upon the epidemiologic factors relative to its transmission cycle. Most diseases transmitted by arthropods are not transmitted from and to man or by the usual vehicles of transmission. Some diseases are under international control as specified in the International Sanitary Regulations. Control measures include the destruction of breeding places and the use of insecticides known to be lethal to the vector.

Rodent control

Rodents and vectors may be one and the same in some instances. However, rodents are generally classified as mammals, wild or domestic, with incisors adapted for gnawing. Chief among common rodents are rats, mice, rabbits, and squirrels. Infected rodents serve as the host for insect vectors in diseases such as bubonic plague, in which the disease is transmitted to man by the bite of the vector *Xenopsylla cheopis* (rat flea).

Rodent control includes poisoning, trapping, rat-proofing of buildings, fumigation, and destruction of breeding places, particularly around docks, warehouses, and places where grain is stored. Proper care and firing of incinerators in residential dwellings and the use of insecticides are important measures in control. The accumulation of garbage in uncovered containers provides a feeding place for rats and mice and encourages their proliferation.

Animal control

Many animals, wild and domestic, may serve as a reservoir of infectious disease. Of primary concern is rabies, which is highly fatal to man and animals. A number of animals are involved in transmitting the disease, including wolves, foxes, skunks, racoons, coyotes, bats, and dogs. Dogs are the most common source of the disease in man, but cats may also be infected. Domestic farm animals are sometimes bitten by a rabid animal. Other diseases such as certain *Salmonella* infections, tularemia, and cat-scratch fever may be transmitted to man. Tetanus may be transmitted through indirect contact, since the tetanus bacillus lives in the intestinal tract of animals and may infect the soil and dust.

The prevention and control of rabies in dogs is by inoculation with rabies vaccine. Some states have laws that require annual vaccination of all dogs 3-6 months of age or older. The control of stray dogs through enforced local ordinances helps in the control of the disease. The use of rubber gloves when dressing rabbits, testing cows for Bang's disease, and pasteurizing milk for the prevention of tuberculosis are also important aids. All wounds and scratches should receive immediate attention, including thorough

A

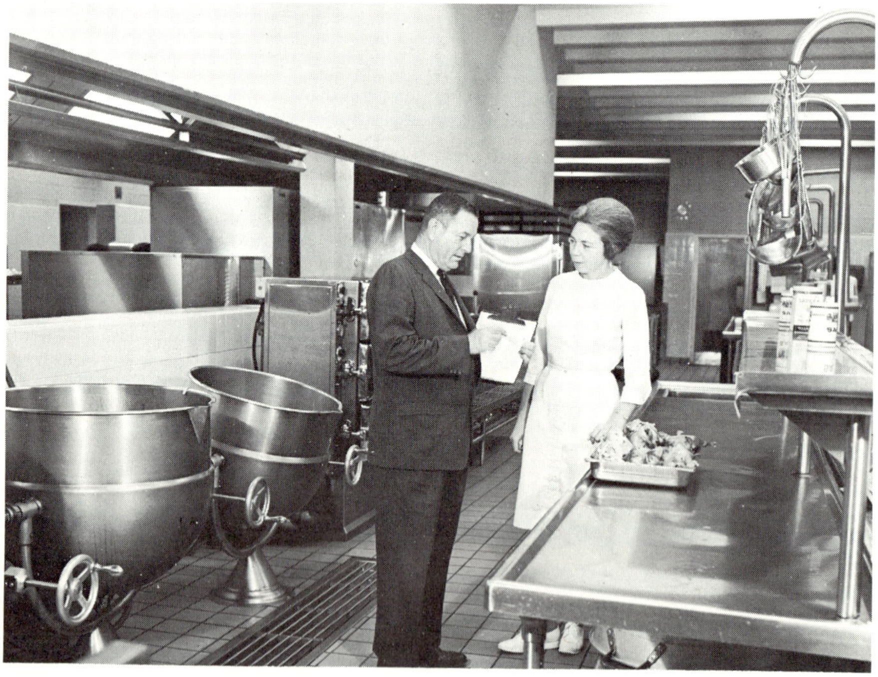

Fig. 3. Inspection of food-handling establishments. **A,** Inspector works with a dietitian on matters of sanitation. **B,** Checking equipment for sanitation. **C,** Inspector stresses the importance of handwashing. (Courtesy Athens, Clark County Health Department, Athens, Ga.)

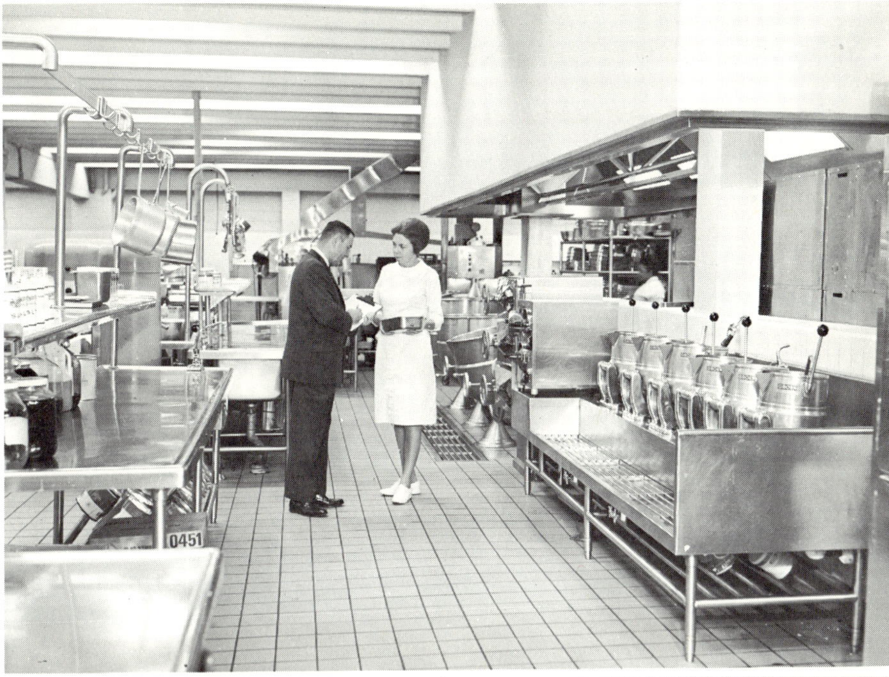

B

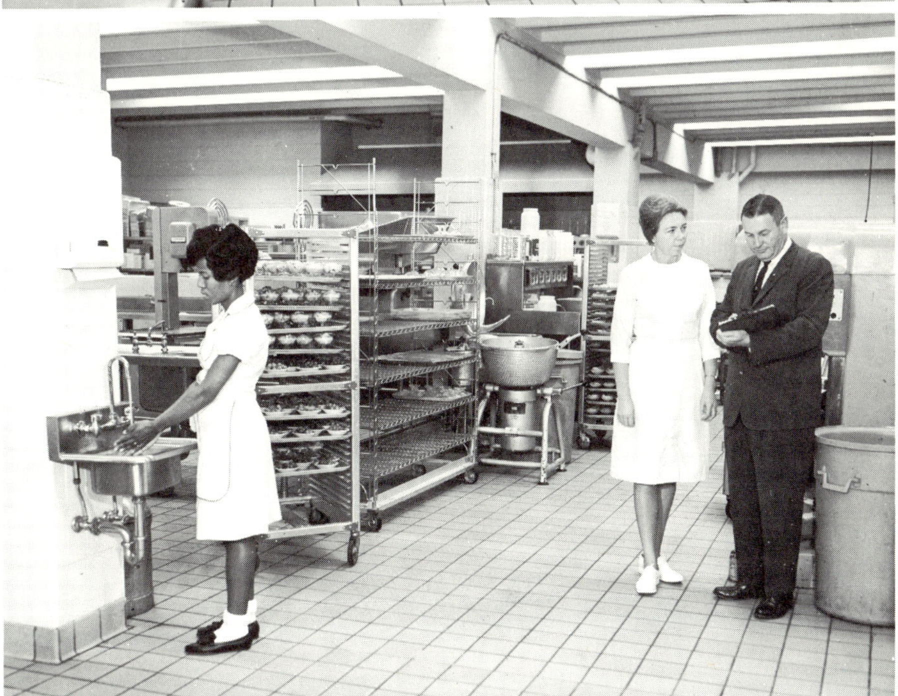

C

Fig. 3, cont'd. For legend see opposite page.

cleansing, and interstate and international control of animal food products should be a part of control methods.

Food product control

Food infection is the commonest disease resulting from contaminated food. However, typhoid fever, paratyphoid fever, and dysenteries may be transmitted through food by carriers. Certain ready-to-eat frozen foods have been incriminated in outbreaks of food infection (gastroenteritis). The control of food infection requires public education in the sanitary handling of food, thorough cooking, and proper refrigeration. The pasteurization of milk and egg products and the international control of food and animal feed are necessary for the prevention of food infection. There is a need for federal regulations concerning ready-to-eat frozen foods.*

Public education

No program, no matter how good, can move faster than the people. Education of the community, large or small, is basic to the control of communicable disease. The health department occupies a strategic place in this important phase of health work. Nurses employed in hospitals and physicians' offices have an equally important responsibility in public education. Hospital nurses have contact with large numbers of people every day, and they may exert considerable influence upon the parents of small children in the prevention of communicable disease. It is not enough to schedule immunization clinics unless the parent understands and appreciates the importance of protection. Physicians and nurses share the responsibility in developing an understanding of why the pregnant woman should not be exposed to german measles, mumps, or hepatitis. What may seem like a simple, routine isolation procedure to the nurse may be a traumatic experience for the patient. It is useless to exclude a child from school because of suspicious communicable disease unless the parent understands the importance of caring for the child and the need to protect other children. Too often it is easy to label a patient as uncooperative when actually someone has failed in some important aspect of education.

Today, as never before, mass communication media make it possible to reach large segments of the population with broad programs of public education. Health departments and professional groups frequently overlook these media, and lay people to a greater extent than at any other time are taking over matters concerning health education.

---

*The student is referred to chapters on specific diseases for more detailed information on prevention and control.

REFERENCES

1. Blake, John B.: Public health in the town of Boston 1630-1822, Cambridge, Mass., 1959, Harvard University Press.
2. Daland, Robert T.: Government and health, Birmingham, Ala., 1955, University of Alabama Bureau of Public Administration.

3. Gordon, John E.: Control of communicable disease in man, ed. 10, New York, 1965, American Public Health Association, Inc.
4. Hanlon, John J.: Principles of public health administration, ed. 4, St. Louis, 1964, The C. V. Mosby Co.
5. Heimann, Harry: Air pollution and respiratory disease, Public Health Service Bulletin no. 1257, Washington, D. C., 1964, U. S. Government Printing Office.
6. James, George: Emerging trends in public health and possible reactions, Public Health Reports **80**:579-586, July, 1965.
7. The Public Health Service today, Public Health Service Bulletin no. 165, Washington, D. C., 1964, U. S. Government Printing Office.
8. Van Avery, Peter, editor: Public Health 31, no. 6, New York, 1959, H. W. Wilson Co.

3
IMMUNOLOGY

The science of immunology is a complex one about which much is still unknown. The immunologic phenomenon goes far beyond the defense against disease, although a significant aspect of it is the prevention of disease. In its simplest terms and for our purpose we may say that immunity is the result of antigen-antibody reaction or the resistance that a person has against disease. The antigen-antibody reaction is the result of many complex physical, chemical, and biologic processes and circumstances. It is not the intent of this chapter to present in detail the numerous complexities of the immune process. The student who desires a more comprehensive review of the subject should turn to the references at the end of the chapter.

History

The earliest effort toward producing immunity in an individual occurred centuries before our present knowledge of immunology. The technique of variolation to modify active smallpox and produce a lasting immunity was introduced into England in 1721 and also into the American colonies about 1721, although it had been practiced in other countries long before. The sciences of microbiology, bacteriology, and immunology were essentially unknown. Without scientific knowledge of these principles, success of the procedure was based upon experience and observation.

Before the end of the eighteenth century Edward Jenner (1749-1823) had discovered that persons could be made immune to smallpox by inoculation with the virus of cowpox. Jenner was the first to use the term *vaccination,* and years later Pasteur extended usage of the word to apply to any vaccine used for immunization against infectious disease.

Nearly 100 years later Louis Pasteur (1822-1895), working with cholera in fowl, discovered that the disease could be prevented by inoculating the fowl with a preparation containing the weakened germ of cholera. From this discovery he conceived the idea that humans could be made resistant to specific diseases by inoculation with harmless germs of the disease. Continuing his investigations, he applied his knowledge to anthrax (a disease of cattle and secondarily of humans) and developed the anthrax vaccine, which with certain modifications is widely used to prevent the disease in animals and man. The most far-reaching work of Pasteur was the development of an antirabic vaccine to prevent rabies. Administration of the vaccine to a person exposed to rabies is called the "Pasteur treatment." Although some changes have been made in the original vaccine, the treatment continues to be used throughout the world.

The period between 1882 and 1910 has been described as the "golden age of discovery." The work of Jenner, Pasteur, and Koch had caught the imagination and stimulated the curiosity of early American bacteriologists, and between these years most of the pathogenic organisms causing disease were identified. The time was emerging when the science of immunology would become a reality. Attention was now being focused toward the development and introduction of antitoxins and vaccines to prevent specific diseases. The concept of immunity, antigens, and antibodies was known to the scientists, but they did not have the tools to investigate the processes that resulted in immunity. Today scientists have at their disposal fluorescent dyes, the electron microscope and radioactive isotopes with which they are able to study the unique phenomenon of antigens and antibodies and the way in which they work in the body to prevent communicable diseases.

Antigens and antibodies

Most antigens are proteins or closely connected protein-polysaccharide substances of microorganisms. Whether or not any nonprotein substance may be antigenic has not been proved. Antigens usually consist of substances that are foreign to the body, and when taken into the body, they stimulate the production of antibodies. However some recent evidence indicates that some antigenic substances are not foreign to the body and that antibodies may be present in the plasma in the absence of any specific disease. Such instances are regarded as a general biologic phenomenon. In general, however, if no antibodies are produced, a substance cannot be considered antigenic. In most instances the production of antibodies by the cells is an effort to reject or resist that which is foreign to the body or not of the body.

The rejection of substances that are foreign to the body may be illustrated by the failure sometimes encountered in tissue grafts and organ transplants. Homographs of skin undergo gradual changes including inflammation, edema, and eventually necrosis. However, when the donor is also the recipient, the graft is usually successful. In the case of identical twins, when the genetic constitution is identical, skin grafts may be successful. Researchers are studying the possibilities of suppressing the immune response through irradiation, radiomimetic drugs, corticosteroids, and antimetabolics. The belief is that by suppressing the immune response it may provide help during the most critical period of homografts.[2]

A more common example concerns the isoantigens of the erythrocytes.

The presence or absence of certain antigens (agglutinins) in the blood of individuals forms the basis for the classification of immunologic groups as A, B, AB, O, and Rh+ or Rh− antigens. The purpose of crossmatching blood, donor and recipient, prior to transfusion is to assure antigenic compatibility. However, it should not be assumed that antigenic compatibility eliminates all danger of a transfusion reaction, since an acute hemolytic transfusion reaction or febrile reaction may occur.

Antigens are classified as complete antigens that are capable of stimulating the production of antibodies. Partial antigens are called haptenes and are incapable of stimulating antibody production, although they are capable of reacting with certain antibodies. In the immunogenic process, differentiation between an antigen and a haptene may be difficult to determine.

Antibodies represent a complex group of related proteins known as immunoglobulins. The formation of antibodies occurs in the tissues and involves the cells of the reticuloendothelial system; however, other cells including lymphocytes, macrophages and eosinophils may be involved directly or indirectly in antibody production. Antibodies are produced whenever any foreign substance is introduced into the body. Numerous factors are involved in the antigen-antibody reaction including the route of administration. If an antigen is placed directly into the bloodstream, there is a rapid dissemination of the antigen throughout the tissues and immediate antigen-antibody response followed by a decline in antibody response. The intravenous injection of an antigen is used primarily in animal studies. When the antigen is injected intramuscularly or subcutaneously, there is a gradual release from the point of injection, which generally results in the effective production of antibodies and appears to prolong the antibody response. Most vaccines and serums designed to produce immunity by stimulating antibody production are administered subcutaneously or intramuscularly. Other related factors include the size of the dose and the use of adjuvants. The precise value of adjuvants in increasing the level of antibody response varies with the substance used, and their general effectiveness is still under investigation.

Resistance

At the beginning of this chapter it was stated that immunity is the resistance that an individual has against a disease. Individual resistance may be nonspecific or may be dependent upon the presence of specific antibodies in the blood or tissues, the action of which prevents or modifies a certain disease. Nature has endowed individuals with certain mechanical and chemical mechanisms that enable them to resist invasion by pathogens. These mechanisms are both external and nonspecific internal defenses. The unbroken skin and mucous membranes provide a formidable barrier to the invasion of pathogenic organisms. Normal body secretions such as the lacrimal fluid that bathes the eyes the acetic acid content or perspiration, the acidity of vaginal secretions, and the acid content of the stomach kill many pathogens before they can produce disease. The sticky mucus secretions of the respiratory passages trap bacteria and may be expelled by coughing and sneezing. The ciliated epithelial cells of the deeper respiratory passages are in a continuous wavelike motion that propels pathogens and foreign particles upward where they may be swallowed or expectorated.

Nonspecific defenses are less well understood. Evidence indicates that the blood and other body fluids offer limited resistance to pathogenic organisms. Intensive research has led to a partial understanding of properdin as a factor in nonspecific resistance. Properdin is a serum protein that is distinct from the serum immunoglobulins but that does participate in immune reactions. Properdin together with other substances, magnesium ions and complement component C3, is known as the properdin system.

Environmental factors such as temperature, humidity, and seasonal and cyclic incidence of communicable disease may have a relationship to individual resistance. These factors are not well understood, but they may affect the susceptibility of the individual to disease by altering the normal physiology of the body.

A number of physical factors are known to influence susceptibility of the individual to disease. Studies have shown that malnutrition resulting from insufficient or inadequate food, extreme fatigue, and exhaustion may decrease individual resistance and render a person more susceptible to diseases such as pneumonia or tuberculosis. However, by the same token environmental factors and repeated pregnancies may increase a person's susceptibility to tuberculosis. Good nutrition and vitamin supplements do enhance a person's resistance to disease. Age appears to play an important role in resistance. Some communicable diseases are most hazardous to infants and young children, whereas they rarely affect elderly persons, or the direct opposite may be true.

The state of a person's health bears a positive relationship to his degree of resistance to communicable disease. Studies have shown that individuals with leukemia, cancer, diabetes, and uremia have an increased susceptibility to infectious diseases.

Phagocytosis

The role of phagocytosis in defense against pathogenic organisms is one of the body's most important defense mechanisms. The defense results from the action of the polymorphonuclear leukocytes that circulate in the bloodstream and have the power to migrate to a focal point of injury. The macrophages (wandering cells) engulf and eventually clear away cellular debris. Although phagocytosis is an important defense against many bacteria, their action is purely defensive and does not result in any immunity. However, specific antibodies are known to act as adjuvants to the phagocytes in the immunologic process, but their specific mechanisms of action are still to be determined.

Classification of immunity

Immunity is a state of defense carried out by specific immunological reactions in the body, and the process needed to induce such a state is called "immunization." Immunity is either natural, such as a species-specific, racial and individual, or acquired, which may be active or passive.

Natural immunity. A natural passive immunity is known to exist in newborn infants. Just how the placental transfer of immunoglobulins from the maternal circulation to the fetus occurs is not completely understood. It is known that not all globulin antibodies are transferred. Antibodies against certain of the bacterial diarrheal diseases such as those caused by *Salmonella typhosa* and *Escherichia coli* are not transferred. The infant is dependent upon his own immunologic mechanisms for the production of antibodies against these diseases. The infant does have globulin antibodies that protect against many bacterial and viral diseases. Many antibodies are present in colostrum and breast milk, but there is doubt concerning their transfer to the breast-fed infant. At present the general belief is that no transfer takes place.[5] This kind of immunity protects the infant for several months. There is increasing evidence that certain vaccines may be safely administered to the newborn or the very young infant and that by doing so the antibody level is increased and prolongs the immune state.

Species immunity involves differences in susceptibility to communicable diseases among species differing from one another. It is known that many diseases of animals are not transmitted to man, while those of man are not transmitted to members of the animal kingdom. However, there are a number of diseases common to domestic animals, rodents, fowl, and insects that may be transmitted to man. In such cases man is usually the innocent bystander, with infection being accidental.

Racial immunity appears to exist among different races and groups of the same species. Such immunity involves some animals as well as man. It has generally been believed that certain races of people have immunity to diseases to which other races are susceptible; for example, Jewish people are more resistant to tuberculosis than the Negro race. There is some belief that the disparity in standards of living may be a factor in the degree of susceptibility.

There is little evidence to substantiate the belief in individual immunity. Since man lives in an environment in which he is frequently exposed to minute doses of infectious agents without his knowledge, it seems likely that inapparent invasion of pathogenic organisms has resulted in antibody production rather than any inherent quality being present.

Acquired immunity. Acquired immunity is the result of natural infection or artificial inoculation against infection.

A typical example of *acquired passive immunity* is the maternal antibodies a fetus receives *in utero,* which help the infant combat infection after birth. Such antibodies usually provide protection for only 3 to 6 months after birth. This type of immunity is also called "naturally acquired passive immunity."

Passive immunity can also be induced by the administration of previously prepared antibodies, such as the use of antitoxin sera in the management of diphtheria and tetanus. Similarly, hyperimmune sera are used in the prophylactic prevention of infectious hepatitis and smallpox vaccination complications.

Acquired active immunity may be acquired either naturally, such as after a subclinical or an overt attack of a disease (smallpox), or it may be induced artificially (immunization programs carried out for children).

Immunization programs are carried out to induce *acquired artificial active immunity*. Immunity may be induced through either the use of dead bacteria, attenuated live organisms, or a modified toxin (toxoid). They all provide protection by stimulating the production of antibodies. Booster doses are needed to keep an adequately high level of these antibodies. The program of active immunization is usually started at about 6 months of age because by this age maternal antibodies acquired *in utero* are at their lowest level, and do not interfere with the active immunization. Moreover, at this age, the child's own antibody-forming system is well developed.

Vaccines and bacterins

Vaccines may be live and when administered produce active immunity by infection. They may also be killed (noninfective) antigens rendered inactive by heat or chemicals. If the antigenic substance has been prepared from bacteria, it is called a bacterin. The vaccine consists of the active agent of the disease or one closely related to the organism causing the disease. Live attenuated vaccines are modified or weakened in such a way that they do not cause serious disease in the host to whom they are administered, but they must be capable of producing an active immunity. Under certain conditions the killed or inactivated vaccine may be reactivated. Vaccines are administered prior to exposure to the disease except in the case of rabies vaccine. (See Table 1.) Almost all vaccines are administered by the subcutaneous or intramuscular route. The Sabin attenuated live poliovirus vaccine is administered orally. Vaccines administered to produce active immunity require several injections spaced at varying intervals; exceptions are measles and smallpox vaccine, which require only one inoculation. The response of the vaccine in producing antibodies depends upon a number of factors, including the particular antigen, the condition of the individual, the route of administration, and the size of the dose. The toxicity of most vaccines is relatively low; however, viruses for vaccine grown on chick embryos may result in a serious or fatal reaction if administered to persons hypersensitive to eggs, chicken, or chicken feathers. Therefore, administration to such persons is contraindicated. Earlier in this chapter we referred to the fact that the immune response may be suppressed by certain drugs and roentgen rays. Considerable research, although not conclusive, indicates that persons with certain malignant diseases tend to be poor producers of antibodies.[5]

Text continued on p. 48.

Table 1. Immunization schedule

Disease	Causative organism	Immunizing agent	Recommended age	Number of injections
Diphtheria	*Corynebacterium diphtheriae*	Triple vaccine—diphtheria toxoid usually combined with tetanus toxoid and pertussis vaccine (DPT)	3 to 6 mo.	3
Influenza	Influenza virus types A, B, A-1, and A-2	Influenza vaccine (CCA)	Annually for high risk groups—elderly patients with chronic disease and pregnant women	2
Mumps	Myxovirus	Live attenuated mumps vaccine	Susceptible children approaching puberty, adolescents, and adults	2 given if skin test is negative
Pertussis (whooping cough)	*Bordetella pertussis*	Triple vaccine—pertussis vaccine usually combined with diphtheria and tetanus toxoids	2 mo. to 6 yr.	3
Poliomyelitis	Polioviruses types 1, 2, and 3	Live attenuated poliovirus vaccine (Sabin Oral) with attenuated live viruses of types 1, 2, and 3	1 to 2 mo. or 4 to 5 mo.	3 feedings of monovalent or 2 feedings of trivalent; trivalent vaccine has now largely replaced the monovalent vaccine—trivalent oral polio vaccine (TOPV)
		Inactivated poliovirus vaccine	1 to 2 mo.	
Rabies	Virus	Rabies vaccine (Semple)	After exposure	14 to 21
		Duck-embryo vaccine	Postexposure	14 to 21

Interval	*Reinforcing doses*	*Side effects*	*Comments*
4 to 6 wk.	Each 3 to 5 yr. until 12 yr. of age.	Minor in children; may produce severe reaction in adults and older children	Adult toxoid or fluid diphtheria tetanus toxoid should be given to persons over 12 yr. of age to avoid severe reactions
2 mo.	1 dose annually—usually in fall	Febrile reaction with aching and malaise	In emergency, primary injections may be given at 2-week intervals; vaccine may also be given to infants and children; the status of immunization schedule and vaccine can change rapidly so recommendations by the Department of Health should be consulted before any procedure is carried out
1 to 4 wk.	None	Minor	Positive skin test with mumps antigen indicates immunity to disease; vaccine may decrease severity of disease and prevent orchitis in adult male; vaccine is contraindicated for children less than 12 mo. of age, and for pregnant women
4 to 6 wk.	Each 3 to 5 yr.	Minor when combined with diphtheria and tetanus toxoids	Pertussis vaccine may be discontinued after 6 to 8 yr. of age; pertussis vaccine administered alone may cause cerebral pathology, although it is rare; babies with a history of seizures or other central nervous system disease should not receive the vaccine
4 to 6 wk.	Variable	Few	Some variations in schedules and ages permitted for all children, also adults; recommended for adults at risk, for overseas travel, to military personnel, and under epidemic conditions; vaccination is contraindicated in patients with severe underlying diseases such as leukemia or generalized malignancy, or those with lowered resistance because of therapy; should not be given to pregnant women especially in the first trimester
1 mo.	7 mo. and 2 to 3 yr.		Use being limited in favor of oral vaccine
Daily	None	Encephalitis possible	In some instances hyperimmune rabies serum may be administered in addition to Semple vaccine
Daily	None	Few if any	

Continued.

Table 1. Immunization schedule—cont'd

Disease	*Causative organism*	*Immunizing agent*	*Recommended age*	*Number of injections*
			Preexposure	4
Rubella (German measles)	Virus	Attenuated live virus vaccine	1 yr. to puberty; should be offered routinely to all girls between the ages of 11 and 14 yr.	1
Rubeola (measles)	Virus	Live attenuated measles vaccine (Edmonson B strain); live attenuated measles vaccine (Edmonson B strain) with immune globulin; Schwarz and Moraten strains	12 mo.	1
Smallpox (variola)	Poxvirus variolae	Smallpox vaccine	After 12 mo.	1
Tetanus	*Clostridium tetani*	Tetanus toxoid combined with diphtheria toxoid and pertussis vaccine (DPT)	2 mo.	3
Tuberculosis	*Micobacterium tuberculosis*	Attenuated Bacille Calmette Guérin vaccine (BCG)	All ages—only if tuberculin negative	1

Interval	*Reinforcing doses*	*Side effects*	*Comments*
3 weekly fourth, fifth, or sixth month	Booster at 1- to 2-yr. intervals	Few	If exposure occurs after preexposure immunization, 1 dose of vaccine is given; if exposure is severe, additional doses should be given for 10 to 20 days
		Mild fever, arthralgia, lymphadenopathy, and variable severity of rashes	Contraindicated for pregnant women—gamma globulin may be administered to exposed pregnant women during first trimester of pregnancy; the vaccine is also contraindicated for individuals with altered immune states—leukemia, lymphoid malignancies, recipients of immunosuppressive therapy
	None	Febrile reaction with temperature; may have skin rash	Vaccine not given to adults as most persons are serologically immune by the age of 15 yr.; gamma globulin will reduce severity of bebrile reaction; not indicated with Schwartz strain; live attenuated vaccine should not be given to pregnant women or to patients being treated with steroids, irradiation, antimetabolics, or agents that depress immunologic capacities
None	Every 5 yr.	Local and occasionally systemic	Public Health Departments are now recommending that primary smallpox vaccination be discontinued on a routine basis; they stress vaccination in the event of exposure and in preparation for foreign travel; personnel in medical and allied health fields should be vaccinated every 3 yr.; vaccination is contraindicated in cases of eczema and skin lesions, in patients with depressed immunologic responses, and in pregnancy
4 to 6 wk.	10 yr. or after injury	Minor	If given alone, administration should begin at 3 mo. of age; may be given to adults at any time
	Repeat after 2 to 3 mo. if tuberculin negative	Local	Administered to persons living or travelling in areas of the world where tuberculosis is a major health problem; and for those likely to be exposed directly to the disease—give 2 mo. before the exposure

Continued.

Table 1. Immunization schedule—cont'd

Disease	*Causative organism*	*Immunizing agent*	*Recommended age*	*Number of injections*
Typhoid fever and paratyphoid fever	*Salmonella typhosa* and *Salmonella Paratyphosa*	Typhoid vaccine (TAB vaccine)	2 yr. and over	3 Primary
Yellow fever, cholera, typhus, Rocky Mountain spotted fever*				

*Vaccines are available and may be required for foreign countries where diseases are epidemic. Vaccine

Table 2. Classification of vaccines

Live attenuated	*Killed noninfective*	*Toxoids*
Bacterial	*Bacterial*	
BCG (bacille Calmette Guérin)	Pertussis	Diphtheria
	Typhoid paratyphoid	Tetanus
Viral	*Viral*	
Measles	Influenza	
Edmonson B strain		
Schwarz		
Poliomyelitis (Sabin)	Poliomyelitis (Salk)	
Smallpox	Rabies	
Yellow fever	Adenovirus (3, 4, 7)	
Mumps	Measles	

Pertussis vaccine and diphtheria and tetanus toxoids combined as DPT.
Quadruple vaccine, diphtheria, tetanus toxoids, pertussis, and Salk vaccine are available.

Toxoids

Toxoids for active immunization are available for diphtheria and tetanus in two forms: an aqueous or fluid preparation and an absorbed or precipitated preparation. Toxoid is an exotoxin that has been detoxified to eliminate the danger from the use of the toxin but it remains capable of stimulating antigen-antibody response. Formalin is used to detoxify the aqueous preparation, while the absorbed toxoid consists of a suspension of the toxoid and is precipitated by adding alum. The preparation known as alum-precipitated toxoid has had wide use in immunization practices. Only two injections are required of the toxoid. A multiple preparation of absorbed diphtheria and tetanus toxoid and pertussis vaccine is administered to infants and children under 4 years of age. Children between 4 and 12 years of age should receive only diphtheria and tetanus if they have been

Interval	Reinforcing doses	Side effects	Comments
Weekly	Every 1 to 2 yr. if travelling abroad	Local and systemic	Routine immunization not recommended; limited to persons exposed and to persons travelling abroad

for Rocky Mountain spotted fever may be given to high-risk groups of persons.

previously immunized. After 12 years of age an adult type of diphtheria and tetanus toxoid is administered.[3]

Booster doses (secondary response)

The primary antigenic stimulus occurs after the initial series of injections of vaccine or toxoid. When the same antigen is reintroduced (booster dose), after a period of time a more rapid and higher antibody level frequently occurs. This antigenic stimulation is the secondary response.

The antigen-antibody response is slow and gradual after the primary stimulus, but after the secondary stimulus a response may be noted in a few hours, reaching a peak level in eight to ten days. Investigation appears to indicate that a latent period between the primary and the secondary stimulus is necessary in order for the booster dose to be effective. Antibody response after the secondary stimulation has been shown to be longlasting, making it possible to delay reinforcing doses. The present system of scheduling injections is based on this principle. If an infant receives three injections of DPT at monthly intervals (primary stimulus), the first booster dose (secondary stimulus) is given about one year later and the second booster or reinforcing dose about four or five years after the first booster dose. The same preparation should be used for the first booster dose (DPT), but pertussis vaccine is eliminated from the second booster and from any reinforcing doses given subsequently.

Antitoxins (antiserums)

Antitoxins are serums administered to neutralize toxins produced by bacteria in certain diseases, primarily diphtheria, tetanus, gas gangrene, and botulism. Antitoxins are prepared in the bodies of animals, usually horses or rabbits that have been sensitized against the disease in question. The administration of antitoxin produces an acquired passive immunity the duration of which is about two or three weeks. Immunologic agents for active immunity are not administered at the same time or immediately following prophylactic or therapeutic doses of antitoxin. Unlike vaccines that are administered prior to exposure to disease, antitoxin is given to persons who are sick with the disease. Exotoxins produced by the bacteria are extremely dangerous, and antitoxin provides readymade antibodies to neutralize the toxin. The exotoxins of tetanus and botulism are similar, since they are produced by organisms related to the same species. Both are protein substances and have a similar affinity for specific tissue. The administration of antitoxin involves a certain degree of risk to the individual. A person hypersensitive to the protein of horse serum may suffer serious serum sickness or anaphylactic reaction. Therefore, it is important that sensitization tests be done before the administration of antitoxin. Antitoxin may be administered intravenously, but the intramuscular route is usually used. Children under 10 years of age who have been exposed to diphtheria and who have no history of active immunization against diphtheria may be given a prophylactic dose of antitoxin.

Gamma globulin (human)

Gamma globulin is one of the immunoglobulins that contains antibody activity. It is derived from the serum of persons who have recovered from the disease. It has also been made from human placentas that contain large amounts of adult serum. The serum from about 1000 specimens is pooled, which concentrates the antibodies and appears to be significant in eliminating the danger of serum hepatitis that may be encountered in unconcentrated gamma globulin. Immune serum globulin produces a passive immunity, and where it has been administered to children with measles the disease has been modified, but a natural active immunity follows the disease. Immune serum is administered with live attenuated measles vaccine to reduce the febrile reaction that may accompany the vaccine. (See Table 1.) Human gamma globulin has been used as prophylaxis in patients with infectious hepatitis and rubella and in adult males with mumps (parotitis).

A tetanus immune globulin has recently been released and is effective prophylactically in patients with wounds that may be contaminated with tetanus organisms. Its primary advantage is that it is free from the risk of inducing hypersensitivity.[6]

Intracutaneous immunity tests

A number of preparations are available for intracutaneous tests. Some tests are diagnostic as in the tuberculin skin test, or they may be for the determination of susceptibility to a disease as in the Schick test in diphtheria. The Schick test consists of 0.1 ml. of diphtheria toxin injected intracutaneously on the flexor surface of the forearm, and a control is placed on the other arm. If an area of redness begins to appear in twenty-four hours, becoming progressively more pronounced within a week and showing some swelling and tenderness, the test is diagnosed positive. A positive test indicates that few, if any, antibodies circulate.

Other tests will be discussed under prophylaxis in the appropriate sections of the book.

Antimicrobial drugs

Many drugs have a place in the prophylaxis of certain communicable diseases. Such drugs probably act in three ways: (1) by preventing the occurrence of an infection, (2) by checking an infection during its incubation phase, or (3) by controlling an infection after it has developed and preventing its progress and complications. Examples of such drugs include the use of sulfonamides to prevent outbreaks of meningococcus meningitis. Studies have been underway for some time in the use of Isoniazid as prophylaxis among contacts of active cases of tuberculosis. Certain antibiotic drugs have been in use for some time to prevent streptococcal infections among persons who have had rheumatic fever. Chemotherapeutic drugs have been used successfully in preventing rickettsial disease, psittacosis, and some respiratory infections. Recently a new drug N-methylisatin β-thiosemicarbazone, has been used to prevent smallpox in exposed persons. The drug appears to have a prophylactic effect regardless of any prior condition such as age, vaccination history, or state of immunity.[1]

Contraindications

The use of antigenic substances for active or passive immunization is a safe procedure for most persons. Under certain conditions their use may be restricted; however, each case must be determined on an individual basis by the physician.

Some antigenic substances have been prepared using chick embryos, or they may contain penicillin. These preparations are generally contraindicated if the individual has a history of hypersensitivity to chicken, feathers, eggs, or penicillin. Physicians generally delay a scheduled inoculation for a child who appears ill at the time of appointment. Research has shown that patients with certain types of neoplastic diseases show a derangement of the immune system. Such persons have a decrease in antibody production, and patients become highly susceptible to infectious disorders. The same is true of patients receiving steroids, x-ray therapy, alkylating drugs, and antimetabolics. Live attenuated vaccines are usually contraindicated during pregnancy. Green and associates have cautioned against vaccination for smallpox during pregnancy because of the possibility of vaccinia in the human fetus. If for any reason the vaccination is required, as in foreign travel, they state that hyperimmune gamma globulin should be given at the same time that the vaccination is given.[4] Vaccination for smallpox is generally contraindicated for children with eczema or other skin disorders until such conditions have abated.

Side effects

Most vaccines are relatively free from any side effects; however, febrile reactions may occur in some children. Reactions in infants may vary from slight irritability to fever, refusal of food, and restlessness. Febrile reactions may follow the administration of live attenuated measles vaccine. The administration of immune globulin at the same time reduces the incidence of severe reactions. Most problems encountered after immunization procedures are complications that may be caused by faulty technic, improper sterilization of equipment, or some factor within the recipient.

Serum sickness and anaphylactoid reaction. Serum sickness and anaphylactoid reaction are manifestations of an allergic response to the introduction of a foreign protein. The use of immune horse serum is largely confined to tetanus antitoxin, botulinus, and gas gangrene, rabies, and snake venom antiserums. However, it should be kept in mind that horse serum is not the only cause of an anaphylactoid reaction. Severe reactions may occur from insect stings, drugs, pollens, or chemicals to which the individual is hypersensitive.

Primary serum sickness is dependent on the size of the dose, route of administration, and purity of the product used. The local reaction occurs about the site of the injection and consists of edema and erythema. At about seven to twelve days after the injection a systemic reaction occurs, characterized by fever, aching, urticaria, and maculopapular eruptions. Severity of symptoms may vary from mild to severe, lasting from days to weeks.

Accelerated serum sickness occurs after a second injection of horse serum. Symptoms appear sooner, and in addition to those in primary serum sickness there may be dyspnea and wheezing.

Atopic serum reaction occurs in persons with known allergy or hypersensitivity to animal dander and horse serum. If horse serum is administered to these persons, generalized symptoms occur with vasomotor collapse and possibly death. Such anaphylactoid reaction occurs immediately following injection of the serum.

While anaphylactoid reaction rarely occurs, its prevention is dependent on obtaining a careful history before the administration of any preparation containing horse serum or antibiotic such as penicillin. When the life of the patient may be dependent on the preparation to be injected, careful preparation should be made for any emergency and should include epinephrine, antihistamines, oxygen, and a tracheotomy set.[5]

Nursing

The administration of immunologic agents is carried out in health department clinics, in outpatient clinics, in hospitals, in physicians' offices, and in mass survey procedures. In all, nurses play an important role. Nurses are responsible for proper care and sterilization of the equipment used. Syringes and needles should be the proper size for the agent used and the route of administration. Intramuscular injections given to children under 3 years of age should be placed in the gluteal muscle, and for children over 3 years of age they may be given in the deltoid muscle. Injections should be alternated from left to right sides in both the gluteal and deltoid muscles. If live attenuated measles vaccine and immune globulin are given at the same time, the vaccine is placed in the gluteal muscle on one side and the immune globulin in the gluteal muscle on the opposite side. The gamma globulin and vaccine should not be mixed in the same syringe.

Nurses should be familiar with the immunologic agent being administered and any possible side effects that may be anticipated. They should also be aware of the possibility of severe reaction, and epinephrine should always be available. A physician should always be present when antitoxin is administered, and blood pressure and pulse should be checked at frequent intervals during and after administration.

Accurate records should be maintained of all primary and reinforcing injections. Many states or cities require such records for children entering school for the first time.

The nurse working in the hospital with mothers of young children has a challenging opportunity to teach, interpret, and encourage primary immunization of all young children and to stress the importance of keeping appointments for booster or reinforcing doses. Nurses in clinics or physicians' offices should be aware of the many visits that are necessary in completing immunizations. Small children become restless and irritable, and arranging visits to avoid long delays is appreciated by most parents.

Investigational vaccine program

On the recommendation of the Public Health Service Advisory Committee on Immunization Practice, the National Communicable Disease Center in Atlanta, Georgia, has announced the establishment of an Investigational Vaccine Program. The first product to be made available is the pentavalent (ABCDE) botulinum toxoid, aluminum phosphate absorbed. The center is expected to announce in the near future the addition of an anthrax vaccine, anthrax protective antigen, aluminum hydroxide adsorbed. Both of these products were developed by George C. Wright and associates at the Army Biological Laboratories at For Detrick, Frederick, Maryland.

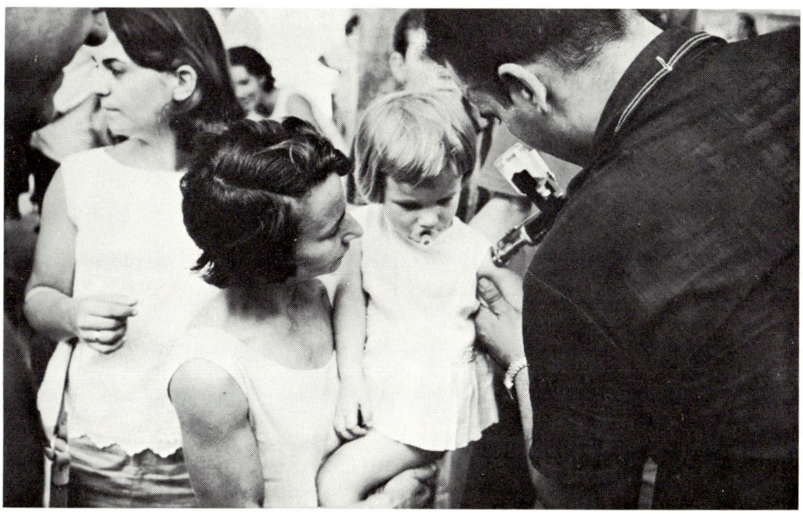

Fig. 4. Small girl, in her mother's arms, being immunized. (Courtesy National Medical Audiovisual Center, Chamblee, Ga.)

The objective of the new program is to provide qualified medical investigators with a source of vaccine whose effectiveness and safety are established but whose applications are too limited to sustain commercial production and distribution.*

Immunization schedule

A survey of the literature indicates that there is some variation in agreement concerning the most desirable schedule for immunizations. Table 1 summarizes some of the recommended procedure.

---

*Magovern, M. Patricia: Personal communication.

REFERENCES

1. Chemical agent may protect against smallpox, Am. J. Nurs. **65**:28, Jan., 1965.
2. Dubos, Rene J., and Hirsch, James G., editors: Bacterial and mycotic infections of man, ed. 4, Philadelphia, 1965, J. B. Lippincott Co.
3. Gordon, John E.: Control of communicable diseases in man, ed. 10, New York, 1965, American Public Health Association, Inc.
4. Green, D. M., Reid, S. M., and Rhaney, K.: Generalized vaccinia in the human foetus, Lancet **1**:1296-1298, June 11, 1966.
5. Smith, Alice Lorraine: Carter's principles of microbiology, ed. 4, St. Louis, 1961, The C. V. Mosby Co.
6. Tetanus immune globulin, Am. J. Nurs. **65**:159-160, Nov., 1965.

4

SOCIAL, PSYCHOLOGIC, AND ECONOMIC FACTORS

The purpose of this chapter is to try to elucidate some of the factors in our society that contribute to the incidence of communicable diseases, what such diseases mean to the psychic constitution, and the economic impact at all levels of society.

SOCIAL FACTORS

Man is a social creature and belongs to a large group that includes men, women, and children of all ages, sexes, and races. The larger society is a complex structure that determines social behavior and the role that each individual member is expected to play. Within certain well-defined limits the individual is expected to conform to the standards established by organized society, and his failure to do so carries a threat of punishment.

Organized society is not perfect and never has been. Within its loosely tied system of values, disorganization and social discontent occur, and established patterns break down because they are no longer compatible with social change. As a result, people begin to view certain aspects of society as undesirable, and what was once accepted is now regarded as untenable, and a demand for change is made. When disorganization and discontent occur, social problems are created.

During the past several decades social change has been rapid, and almost every facet of American and Canadian culture has been affected. Society demands more and better education, more and better health services, elimination of slums, and better housing. It demands better care for the aged and increased control of the nonconforming members of society.

Today the social problems loom as a giant kaleidoscope, and no matter what way it is turned society is made aware of the need for amelioration and elimination of the undesirable and intolerable patterns of American and Canadian culture (Fig. 5).

Many communicable diseases fall into the realm of social problems, in-

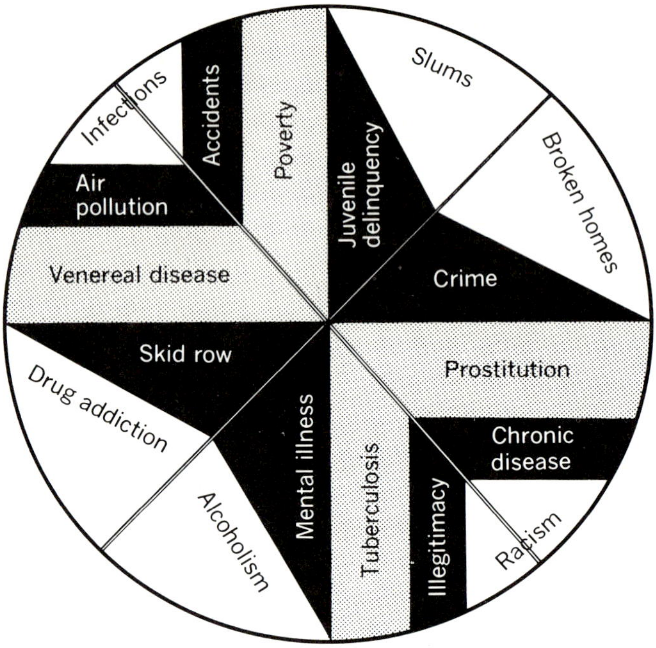

Fig. 5. The kaleidoscope of social problems.

cluding tuberculosis, venereal disease, and hospital-acquired infections. There are those in society who envision a world free of tuberculosis, smallpox, measles, diphtheria, venereal disease, and pertussis. Countless hours of labor have produced the weapons aimed at eradication. A sterile world in which pathogenic microorganisms are reduced to the irreducible minimum must be viewed as visionary rather than realistic. The production of preventive and therapeutic agents for the eradication of communicable disease is a noteworthy achievement. However, when segments of the world's population live in hopeless dejection, devoid of the essentials to sustain life, and without accessibility to medical services, it is fallacious reasoning to believe that eradication is just around the corner.

Communicable disease is not an isolated entity peculiar to only one segment of society, but too frequently its propagation is nourished and kept alive by an increasing segment of underprivileged society.

Poverty

Within the framework of American culture several million men, women, and children live in poverty. Poverty is not new, and it is a worldwide problem. There is ample evidence that it has existed for thousands and thousands of years. The Old Testament is filled with references to poverty and its causes. Jesus said "for the poor always ye have with you."* Poverty rep-

*St. John 12:8.

resents differences in class structure. To be poor means to lack adequate food, clothing, housing, medical care, and a host of ordinary necessities of contemporary living. In some countries to be poor means the likelihood of typhus, smallpox, malaria, and death by starvation (Fig. 6).

It is not easy to define poverty because there are different kinds of poverty, and people view poverty in different ways. The United States Government has attempted to define poverty in terms of financial income, however, income is a poor criterion for determining poverty.

Many nurses in hospitals, public health agencies, nursing homes, and schools see the results of poverty while engaged in their daily activities. It may be poliomyelitis or diphtheria because of the lack of immunization, or it may be severe infantile diarrhea, tuberculosis, infections of worms, or skin infections. In a study made by Yow and associates, of infantile diarrhea among 170 children under 2 years of age it was shown that all came from low socioeconomic families.[5] Since the same conditions may exist among the more affluent population, we need to consider the factors that differentiate the higher strata of society from the lower strata.

Slums

Slum living is a way of life for millions of American citizens. It is a world apart and unknown to the larger society, and a part that most would

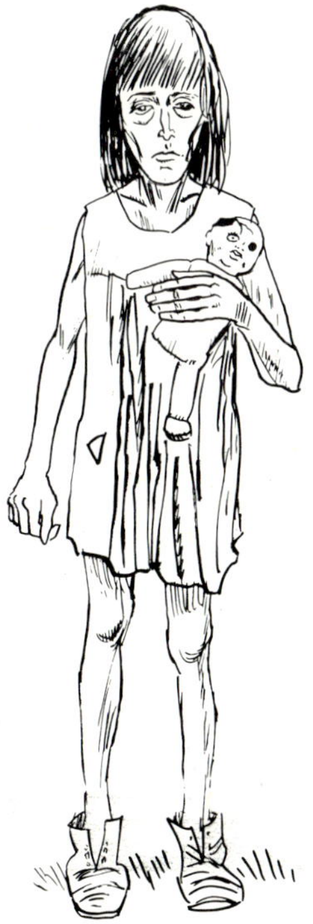

Fig. 6. Poverty wears many faces.

rather forget. Slum dwelling is a world of rickety stairways, falling plaster, high rents, broken windows, evictions, and rodents. There are no bathrooms, or at best one shared by many persons, no hot water, no flush toilets, and many persons crowded into few rooms. Slum living is a world of homeless men. "Skid row" is a district of cheap flophouses and bars, in which chronic unemployment, alcoholism, malnutrition, drug addiction, and chronic disease abound.

Slum living characterizes poverty at its worst. Few of the residents have any knowledge about disease, and few are motivated to secure medical services. However, a great gulf exists between the availability of care and the need for health services. The reason why some health needs are not met is well summed up in the following statements (see also Fig. 7):

> How important does a trip to a well-child conference for medical appraisal of the new baby and booster shots for two preschoolers seem to a mother whose husband has been dropped from his third job in less than a year, whose rent is two months overdue, and who has three dollars on which to feed her family for the next four days until the unemployment check comes through?*
>
> It is particularly difficult to interest the poor in immunizations or other preventive measures both because they do not think in terms of future benefits and because of their fatalistic attitude. If you are going to get sick, you are going to get sick, and there is no use worrying about it.†

Cooley has pointed out that the poor who suffer from malnutrition lack physical energy, cannot think clearly, and cannot plan for work and the future.[1]

A public health nurse may have made an appointment for the new baby

*Keller, Jane D.: The nurse and urban renewal, Am. J. Nurs. **65**:91-93, Feb., 1965.
†Low-income life-styles, Welfare in Review **4**:13-14, Sept., 1966.

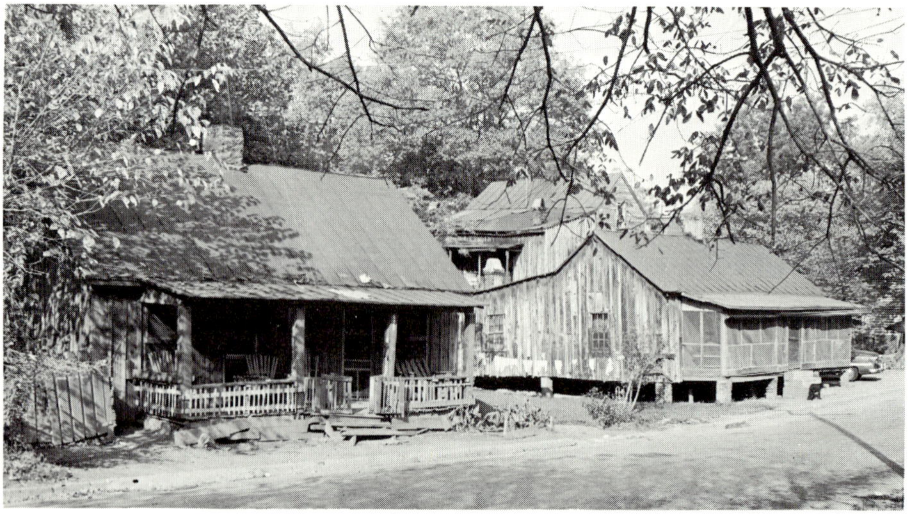

Fig. 7. Slum environments foster and disseminate communicable diseases.

to begin immunizations, but a mother weak from too many pregnancies and suffering from insufficient and inadequate food may not have the physical energy to make the trip, perhaps across town, to keep the clinic appointment.

Against this background there is more tuberculosis, pneumonia, veneral disease, and infectious diarrhea and less protection against preventable diseases. In one midwestern city an epidemic of diphtheria occurred among a group of men in skid row, with six cases and one death. These homeless men drift about the country from city to city and are a constant threat to public health.[2]

Studies have shown that the incidence and fatality rates from tetanus are higher among users of heroin, whose habitat is frequently the skid-row district.

Migrant workers

The world of the migrant farm laborer is one of malnutrition, diarrheal diseases, infectious skin diseases, parasitic infections, and sporadic outbreaks of typhoid fever and diphtheria. Every spring more than 2 million men, women, and children, from infants to grandparents, begin the long trek that will take them from county to county, state to state, and province to province to work in the crops. Children from 10 years of age work as farm hands to help the meager family income.

Most housing is poor and crowded and lacks adequate sanitary facilities. While en route, there is little money and food consists for the most part of lunches. When the last of the crops has been harvested, families begin the long journey back to areas along the southwest and southeast United States to await another spring.

Most communities are not prepared for the sudden influx of 100 to 10,000 economically depressed persons. Each family brings to the community public health problems and the threat of outbreaks of communicable disease. They also bring pregnant women for whom antenatal care is unknown. Chronic disease and a host of other health problems exist. The children are poorly immunized against preventable diseases, and many children receive little education.

When illness occurs requiring medical and hospital care, another problem is created, since few have any hospital insurance, and as nonresidents they are ineligible for public assistance. Many are Spanish-speaking persons from Mexico or Puerto Rico, and language problems are created. Local philanthropic agencies have given assistance, and public health nurses have tried to cope with the many health problems. Although local, state, and federal governments have been cognizant of the problem for decades, nothing was done until 1963, when the United States Congress passed the Community Health Services Act. The act provides for grants to public or private nonprofit agencies to assist in the cost of providing family health service clinics or other activities to prevent disease and improve the health of migrant workers.

The social problems of the migrant workers are far from solved, and the potential threat of epidemic disease continues to exist.

Unemployment

Unemployment characterizes certain segments of the population and in many instances must be regarded as a chronic affliction. However, unemployment resulting from labor-management conflict, seasonal layoffs, and technology reduces the family budget, and when income is reduced, health services are among the first to be cut. When a decision must be made between payment on the family automobile and booster shots for the children, the decision is usually in favor of the automobile.

Religious groups

Almost all persons today recognize the communicability of many diseases. However, the belief still exists among some religious groups that they will be protected if it is God's will, and, therefore, immunization is unnecessary. Such religious beliefs may be found among the most intelligent persons in upper class society. In contrast, social stratification has placed near the bottom a group who interpret Bible statements in a literal sense and reject all scientific medical care. Since states and school districts have made immunization mandatory for school attendance, religious groups who have opposed such procedures have become increasingly few. However small the minority may be, they constitute a potentially susceptible reservoir for epidemic disease.

Politics

Political factors in organized society exert tremendous influence on the control of communicable disease. Organized medicine may oppose immunization clinics, while political subdivisions may deny funds for a public health nurse, health officer, or clinic. The same state or province that may require and conduct clinics to protect dogs from rabies may fail to provide immunization facilities for the immunization of children against diphtheria. State and provincial laws may require physicians to report certain communicable diseases and provide penalties for failure to do so, but it is well known that only a fraction of some communicable diseases cared for by physicians are reported. Large urban centers may do little to provide relief from the slum areas that propagate communicable disease, while spending millions for recreational and cultural centers that benefit the more affluent of the society. Modern communication media do much to inform the public if an epidemic of disease exists, while at the same time governmental officials deny the existence of epidemic disease for fear that knowledge of it will harm the tourist trade.

The foregoing represent only a fraction of the factors in society that contribute to the incidence of communicable diseases. To these may be added the lack of health education and teaching of sex education in the home or school, apathy and indifference, ethnic and cultural differences, illiteracy, high mobility of the population, and lack of medical facilities. The cost of medical care continues to increase, while millions of people continue to subsist on minimum wages, making it impossible to meet the cost of numerous injections for a family of children. All of these problems are interrelated, and no matter how small a part each may play, when taken together they represent a total problem requiring continuous appraisal and surveillance.

PSYCHOLOGIC FACTORS

What communicable disease means to an individual or a family depends on numerous factors, including all that have been reviewed in this chapter, and in addition the particular disease involved, the family member affected, individual status and self-image, security, and loss of freedom. Whether caring for patients with communicable disease in the hospital or in the home, nurses are constantly confronted with emotional factors. The public health nurse spends hours in convincing a patient seriously ill with tuberculosis of the benefits of hospital care, only to have him leave the hospital against medical advice. When long periods of hospitalization were required, patients frequently left the hospital and a common reason was worry about their families. Few persons who contract serious communicable disease are psychologically prepared to accept it with any degree of equanimity. The mother is emotionally involved and anxious over the recovery of her child. The head of the household may be worried about the loss of his job, while the adolescent is concerned about loss of school and falling behind in class. The stigma attached to certain diseases such as tuberculosis and venereal disease still clouds many minds.

Anxiety and fear

Anxiety is an emotional feeling indicating a state of uncertainty, fear of outcome, or apprehension over a given situation. Anxiety is a component of many illnesses, and the extent of the anxiety may be related to the disease or condition and the individual's ability to accept stress situations. There are differences among persons in their ability to accept stress, and differences may occur in the same individual in different situations. For example, a parent may have little concern over a child with a mild case of chickenpox, but when a child dies from diphtheria because of lack of immunization, a profound stress situation is precipitated in the same parent. There may be anxiety over the child's chance for recovery, and if the child dies, there may be feelings of remorse and guilt.

When a husband and father is found to have tuberculosis, anxiety may play a major role in his recovery from the disease. His anxiety may be manifest in fear that he may have infected members of his family. He may worry about loss of income, the security of his job, and his status among friends and coworkers. When his wife goes to work to support the family, his self-image changes to feelings of inadequacy in not being able to fulfill his role as head of the family. This in turn may lead to anxiety about his status in society. Feelings of inferiority may lead to irritability; he may be overcritical and have periods of depression. The nurse who is caring for such a patient needs to understand that the external manifestations are only a reflection of the anxiety within.

A mother whose hospital discharge has been delayed because of a hospital-acquired infection may worry about the welfare of her family and the increased costs. Her anxiety may lead to feelings of resentment toward the hospital and nurses and may be expressed in sullenness and undue demands upon nursing service.

The way in which an adolescent may react to a crippling condition from poliomyelitis is exemplified in the following case. John had poliomyelitis at the age of 7 years, which left him with a severely crippled left leg. As he grew older, the deformity became more apparent and prevented him from participating in many activities of his age group. Through the years the public health nurse had tried to get the family to consent to the physician's recommendations for surgery. However, they would never agree. When John was about 14 years old, he began to transfer his feelings of hostility to his parents, the school, and society. He was unable to control his emotional feelings and became a disciplinary problem. He made failing grades in school and ignored the admonitions of his teachers and parents. His basic argument was that he could do anything that anyone else could do. To prove his point he would ride his bicycle rapidly up and down the street and into dangerous situations. He openly admitted his resentment over his handicap and his feelings of hostility, believing everyone was against him because of the handicap. John accepted one person in the community, a clergyman. Ultimately through counseling and individual work the clergyman was able to help John to accept his handicap and to redirect his feelings toward socially acceptable channels.

Fear has been associated with epidemics and pandemics of disease throughout history. During the plague years in Europe and the British Isles, fear was so great that people fled their homes. Fear of smallpox and the disfiguring that often followed led many persons to resort to inoculation. In more modern times the pandemic of influenza that occurred in 1918 and 1919 might have resulted in fear among the population. Today a single case of meningitis or encephalitis will result in fear and anxiety among persons in the community. Parents request the schools be closed. Not many years ago when several cases of poliomyelitis occurred in a community, schools and theaters would be closed and the population warned to avoid crowds. Today an epidemic of rubella may spread fear among pregnant women because of the defects that may be produced in the fetus.

Stigma

At the beginning of the century, stigma was attached to many diseases, and while public health education has done much to influence attitudes, all feelings of stigma have not been eradicated. Some persons still attach stigma to tuberculosis, and it is not uncommon to find a family who does not want it known that a member has cancer. While progress has been made in the open and frank discussion of venereal disease, stigma is invariably attached to a person who contracts syphilis. To contract syphilis or gonorrhea frequently means the violation of moral codes of behavior that have been established by society. Although most persons will readily admit past or present tuberculosis or typhoid fever, few, if any, will admit having had syphilis or gonorrhea. Most laws require that venereal disease be reported but hold that reports are confidential. Infection with syphilis and gonorrhea may result in feelings of guilt and frustration in the individual concerned.

Isolation

The isolation and quarantine of persons with communicable disease restrict their freedom of movement. Isolation sets the individual apart from the larger society and imposes certain restrictions upon his individual liberty. The right to make decisions and execute them has its origin in the psychologic mechanisms, and isolation restricts these rights. Thus, the patient becomes isolated psychologically as well as physically. Failure to prepare the patient emotionally for isolation may result in feelings of anxiety or even panic. The following example occurred. A patient who was suspected of having tuberculosis was admitted to the medical service. The physician ordered isolation. However, nothing was said to the patient. When a member of the family came to the hospital and found the patient isolated, he was greatly disturbed. The patient became emotionally upset and began to cry. The entire situation was so frustrating to all concerned that the physician requested that the isolation be terminated.

The need for proper emotional response and interpersonal relationships is a basic individual need. Often isolation deprives the person and prevents fulfillment of this need. The result may be that the patient becomes depressed, isolates himself from others, and withdraws into a world of his own.

THE NURSE

The attitudes of nurses toward patients with communicable disease may be one of acceptance or rejection. The nurse may view the patient as unclean and wish to spend as little time as possible with him. The nurse may avoid caring for the patient because of fears of contracting the disease. Behavior patterns may be the result of conditioning earlier in life, or they may be from lack of understanding and training in communicable disease nursing. The nurse cannot strengthen and support the patient unless she is free of fear and able to accept the patient and the disease.

ECONOMIC FACTORS

Although social and economic factors are separate entities, their interdependence is clearly evident in many illness situations, including those of communicable disease. It is well known that the incidence of communicable diseases is greater among economically deprived families. It has never been determined with any degree of certainty whether disease is the cause of economic deprivation or whether lower socioeconomic standards result in a greater incidence of disease. Environmental factors previously mentioned may have a positive relationship to the economic aspects of communicable disease, for example, typhoid fever among migrant farm workers.

Communicable disease is not confined to the economically deprived, but it also affects higher social and economic levels of society. However, the lower economic groups are less able to cope with the economic problems. Therefore, most of the financial responsibility for these groups must come from public and private sources.

It is impossible to determine with any degree of accuracy the total economic effect of communicable disease in any given situation. If a mother develops poliomyelitis and as a result must spend the rest of her life in a respirator, there is an economic loss in wages if she was employed or in services if she was a housewife. There is also the cost of hospital and medical services and respiratory care. If there are children, there is the additional cost of a mother substitute. If a father contracts tuberculosis and spends six months in the hospital, there are problems of a loss in wages, cost of hospitalization, and cost of posthospital medication, while the family may be dependent upon public relief. If a 2-year-old child dies from diphtheria, his life-time earning potential is a total loss. It is estimated that the cost of caring for the syphilitic insane in institutions is costing millions annually. Millions of dollars have been spent in rehabilitation of persons crippled by poliomyelitis. The economic cost of communicable disease touches many facets of individual and community life, and it involves more than loss of wages or interruption of a child's education.

On the other side of the economic ledger are public health expenditures for the prevention and control of communicable diseases. The cost of maintaining immunization clinics may be balanced by saving lives that otherwise would be lost from preventable disease. The cost of epidemiologic investigations of typhoid fever, or of malaria control programs, or of smallpox vaccination in Tonga, without which severe economic burdens could be realized by individuals, families, and communities, are difficult to evaluate in terms of economics.

SUMMARY

Social progress brings improvement in many social conditions believed undesirable, at the same time creating new problems. Stratification in employment creates more jobs at the top of the occupational ladder, leaving a larger number of unskilled workers at the bottom of the ladder. The economically deprived family tends to gravitate toward the depressed environmental areas characterized as "slums." The deficiencies of the area create conditions in which the microorganisms of communicable diseases find optimum conditions for their growth and dissemination (Fig. 8).

The most affluent of society frequently avail themselves of protective vaccines to a greater extent than persons or families who are economically or intellectually deprived. However, epidemic disease such as outbreaks of

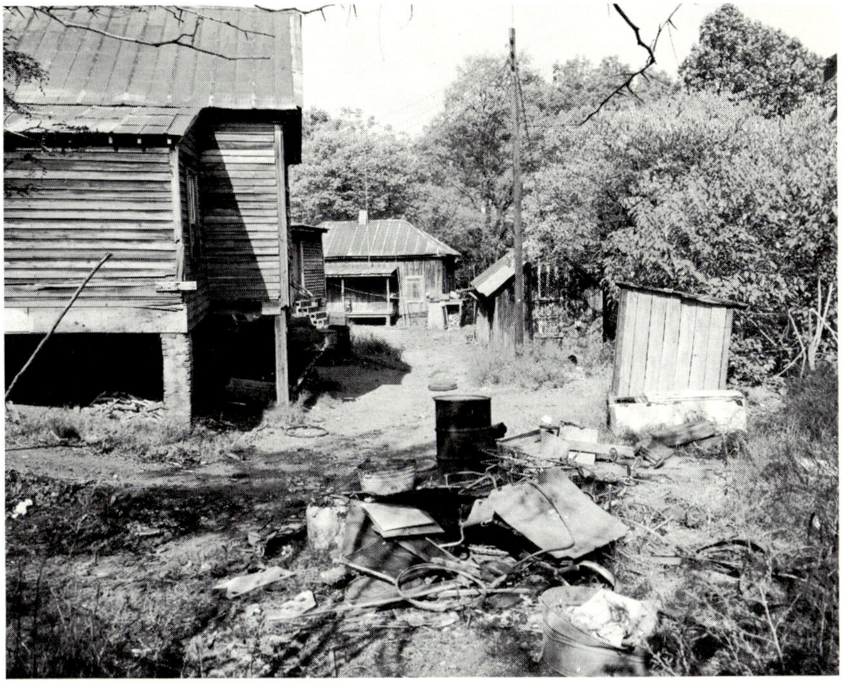

Fig. 8. Slums continue to exist in an affluent society.

meningitis or encephalitis may produce fear and anxiety at all levels of society. Nurses who are well trained in communicable disease nursing are in a better position to understand the patient's feelings and behavior and provide psychotherapeutic nursing care.

When people lead a day-to-day existence, they are not likely to see the benefit of immunization or public health programs. To sustain human motivation requires patience, effort, and ingenuity.

REFERENCES

1. Cooley, Charles Horton: Social organization, New York, 1962, Schocken Books, Inc., Chap. 26.
2. Heath, Clark W., and Zusman, J.: An outbreak of diphtheria among skid-row men, N. Engl. J. Med. **267**:809-812, Oct. 8, 1962.
3. Keller, Jane D.: The nurse and urban renewal, Am. J. Nurs. **65**:91-93, Feb., 1965.
4. Low-income life styles, Welfare in Review **4**:13-14, Sept., 1966.
5. Yow, Martha D., Melnick, Joseph L., Phillips, Charles A., Lee, L. H., Smith, Mary A., and Blattner, Russell J.: An etiologic investigation of infantile diarrhea in Houston during 1962 and 1963, Am. J. Epidem. **83**:255-261, 1966.

5

JET-BORNE COMMUNICABLE DISEASES

INTERNATIONAL TOURISM

The jet plane has become a major source of world transportation. The volume of international travel is growing steadily. In 1962 international air line passengers numbered 28 million. In 1970 there were 350 million. What will it be in 1980? As a result diseases imported by these international travelers present a growing challenge to public health. When voyages were made by ship, the return voyage home was usually longer than the incubation period of most infectious diseases the traveller may have contracted. By the time the traveller disembarked, the symptoms of the disease were present, and the Public Health authorities could identify and deal with it.

Today, a traveller from British Columbia may become infected with smallpox in India or malaria in Africa and be home on the same day. The tourist now often returns home during the incubation period feeling well and presenting neither signs nor symptoms. Thus, he passes freely through the Public Health barriers, which are designed for the purpose of detecting overt disease. Days or even weeks later the disease will develop fully, and its true identity may be overlooked.

In December 1970, a German citizen returned home by air from Pakistan. He was recovering from infectious hepatitis, but otherwise appeared well. Eleven days later he became ill and feverish, and was admitted to the hospital for observation. A few days later smallpox developed. In the following weeks twenty more cases developed with four deaths. The usual rush for vaccination took place, and finally the outbreak was controlled. This incident was typical in two respects. First, the disease was introduced by an international traveller into his own country. Second, the disease did not become overt until well after his return, meaning the present-day public health barriers being enforced had failed.

The whole problem is complicated by the boon in travel and tourism. Mass media exhort people to travel to exotic places to escape everyday cares and worries; no one, however, takes the time or effort to point out the dangers that are frequently involved, such as eating infected foods or being bitten by a malaria-carrying mosquito. The hazards for ordinary tourists are slight, it is true, because they stay in regular tourist areas, but for those who wander off the beaten track the dangers increase immensely. Recently sleeping sickness was discovered in a group of American tourists who had been on a trip to the bush. Typhoid fever and bacillary dysentery are other risks. The world traveller must be taught to find out for himself what to do to protect himself against diseases he inevitably contacts.

IMMIGRATION

Immigration patterns have also presented new problems. New arrivals may enter a country with undetected acute or residual infections such as typhoid fever, which constitute a danger to public health. On the whole, however, they usually suffer from chronic conditions such as schistosomiasis (snail fever). But many of the conditions are not notifiable.

Schistosomiasis is one of the world's most important medical problems. As a global disease, it is second only to malaria in the geographic extent of the incapacity and morbidity produced. It has been estimated that in 1971, 25,000 cases were imported into the United States from Puerto Rico.

To most people, the most alarming disease imported by immigrants is probably leprosy. This disease may remain undiagnosed for months or even years after entry into a country. Nevertheless, despite emotional and unrealistic attitudes about this disease it is really a minor public health problem; in fact, only three secondary cases have appeared in England in this century.

Much more significant as a public health menace from immigrants is pulmonary tuberculosis, which can readily be spread in communities in which the immigrants settle. The disease is usually successfully confined and controlled because public health workers and doctors are conscious of it, and the Public Health Department has set up certain routines around it.

Certain worldwide infections such as influenza are constantly in the minds of health workers, but many others are not, such as malaria, trypanosomiasis (sleeping sickness), and schistosomiasis (snail fever). This lack of awareness is a real danger. The failure to detect imported diseases really lies in the fact that the public, doctors, nurses, families, friends, and employees are unaware of the risks of travel abroad and, therefore, are not aware of the possibility of such conditions.

Ways must be found to educate both the medical profession and the public. The problem is global. The movement of a single tourist, a group, or a labor force of immigrants may result in the reintroduction of a disease into an area where it had been eliminated, and where public health protective measures have thus become lax.

SUMMARY

The medical profession and the public must be educated to think in terms of imported diseases. Each individual must be made aware of the medical significance of his travels, and the importance, in the event of illness on returning home, of reporting the illness and of telling the doctor where and when he has been travelling. Similarly, doctors and nurses must be educated to ask pertinent questions regarding the patient's recent travels. There must be internal national surveillance and improved public health regulations to keep jet-borne diseases controlled.

6

CARE OF PATIENTS WITH COMMUNICABLE DISEASES

THE NURSE AND COMMUNICABLE DISEASE

As a member of the team, the basic function of the professional nurse is the nursing care of the patient with a communicable disease. However, a nurse's responsibilities extend beyond the immediate care of the patient. The nurse must be knowledgeable about the following:

1. The nature of the specific microorganism and its capacity for survival both within and without the body
2. The most effective methods for destruction of the specific organism
3. How the organism invades the host and its route of escape from the body
4. The incubation periods, prodromata, and length of communicability
5. How specific drug therapy may alter the clinical signs and the infectious course of the disease
6. The most recent methods and concepts of prophylaxis for communicable diseases
7. The rationale of control measures, including isolation technic
8. The assignment of duties and supervision of nonprofessional persons who participate in patient care

All nurses should appreciate the incidence of worldwide communicable disease and the constant threat of epidemics in the United States and Canada brought about by modern means of transportation. The nurse should also be sensitive to the community problems that contribute to the incidence of communicable disease and to the problem of surveillance and control. Above all, the nurse should be cognizant of the emotional problems of patients with communicable disease and the early rehabilitative efforts in helping the patient toward a healthy and meaningful life.

THE PATIENT AND COMMUNICABLE DISEASE

The incidence of communicable disease has been declining over the years. Immunization programs have reduced the size of the reservoir of active, subclinical cases and carriers of several diseases such as diphtheria. At the same time the programs have created a large segment of susceptible adult population. Sporadic cases of communicable diseases continue to occur, frequently accompanied by mortality.

Most patients with minor communicable diseases such as chickenpox, mumps, whooping cough, and scarlet fever are cared for at home. However, if complications occur, they may be hospitalized. Other patients with serious diseases such as meningitis, bacterial pneumonia, poliomyelitis, and typhoid fever may be admitted to the hospital. These patients are usually seriously ill and require highly skilled nursing care.

THE PATIENT'S ENVIRONMENT

Communicable disease hospitals are gradually being discontinued, and patients are being admitted to short-term general hospitals. With the development of intensive care units, facilities may be provided for patients in need of continuous observation and nursing care. However, in most situations the patient will be admitted on a regular medical unit. Depending on the disease, its infectiousness, and the specific needs of the individual patient, he may be placed in a private room, cubicle, or ward. For patients with diseases such as rabies, encephalitis, and tetanus, the need for absolute quiet is important, and such patients should be placed where environmental manipulation can be controlled. The patient area should be bright, pleasant, and cheerful to add much to the patient's comfort and acceptance of hospitalization, especially if convalescence is prolonged. The room should be well ventilated and free of drafts, and for some communicable diseases should be located away from the main flow of traffic.

ISOLATION

Many hospitals need to review critically their policies and procedures for isolation. Research is constantly finding out hitherto unknown facts about microorganisms, and isolation should be based on scientific facts rather than unproved opinions. The development of sulfonamide and antibiotic therapy has drastically shortened the period of communicability of many diseases, and thereby decreased the period of isolation. An isolation procedure may be so rigid as to cause the patient undue emotional tension and retard his physical progress or recovery. Also, isolation may be hurriedly set up without definite policies and be so loosely conceived that it has little effect and gives only a false sense of security.

Purpose of isolation

The basic purpose of isolation in the hospital is to confine the infectious agent to a circumscribed area and to prevent its escape from that area. To accomplish this the nurse must understand the principles of medical asepsis, concurrent disinfection, and clean as opposed to contaminated areas. Strict isolation is required for some diseases, while for others a modified form of isolation may be instituted under the direction of the physician.

Order for isolation

An order for isolation should be written by the attending physician. Many hospitals require that a consent form be signed by all patients on admission. The nurse should be sure that a form signed by the patient or a responsible member of the family is on the patient's record. It is the duty of the physician to prepare the patient for isolation[4]; however, the sick person does not always comprehend or understand the significance of the restrictions imposed by isolation. The nurse must share in interpreting to the patient the reason why the procedure may be necessary and in teaching the patient the precautions that he should take to prevent the spread of his infection. The patient's family may be just as confused as the patient, and the nurse's responsibility extends to teaching and interpreting the isolation procedure to the family and friends.

Duration and termination of isolation

Theoretically the patient should be isolated as long as he is infectious. There are two methods by which this may be determined. The oldest method is based on a predetermined period of time and makes no provision for individual differences, but on the basis of past experience it assumes that after a given number of days all patients with the same disease are no longer infectious. The other method is by bacteriologic examination of body fluids or feces. Although the margin of safety may be somewhat greater, this method also has limitations. The duration of isolation for diphtheria is usually specified until two cultures from the nose and throat taken twenty-four hours apart are negative. Experience and skill are necessary to secure material satisfactorily from these areas, especially if the patient is a screaming child. It is entirely possible for the organism to be absent from the specimen obtained, while still being present in a tonsillar crypt. Also, since minute amounts of the specimen are examined in the laboratory, the organism may be missed in the particular examination.

Another factor that may affect the duration of isolation concerns the administration of chemotherapeutic drugs. For example, patients with pneumococcal pneumonia or scarlet fever may be released from isolation after twenty-four hours if they are receiving penicillin.[6] In contrast a patient with typhoid fever may be clinically well in a few days after the administration of chloramphenicol or a tetracycline, but he will continue to discharge the infectious organism, *Salmonella typhosa* for weeks or months.

After a careful consideration of all factors the physician should determine when isolation may be terminated. An order for the patient's release should be written.

Hospital policy

Policies for the care of communicable diseases vary widely among hospitals. However, every hospital should have its policies in writing, and all members of the medical and nursing staffs should be familiar with them and adhere to them. Policies should be reviewed at intervals to keep them consistent with the most recent findings of scientific research. Formulation and review of policies should be a joint responsibility of the medical, nursing, laboratory, and administrative personnel. Many hospitals have organized a surveillance or infection committee, which maintains a constant alert for conditions or situations that may result in hospital-acquired infection.

REVERSE ISOLATION

Reverse isolation is now a commonly accepted concept in isolation practice. Under usual conditions the patient with a communicable disease is isolated to prevent the spread of the pathogen to the environment. Reverse isolation seeks to isolate the patient from environmental microorganisms. It has been used for patients with leukemia whose resistance is very low because of intensive treatment with chemotherapy.[9] The application of the technic has increased as investigation continues in the use of radiation therapy and various agents to suppress the immune response in order to enhance the success of homografts and transplants.

NURSING CARE

Care of patients with communicable diseases involves the following:

1. Self-protection
2. Preventing spread of the infectious agent through medical asepsis and concurrent disinfection
3. Physical care of the patient
4. Emotional support of the patient

Protection of the nurse

Nurses who care for patients with communicable diseases should avail themselves of the prophylactic agents recommended for their age groups. As a rule these include vaccination for smallpox every three to five years, annual booster doses of tetanus toxoid, and annual chest x-ray examination if the nurse is tuberculin reactive. If the tuberculin test is negative, it should be repeated every three months. For the tuberculin-negative person bacille Calmette-Guérin vaccine may be given. Conscientious medical asepsis is the surest method of self-protection when immunization is not advisable.

It is a general policy that a gown should be worn by persons who give direct nursing care to isolated patients. The practice of folding and hanging the used gown for reuse is now obsolete. A clean gown should be used each time when patient contact is necessary and discarded following use. The purpose of the gown is to avoid soiling the uniform, which in some situations might result in danger to the nurse or to other patients for whom the nurse may care. A gown worn in the isolation unit should be long enough to cover the uniform and should lap at least twelve inches in the back.

There is no consistent policy concerning the use of masks. It is believed that in the past too much emphasis has been placed on masks that were poorly fitting and improperly used. A mask that becomes wet provides no protection. A mask should meet the following minimum requirements. It should fit sufficiently well to exclude any air that might enter around the edges, and it should be constructed of material having the greatest filtering efficiency possible.[2] Masks should be discarded the same as gowns, and a clean one should be used with each encounter with the patient.

One of the most important safeguards in preventing the transmission of pathogens is proper handwashing. The hands should be washed thoroughly after contact with the patient or any article in the contaminated unit. Handwashing facilities should include warm running water. If automatic foot or knee controls are not available, hand faucets may be used satisfactorily with the following procedure. After turning the water on, the faucet should be lathered and washed while washing the hands. The clean spigot may then be closed with the clean hand. Another method for turning off the faucets involves the use of paper towels. The towel acts as a protective barrier between the hand and the faucet. Soap may be in liquid form with an automatic dispenser or bar soap placed in a drainable soap dish. Contrary to some opinions, research has shown that bar soap does not support bacterial growth.[1] An ideal situation is a warm air blower for drying the hands, but the most commonly used method is with paper towels. The nurse should avoid cuts and abrasions on the hands through which some pathogens could enter. The use of a hand lotion to prevent chapping and irritation is desirable.

Concurrent disinfection

Pathogenic organisms escape from the body by way of the respiratory, gastrointestinal, and urinary systems. They may also be released from draining wounds, skin lesions, or body cavities. Depending on the disease, secretions and excretions may be teeming with the causative organism. Concurrent disinfection utilizes various methods such as burning, autoclaving, or chemical substances for the destruction of pathogenic organisms. It requires the immediate care and disinfection of objects and materials that are contaminated by contact with the patient.

Dressings from boils, abscesses, and various hospital-acquired infections should be wrapped securely in paper and burned immediately. Discharges from the nose and throat (respiratory passages) are collected in tissue wipes deposited in a paper bag attached to or placed near the patient's bed. The patient should be taught to fold several thicknesses of tissue and place them in the cupped hand to receive sputum. All disposable items such as paper drinking cups, drinking straws, paper dishes, syringes, disposable needles, dressing sets, catheter sets, and solid food waste should be placed in large paper bags, closed tightly, and burned.

Nondisposable articles such as emesis basins, washbasins, water carafes, and instruments should be washed in warm soapy water, rinsed, dried, and autoclaved after the termination of isolation. Bedpans and urinals should be sterilized following use.

Most hospitals are connected to public sewage systems, and excreta, vomitus, and liquid wastes such as bath water and irrigating solutions may be deposited in the regular sewage system without prior disinfection. In the absence of public sewage systems such wastes must be placed in a large container and disinfected before placing them in the disposal system. A 2% to 5% solution of cresol is commonly used for disinfection purposes. Corrosive substances such as chloride of lime should not be used in any type of system that utilizes plumbing.

Contaminated bed linens, towels, and gowns should be placed in a laundry bag and tied securely. The bag should be labeled "contaminated," or special colored bags to indicate contaminated linen may be used. If washed separately, contaminated linen may be placed in the washer without prior sterilization, except in the case of infectious hepatitis and when spores are present. The temperature of the water and the detergent are sufficient to kill most pathogenic organisms. If linens are to be laundered with other hospital laundry, they should be autoclaved and may then be placed in the regular laundry chute.

Plastic covers should be placed on all mattresses and pillows in the communicable disease unit. Many of the covers in use are made of materials that may be laundered with other linens.

Clinical thermometers should be wiped free of mucus and disinfected in one of the following solutions. Buffered glutaraldehyde (Cidex) will kill pathogenic organisms, except spores, in ten minutes and will kill spores in three hours. Ethyl alcohol, 70% or 80% with 0.2% to 0.5% iodine or any of the several iodophors on the market including Isoprep, Weladyne, Betadine, and Virac[10] will kill pathogenic organisms. Iodophors also provide satisfactory disinfection for nondisposable items. A water-soluble lubricant should be used for rectal thermometers, and all thermometers used for patients with infectious hepatitis should be destroyed upon termination of the disease. At the present time there is no disinfectant known that will kill the hepatitis virus. The use of a few thermometers to take many temperatures and inadequate sterilization between patients has been cited as a cause of cross-infections in hospitals and may lead to the spread of various pathogenic organisms.[3] It is preferrable to use disposable thermometers.

Terminal cleaning

If the nurse has been conscientious and thorough in carrying out concurrent disinfection during the course of the disease, routine cleaning and airing of the room by the housekeeping department is considered adequate. After the recovery, transfer, or death of a patient from smallpox, the mattress, pillows, and bedding should be autoclaved.[5]

Physical care of the patient

The nursing care of patients with communicable disease is physical, psychologic, and rehabilitative. The extent of care depends largely on the disease and the patient's ability to accept and adjust to the restrictions placed on his individual liberty. Some patients require only basic nursing care, while others may require intensive care and complicated nursing skills and procedures. Each patient must be cared for as an individual and his individual needs met. Special considerations for each disease will be reviewed in subsequent chapters of this book. Basic care will be reviewed briefly here.

Nursing care of the patient with communicable disease is essentially the same as the care given to any sick person. The specific care includes the following:

1. Bathing and skin care
2. Oral care
3. Attention to elimination
4. Diet and fluids
5. Observation of vital signs
6. Administration of medications

Bathing and skin care. Unless contraindicated, the patient should be given a warm cleansing bath daily. Besides providing soothing comfort and relaxation for the patient, it gives the nurse the opportunity to observe the skin for pressure areas, skin rashes, and the like. When there is severe diaphoresis, several sponges a day may be necessary, and the bed should be kept dry by frequent changes of linens. Tepid or alcohol sponges may be required for elevation of temperature. If itching of the skin occurs, a topical lotion may be ordered by the physician. In febrile conditions the patient should be turned at frequent intervals and positioned to relieve pressure and maintain the body in normal alignment.

Oral care. Patients with communicable diseases that involve the respiratory system need meticulous mouth care, which should include brushing the teeth and using mouthwashes. When lesions are present in the mouth, cotton swabs should be used to prevent injury to the mucous membrane. In some diseases warm throat irrigations may be ordered. When there is a high fever, special care is necessary at frequent intervals with a mild lubricant such as petroleum jelly applied to the lips.

Attention to elimination. Normal elimination may be interfered with when the patient is on bed rest. Constipation may be present in some diseases, while in others there is severe diarrhea. The physician should leave a written order for each individual patient. When the pathogenic organism is in the bowel and bladder excretions the nurse should be especially careful to avoid contaminating the hands. In some situations the use of gloves may be indicated. When diarrhea is present, the frequency, amount, and character of each stool should be noted and recorded on the patient's record. In some diseases laxatives may be contraindicated, but small enemas may be ordered. The use of a room deodorizer will help to disperse unpleasant odors. If indwelling urinary catheters are used, the nurse is responsible for maintaining a sterile closed system that will prevent urinary infection.

Diets and fluids. The diet for communicable disease patients depends on the specific disease. During the febrile state of the disease a liquid diet is usually offered, with gradual return to a regular diet during the convalescent period. In some diseases diets that may cause irritation in the intestinal tract are avoided. Diets that are high in proteins, vitamins, and minerals are important in diseases that cause debilitation of the patient. Vomiting and diarrhea result in the loss of electrolytes and replacement is frequently necessary through the use of intravenous fluids. When vomiting has ceased, oral fluids should be encouraged. Feeding by gavage may be required for some serious communicable diseases.

Observation of vital signs. The temperature, pulse, and respiration should be taken and recorded at four-hour intervals unless ordered otherwise. When the patient's temperature is very high, it may be desirable to take the temperature every two hours. Any sudden drop or rise in temperature should always be reported at once. The pulse should be checked frequently, and a change in rate or volume may be the first sign of serious complications. Depending on the patient's condition and the disease, blood pressure readings may be ordered.

Administration of medications. The nurse should respect the basic rules for the administration of all medications. The specific therapeutic agents used depend on the disease and the individual physician's orders. In some diseases penicillin is the drug of choice, and it is very important to determine the patient's sensitivity before administering the agent. If the nurse is in doubt concerning the patient's sensitivity to any drug, the physician should be consulted before administering it. Few patients experience confirmed allergic reactions to most drugs; however, some patients may suffer from the side effects common to some agents. The nurse should observe the patient carefully and report to the physician any unusual reaction. In some diseases chemotherapeutic drugs render the patient noninfectious in a matter of hours, and the patient becomes asymptomatic, while in other diseases medications may have no effect on the disease process but may make the patient more comfortable.

Psychologic care of the patient

Research into the behavior of microorganisms and in current therapy has done much to change the concepts of caring for patients with communicable disease. Frequently nurses and hospitals cling to obsolete practices that may lead to emotional tension for the patient. Patients who are isolated are deprived of much of their personal liberty, and when family and friends are excluded, the loneliness from lack of companionship may be overwhelming. Patients should not be isolated for longer than absolutely necessary, and in most diseases it is unnecessary to exclude visitors. The nurse helps to provide emotional support by occasional stops at the patient's door with a kind word of encouragement and reassurance. The social worker in the hospital may help to relieve the patient's anxiety by keeping him informed about the welfare of his family. Anxiety and apprehension may be relieved when the patient's employer provides assurance that the patient's job will be waiting for him on his recovery and return to employment. The small child separated from his mother may not adjust readily to the hospital situation and strange environment. The experience may be traumatic and affect the child's future adjustment; however, as an individual, each child will react differently to the situation. The parents of the child may be worried, and the nurse may help to sustain them by giving assurance that everything possible is being done for the child. Parents wish to see that good nursing care is being given their child and to understand why certain procedures are necessary. When children are involved, parents are almost as important as the child.

Rehabilitation

Several communicable diseases carry the threat of major and often permanent disability. Such disability may involve the neuromuscular system, as in poliomyelitis, or the heart, as in diphtheria, scarlet fever, or rheumatic fever. Rehabilitation begins with the acute phase of the disease. The need to recognize early changes in the pulse may be important in minimizing cardiac complications. Proper positioning with support may prevent contractures and minimize orthopedic handicaps. In all communicable diseases, observation of the patient to detect early significant signs of complications is important, and prompt therapy may prevent permanent disability. During prolonged convalescence passive and active exercise may be indicated, and the patient should be encouraged in self-help activities. As the patient improves, evaluation of the disability will be made and plans outlined for restorative care. After the acute phase of the disease various forms of diversion suitable for the age group should be provided. This may be done through an occupational therapy department; auxiliary or volunteer personnel may be helpful. Most often it will be the nurse who responds to the patient's need for diversional activity. The nurse should assist in coordinating the activities of members of the rehabilitative team and be familiar with the services within the hospital, as well as in the community, to assist the patient and his family.

LEGAL ASPECTS OF COMMUNICABLE DISEASE CARE

Laws to prevent and control epidemics of communicable diseases are among the oldest of legislative acts. Some date back to the colonial period, when epidemics of yellow fever and smallpox were prevalent. The legal authority has passed from the town selectman and lay boards of health to the present-day health department. Public health law has invested in the health officer certain legal obligations to guarantee certain rights to all citizens. However, public health law is intricately related to state, provincial, and federal laws.

Public health laws are aimed at protecting the public, and most states and provinces have enacted laws that are mandatory in both prevention and control of communicable diseases. Today most states and provinces have laws requiring children to have had smallpox vaccination in order to enter public schools. This has been extended to include immunization for other preventable diseases. Immunization has become so common that compulsory methods are rarely needed today.

Modern tuberculosis therapy has eliminated most of the so-called "problem patients," that is, patients who are infectious, who for various reasons refuse to protect their families or the public, and who refuse treatment. A number of states and provinces and some cities have enacted compulsory hospitalization laws that make it possible to detain persons with infectious pulmonary tuberculosis.

Usually compulsory methods must be predicated upon the fact that the individual is infectious and is dangerous to the public health. However, physical examination may be necessary to determine infectiousness, and the individual has the right to refuse examination. Prior to examination the belief that a person is infectious must be considered an assumption, and frequently it is difficult to secure a court order to enforce examination.

A number of states and provinces have enacted laws aimed at the prevention and control of certain communicable diseases. Included among these laws are the following:

1. Premarital laws, which require a serologic test for syphilis prior to marriage
2. Prenatal laws, which require the physician, hospital, or clinic to secure a serologic test for syphilis on pregnant women
3. Laws that require the treatment of newborns to prevent gonococcal ophthalmia neonatorum
4. Examination of food handlers and in some cases persons such as teachers who are in contact with young children

In most states and provinces the health officer has the power to order isolation and quarantine, providing there is sound evidence of a communicable disease or suspected disease; however, at times isolation as a form of compulsory detention has been challenged by the courts. As a rule the health officer or a private physician must examine the suspect before ordering isolation or quarantine.

Patients admitted to hospitals with a communicable disease generally will not question the legality of isolation. If the patient is isolated because he is suspected of having a communicable disease with no confirmed diagnosis, he is being denied his constitutional right to liberty, and if he so desires, he may seek protection from the courts.

Patients have the right to privacy, the most cherished right of our age. Nurses should realize that the patient with a rare or unusual communicable disease has the legal right to be left alone. He should be protected from the scrutiny of all persons except those intimately concerned with his care. He should be protected from photographers or interviewers that will in any way place him as a citizen before the public eye.

Throughout this book nurses will be cautioned that in certain diseases the patient must not be left alone and that in some instances restraints may be necessary. The patient has a legal right to freedom of movement, and care and caution must be exercised by the nurse in restraining the patient. Restraints should not be used longer than absolutely necessary to provide safety for the patient. It should also be remembered that if injury to the patient occurs because of the use of restraints, or the lack of restraints, the patient may have the right to legal recourse.

More litigations based on negligence have involved hospitals, physicians, and nurses than for any other reason. "A nurse who is herself careless, or who permits faulty technique in those working under her, not only may be jeopardizing her patients, but may find herself a defendant in court."* Today when so many nonprofessional persons and volunteer workers are participating in patient care, the professional nurse must assess carefully duties assigned to other workers.

As a member of the health team, a nurse shares in patient care and a share in the responsibility for it must be expected.[10] When the patient enters the hospital, he has the right to be protected from mechanical injury and also the right to be protected from infection. When caring for patients with communicable diseases or infectious conditions the nurse has the responsibility to see that the infection is not transmitted to others, that thorough concurrent disinfection is carried out, and that employees with infectious disease are reported to the administrator of nursing service or to the hospital administrator.[7]

In view of court decisions in one of the most publicized cases of recent times, Darling versus Charleston Memorial Hospital, a new concept of the legal responsibility of nurses has emerged.

> The nurse who tries to see that regulations are respected and reports departures from them is no different from the medical record librarian who is responsible for notifying the hospital administrator or the Chairman of the Medical Staff's Medical Records Committee of any failure to complete records within the time prescribed by rules and regulations.†

By the same ruling if there are willful violations of hospital policies concerning the care of communicable disease, including hospital-acquired infections, the professional nurse has the responsibility to report the violation to the nursing service administrator or to the hospital administrator.

> In coping with what may be increased demands on nurses in view of the Darling decision, the staff nurses in the hospital will need the active support of the hospital nursing service administrator, the medical staff, and on occasion, the support of the local and national nursing organizations.†

The legal aspects of nursing patients with communicable diseases differ only slightly from those of nursing patients with other diseases.

---

*Hershey, Nathan: Infection control, American Journal of Nursing **65**:103-104, Nov., 1965.

†Hershey, Nathan: Hospitals' expanding responsibility, Am. J. Nurs. **66**:1546-1547, July, 1966.

REFERENCES

1. Bannan, E. A., and Judge, L. F.: Bacteriological studies relating to handwashing. Part I. The inability of soap bars to transmit bacteria, Public Health Reports **55**:915-922, June, 1965.
2. Blair, Esta H. Menett: Oh, for a mask—effective, comfortable, inexpensive, and disposable, Nurs. Outlook **7**:40-42, Jan. 1959.
3. Editorial: Cross-infections from thermometers, J. Am. Med. Assoc. **164**:669, June 8, 1957.
4. Foster, M.: A positive approach to medical asepsis, Am. J. Nurs. **62**:76-77, April, 1962.
5. Gordon, John E.: Control of communicable diseases in man, ed. 10, New York, 1965, American Public Health Assn., Inc.
6. Hershey, Nathan: Hospitals' expanding responsibility, Am. J. Nurs. **66**:1546-1547, July, 1966.
7. Hershey, Nathan: Infection control, Am. J. Nurs. **65**:103-104, Nov., 1965.
8. Pinpointing your liability for the hospitalized patient, Hospital Physician **2**:55, July, 1966.
9. Seidler, Florence M.: Adapting nursing procedures for reverse isolation, Am. J. Nurs. **65**:108-111, June, 1965.
10. Taylor, Joyce W., Smith, Veneta M., and Zacher, Jane L.: For effective thermometer disinfection, Nurs. Outlook **14**:56-58, Feb., 1966.

7

RASHES

A regular feature of many infectious diseases is skin eruptions. A rash appears in diseases such as measles, rubella, chicken pox, scarlet fever, and smallpox. Such eruptions may or may not be present in other diseases such as infectious mononucleosis and typhoid fever. Skin eruptions in conjunction with an infectious disease are called "exanthem." Similar changes in the mucous membrane are termed "enanthem."

Pathology

The exact mechanism of how a rash occurs is not fully understood, but it is known that two basic changes are involved:

1. Damage to capillaries caused either by toxins, infective agents, or antigen-antibody reaction
2. Damage to skin cells

The evolutionary changes seen in many skin rashes (exanthemas) probably results from the inflammatory reaction at the site of damage.

In order to make a sound clinical diagnosis of the rash, it is necessary that the rash be considered in conjunction with the whole disease, and not as an individual entity. The rash merely represents one facet of the disease. When attempting to recognize the rash, the following points must be considered.

Time of onset of the rash

The interval between the onset of symptoms and the appearance of the characteristic rash is an important point. This is called the "prodromal period." For example, the rashes of rubella, chicken pox, and scarlet fever have a prodromal period of twelve to forty-eight hours. In measles and smallpox the prodromal period is three to four days. Typhoid and paratyphoid fever have a prodromal period of five to seven days; while infectious mononucleosis has a period of seven to nine days.

Site of onset of rash

In rubella (German measles) and rubeola (measles) the rash first appears behind the ears and on the face, and then spreads downward in an orderly fashion, to the trunk, arms, and finally to the legs.

Toxic and allergic rashes are usually more marked on the extensor surfaces.

Distribution of the rash

Why a rash distributes itself across the body in a certain pattern and has a predilection for certain parts of the body is not fully understood. For example, the rose spots in typhoid fever are mainly on the abdomen and the lower chest; while the herpes zoster rash has a unilateral segmental distribution.

Components of a rash

Every rash has a principal initial component that may remain the same and evolve simultaneously (monomorphic) or components that may appear and evolve at different rates and times (pleomorphic).

The basic components of a rash are the following:

erythema a patch of redness that may blanche on pressure.
herpetiform localized groups of vesicles.

Table 3. Salient features in common exanthematous diseases

Disease	*Enanthem*	*Exanthem*	*Duration*	*Remarks*
Chickenpox (varicella)	Vesicles in mouth	Pleomorphic rash with cropping; rash mainly centripetal	7 to 12 days	Post crust; scarring is rare
Glandular fever (infectious mononucleosis)	Petechiae on the hard palate	Fine maculopapular rash over the trunk	2 to 3 days	Associated with a sore throat
Herpes zoster (shingles)		Unilateral segmental distribution; vesicles are in groups	2 to 4 wk.	Postherpetic neuralgia; vesicles heal like those of chickenpox
Measles (rubeola)	Koplik's spots	Maculopapular rash on face, trunk, arms, and legs; dusty red in color	3 to 5 days	Leaves a brown stain when rash disappears
Rubella (German measles)		Maculopapular rash on face, trunk, arms, and legs; rash is pink in color	2 to 3 days	No staining of skin or peeling; painful post-cervical nodes
Scarlet fever (scarlatina)	Strawberry tongue	Lobster-red face and punctate, erythematous rash on the trunk	2 to 3 days	Fine powdery peeling of skin

macule a flat, circumscribed area of skin discoloration.
papule circumscribed area of raised skin varying from a few millimeters to a centimeter.
petechia a small hemorrhage (pin-head size) beneath the epidermis; if it occurs in larger patches it is called "ecchymoses."
pustule a small elevation of the skin formed when the clear vesicular fluid becomes pus.
vesicle sharply circumscribed collections of clear fluid in the skin; when vesicles are larger they are called "bullae."

There are many other names used for other components that have been omitted, but, if the basic components mentioned here are remembered, they will suffice to describe most rashes.

Evolution of a rash

In many unmodified infectious diseases the rash progresses in an extremely orderly manner. The recognition of these evolutionary steps are valuable in differentiation and diagnosis of many infectious diseases. For example:

measles the maculopapular rash on the third to fourth day becomes confluent, and when it disappears a few days later it leaves a brownish stain.
rubella papules disappear in forty-eight to seventy-two hours without any staining of the skin.
smallpox the evolutionary changes progress from erythema to macule to papule to vesicle to pustule to scab; every stage takes approximately seventy-two hours; the whole rash evolves simultaneously.
chickenpox when compared with the smallpox rash, the evolutionary stages are the same, but the time interval between each stage is twenty-four to forty-eight hours.

SECTION TWO

Bacterial diseases

PART A

INFECTIOUS DISEASES CAUSED BY BACTERIA

THE NATURE OF BACTERIA

As early as the fifteenth century there was a belief in the existence of bacteria among various theories concerning the cause of disease. It was the seventeenth century before bacteria were actually observed and an attempt made to classify them. From early times to the present day many persons have contributed to the sciences of bacteriology and microbiology. Research scientists continue to discover hitherto unknown characteristics among these minute microscopic living forms. The destiny of man has been intricately related to his ability to control and manipulate environmental microorganisms.

Bacteria are unicellular organisms, each with the capacity for independent survival and the ability to adapt to a variety of environmental factors. The form of bacteria may be round, cylindric, or spiral. Among each form there is a wide variation in both shape and size. Some bacteria are motile, whereas others are nonmotile. Some form spores, others form capsules, and some form flagella. Certain bacteria have the capacity to form powerful toxins that gain entrance to the bloodstream. Bacteria that live and multiply in body fluids are called extracellular, while those that gain entrance to the tissues are known as intracellular. Some bacteria survive only in the presence of free oxygen (aerobic), whereas others survive and multiply in almost complete absence of oxygen (anaerobic). Bacteria may be differentiated by the way they stain in the laboratory. They may be identified as gram-positive or gram-negative, depending upon the way the cells stain with the gram stain. However, again, several factors may result in variation or reverse a previous staining phenomenon. The behavior of bacteria and the variations are so numerous that volumes have been written about them. In general, we think of bacteria as the genus bacilli, cocci, spirilla. In turn each genus has many species, each of which possesses certain specific characteristics.

Many communicable diseases that are pathogenic for man are caused by one of these microscopic forms of bacteria. A review of the cause of disease demonstrates the wide variation among the different species of pathogenic microorganisms.

8

DIPHTHERIA

Etiology

Diphtheria is an acute communicable disease caused by the extracellular toxin of the *Corynebacterium diphtheriae*. The specific strain of bacteria is commonly called the *diphtheria bacillus*. An older name "Klebs-Loeffler bacillus," after the men who identified and established it as the causative organism of diphtheria, is rarely used at the present time.

The diphtheria bacillus appears as club-shaped rods, which during the process of cell division characteristically arrange themselves in various patterns with the rods at angles to each other. The organism is gram-positive, nonsporulating, and generally aerobic. It does not form capsules or have flagella. Some species of the organism form a powerful soluble toxin, which rapidly gains entrance to the bloodstream and is carried to every tissue of the body. In the past, strains of the organism were classified as gravis, mitis, and intermedius, and it was believed that each strain was related to the severity and fatality of the disease. Research has found that this relationship does not exist, and the present terminology classifies the organism according to the type of colonies that it forms, that is, rough, smooth, or minimus.

The diphtheria bacillus invades superficial tissue with very limited extension beyond the mucous membrane, but the soluble toxin is capable of producing severe or fatal sequelae. What the toxin is or why it is formed is not understood, but the result of its action in the body clearly attests to its destructive nature.

Several species of nonpathogenic corynebacteria are found in man and are called diphtheroids.

Epidemiology

The near eradication of diphtheria represents one of the highlights of medicine.[1] Prior to the beginning of immunization programs hundreds of cases of diphtheria with many deaths occurred in every city and community. The gradual decline of cases is nothing less than phenomenal. In 1875 in

New York City mortality from diphtheria was 300 per 100,000 population. During 1956 to 1960 only fifty-four cases and one death occurred.[1] In 1963, 314 cases, in 1964, 306 cases, and in 1966, 160 cases were reported to the World Health Organization.[3] In 1971, the U. S. Department of Health, Education, and Welfare reported 215 cases; while Statistics Canada reported seventy-five cases. In 1972, 152 cases were reported in the United States, and sixty-nine cases in Canada. In 1973, the number of cases in the United States was 228, while Canada had a total of 174 cases reported. During 1974, 240 cases were reported to the U. S. Communicable Disease Center, and in Canada 174 cases were reported by the Public Health Section, Health and Welfare Division, Statistics Canada. The average annual death rate in the U. S. for the 10-year period between 1960 and 1969 was thirty-nine persons yearly. During 1971, four deaths were reported by Statistics Canada. However, not all parts of the world were so fortunate. In many areas the disease remains endemic and epidemic.

Age and seasonal factors

Diphtheria has been considered a disease of children under 15 years of age. In the early history of the disease most of the cases and deaths did occur in this age group. Studies show that the disease can no longer be considered one of children. Prior to and during the early years of largescale immunization programs, most adults were immune to the disease. The immunity was acquired through contact with known or unknown cases, with carriers and subclinical cases, or by having mild undiagnosed cases. Since the incidence of the disease has declined through widespread immunization, there is no active reservoir of infection; therefore, there is a corresponding decrease in the number of adults with circulating antibodies against the disease and a large adult population who are susceptible to diphtheria.

Diphtheria is primarily a seasonal disease; while sporadic cases occur during the summer months, an increase in cases begins in the fall and continues through the winter months into spring.

Transmission

The sources of infection are persons with typical cases, persons with mild undetected cases, and carriers. It is a typical disease of the respiratory tract.

The transmission of diphtheria is by direct or indirect contact. Most cases result from droplet or droplet nuclei infection resulting from contact with a case or carrier. The organisms are present in the saliva and nasal discharges of patients and carriers and have been known to survive for weeks in accumulated dust near a case. Transmission through fomites and other indirect contact has been cited as a possibility.

Incubation period

The incubation period of diphtheria is usually from two to six days, but may be slightly longer.

Table 4. Chronology of diphtheria

Year	*Scientist*	*Contribution*
1826	Bretonneau	Recognized and diagnosed diphtheria as infectious
1883	Klebs	Saw and described the diphtheria bacillus
1884	Loeffler	Established diphtheria and etiologic agent causing diphtheria
1888	Roux and Yersin	Discovered diphtheria toxin
1890	von Behring and Kitasato	Discovered that toxin caused production of antitoxin that neutralized toxin
1894	Roux and Martin	Immunized horses to produce antitoxin to treat diphtheria
1896	Ehrlich	Developed methods for standardizing toxins and antitoxins
1913	von Behring	Used toxin-antitoxin to immunize humans
1913	Schick	Perfected Schick test to determine immunity or susceptibility to diphtheria
1914	Park	First large-scale immunization program with toxin-antitoxin
1922		State Serum Institute established at Copenhagen, Denmark, to standardize diphtheria antitoxin
1923	Ramon	Developed diphtheria toxoid for active immunization
1933	Havens and Wheeler	Developed alum-precipitated toxoid
1958	Pope and Stevens	Isolation of crystal form of diphtheria toxin

Communicability period

The period is several hours before the onset of the disease, until the organisms disappear from the respiratory tract.

Clinical manifestations

The onset of the disease is insidious, with feelings of fatigue, malaise, slight sore throat, and elevation of temperature from 100° to 102° F. As the disease progresses, there is considerable prostration. Typically, diphtheria starts with an acute inflammation of the pharynx caused by the diphtheria bacillus. The bacilli usually remain localized in the tonsils (if present), and in the upper respiratory tract. The bacilli secrete a toxin that irritates the tissues. The tissues give forth a fibrinous exudate that coagulates into a tough, leathery, greyish-white "pseudomembrane." This membrane is not always present or typical in color or consistency. This membrane along with swelling may occlude the air passages. Any attempt to remove the membrane exposes a red bleeding surface over which a fresh exudate is replaced. Cervical adenitis with tenderness of the glands occurs, and in severe cases the entire neck may become swollen with the edema extending into the chest. The extensive swelling of the neck has given rise to the term *bull-neck form.* If the membrane forms in the larynx, it may extend into the trachea, resulting in respiratory embarrassment and a hoarse, brassy cough with stridor. In this event a tracheotomy may be necessary. After the administration of antitoxin the membrane begins to curl at the edges, separates, and flakes off in large pieces. When the bacillus grows on the tonsils and pharynx it is called "pharyngeal" diphtheria. If the organisms grow in the nose it is referred to as "nasal" diphtheria, and if in the larynx it is known as "laryngeal" diphtheria.

Diagnosis

Clinical diagnosis may be tentatively made from the signs and symptoms, but bacteriologic confirmation should follow. The diphtheria bacillus is present only in the lesions of the disease. Cultures should be taken from the throat and nose and sent immediately to the laboratory. It is important that cultures be taken very carefully to include exudate from the lesions. It is usually possible to tell within four to twenty-four hours from the time a throat culture is started whether diphtheriae-like bacilli are present in the patient's throat. Pure cultures of *Corynebacterium diphtheriae* are necessary for a conclusive diagnosis. Failure to identify the diphtheria bacillus bacteriologically does not always rule out the presence of a diphtheritic infection.

A number of diseases present a problem of differential diagnosis, including Vincent's angina, infectious mononucleosis, acute tonsillitis, streptococcal sore throat, scarlet fever, and catarrhal laryngitis. Gordon believes that in any of these diseases physicians should suspect diphtheria and treat the patient accordingly.[3]

Treatment

The aims of treatment are to inactivate toxins, to kill the organism, and to prevent respiratory obstruction. The specific treatment for diphtheria or suspected diphtheria is antitoxin. A skin test for sensitivity to the protein in antitoxin precedes its administration. The amount of antitoxin administered depends on each individual case. The basic principle is to give enough as quickly as possible, with a tendency to give a large dose in order to raise the blood level as high as possible for an immediate therapeutic effect. Toxin that has permeated the tissues is not affected by the antitoxin. Except in very mild cases antitoxin is administered intravenously in isotonic saline solution or 5% dextrose in a 1:20 dilution. There is a direct relationship between the length of time elapsing between the onset of illness and administration of antitoxin and the case fatality rate.

There are differences of opinion concerning the administration of antibiotic therapy. Some physicians believe that penicillin should be given early and continued for seven to ten days. In general, it is agreed that antibiotics do not alter the clinical course of the disease and that they are no substitute for antitoxin. It is believed that they may have some benefit in shortening the carrier state. Toxoid is given to immunized contacts.

Strict isolation followed by bed rest for two to four weeks with a gradual resumption of activity is indicated for all patients with diphtheria. The diet should be high carbohydrate and high calorie, and extra vitamin C may be advisable. Mild analgesics such as aspirin may be required for relief of pain. An electrocardiogram and serum glutamic oxaloacetic transaminase (SGOT) test, blood urea nitrogen (BUN) test, and urinalysis are done weekly.

Nursing care

In caring for the patient with diphtheria the nurse must recognize the extreme prostration that may accompany the disease. Every effort should be made to provide strict rest, and only essential nursing procedures should be performed in order to prevent exertion on the part of the patient. The patient is isolated, and medical asepsis and concurrent disinfection must be carried out. The room should be well-ventilated with fresh air and the patient protected from drafts.

During the administration of antitoxin the pulse, respiration, and blood pressure should be checked frequently. An emergency tray with epinephrine and hydrocortisone should be available. A tracheotomy tray, suctioning equipment, and oxygen should be kept available during the acute stage of the disease. Temperature, pulse, and respiration are taken every four hours, and the respiration and pulse are taken at frequent intervals with careful attention to rate, volume, and character. The mouth and teeth should be kept clean with cotton swabs and saline solution or a mouthwash. Warm throat irrigations may be ordered, or an ice collar may provide comfort for the patient.

A record of intake and output should be maintained. The patient should be encouraged to take sufficient fluid by mouth, but it may be necessary to administer fluids intravenously. Diet should be liquid, soft, or as may be tolerated by the patient. If the patient is very ill gavage feedings may be necessary.

The patient should remain flat in bed but should be turned at frequent intervals. An important aspect of nursing care is to watch for signs that may indicate complications. Any change in pulse rate or its character should be reported immediately. Vomiting, pallor, abdominal pain, or indication of palatal paralysis should be watched for. The appearance of cyanosis, stertorous respiration, restlessness, and labored breathing may indicate respiratory complication. If a tracheotomy is performed, suctioning secretions, cleansing the inner cannula, and applying sterile dressings as necessary should be done.

In nasal diphtheria, secretions are very irritating to the skin, and excoriation may occur. Careful and frequent cleansing, with the application of a mild lubricant such as petroleum jelly may help to prevent undue irritation.

If the patient is a child, the nurse must be prepared for diversional activities such as reading or telling stories. All activities must be such that the child can be kept quiet.

Complications

The really serious effects of diphtheria stem from the action of the toxin that has an affinity for renal, nervous, and cardiac tissue. Complications vary with the severity of the disease. The most serious complication is myocarditis. This is caused by the action of the diphtheria toxin on the heart muscle. Top differentiates between myocarditis that occurs early during the disease, usually during the first week, and myocarditis that occurs after the acute phase of the infection, but within the first two weeks. When myocarditis occurs early, death may ensue quickly from circulatory collapse. Symptoms of approaching crisis are few, with changes in rhythm, rate, and volume of the pulse being most significant. When the complication occurs later, the symptoms appear gradually with acute abdominal pain, vomiting, pallor, and restlessness. The pulse becomes slow, weak, and thready, blood pressure falls, cyanosis may or may not be present, and death from circulatory collapse may occur suddenly.[4] Not all heart damage results in death, and it may not appear until late in convalescence. The periodic electrocardiogram and SGOT test are valuable aids in detecting cardiac damage and its extent.

Complications involving the peripheral nerves are related to the severity of the disease and vary in their location and time of occurence. Paralysis of the soft palate may occur early in the course of the disease, while respiratory paralysis may occur as long as eight weeks after onset. There may be paralysis of the ciliary muscles of the eye, pharynx, larynx, or extremities. Paralysis of the soft palate interferes with the patient's ability to swallow, and careful feeding is necessary. Foods should be pureed, or gavage may be a safer method of feeding. In pharyngolaryngeal paralysis, suctioning pooled secretions is an important procedure to prevent aspiration. Patients with respiratory paralysis frequently need respirator care.

A small number of patients may develop a mild nephritis during the acute phase of the disease, but permanent damage rarely occurs. Otitis media may occur, but is considered rare.

Carriers

There are three kinds of carriers of diphtheria bacilli:

1. Convalescents—"convalescent carriers"
2. Those who have contact with diphtheria patients—"contact carriers"
3. Those who are not known to have had any association with the disease—called "casual carriers"

The existence of diphtheria carriers poses one of the most difficult problems with which health department personnel have to cope. Carriers may exist among apparently healthy individuals as subclinical cases. However, since mass immunization programs, such carriers have almost disappeared. The convalescent patient may continue to harbor the diphtheria bacillus for weeks. The administration of penicillin, erythromycin, or one of the tetracyclines appears to shorten the duration of the carrier state. For a small number of patients who continue as chronic carriers after three months, a tonsillectomy may result in the disappearance of the organism. Most states require that isolation and quarantine be continued until three cultures taken from the throat and nose twenty-four hours apart are reported negative.

Immunity to diphtheria

Immunity depends to some extent on the presence of antitoxin in the blood, and in part on the ability of a person to manufacture such antitoxin quickly. This ability usually results from previous active immunization by either natural infection or artificial injection of toxoid. The test used to determine the presence or absence of significant antitoxin in the blood is the "Shick test." If the person has no antitoxin in his blood (not immune), within twenty-four hours a small red area appears. The test is read on the fifth day. An area that persists is a "positive" reaction, and means that the person is susceptible to diphtheria. If the Shick test shows no reaction, the person will not contract diphtheria under ordinary conditions of exposure. Newborn babies of immune mothers receive a "passive" immunity because of the transfer of antitoxin from the maternal to the fetal circulation via the placenta. In breast-fed infants, this immunity is augmented by antibodies in the milk of the mother. This immunity is lost by the end of the first year, and from this time to the sixth year most children are susceptible.

Prevention and control

Mandatory reporting of cases of diphtheria is required in nearly all countries. All carriers must be reported and treated. Information concerning the incidence of diphtheria is exchanged through the World Health Organization.

Patients are isolated for a minimum of fourteen days from the onset of the disease or until three cultures from the nose and throat are reported negative. The isolation procedure should include strict medical asepsis and concurrent disinfection. If these responsibilities are properly executed, the need for any extensive terminal cleaning should be reduced.

Nose and throat cultures on all household and close contacts should be taken. Contact with children and food handling should be restricted until bacteriologic examination of cultures are reported negative. Children under 8 years of age who have had previous immunization may be given a booster dose of diphtheria-pertussis-tetanus (DPT) vaccine. Older children and adults may be given diphtheria tetanus toxoid. The present trend is not to give prophylactic antitoxin to contacts but to follow them closely. Every effort should be made to locate the source of the infection.

Active immunization or reinforcing injections of diphtheria toxoid are recommended for all persons traveling to countries where diphtheria exists, and for members of the health team, whether their work includes the care of contagious diseases or not.

REFERENCES

1. Craig, John: Diphtheria: prevalence of inapparent infection in a nonepidemic period, Am. J. Public Health **52**:1444-1451, Sept., 1962.
2. Epidemiological and vital statistics report 19, nos. 7 and 8, Geneva, 1966, World Health Organization.
3. Gordon, John E.: Control of communicable diseases in man, ed. 10, New York, 1965, American Public Health Assn., Inc.
4. Top, Franklin H., and Wehrle, Paul F.: Communicable and infectious diseases, ed. 7, St. Louis, 1972, The C. V. Mosby Co.

9

HANSEN'S DISEASE (LEPROSY OR HANSENOSIS)

Etiology

Leprosy is a chronic communicable disease caused by the *Mycobacterium leprae,* also known as Hansen's bacillus. It involves skin, mucous membranes, and nerves. The disease is also known as hansenosis after Gerhard Hansen of Norway, who discovered the organism in 1871 and published his findings three years later. The organism appears as straight or slightly curved rods with a tendency to form globe-shaped masses or to form groups of parallel rods. *M. leprae* is an acid-fast bacillus that resembles the tubercle bacillus. The organism may be found in the leprous tissue of man, but attempts to grow it or to produce the disease in animals have been unsuccessful.

Epidemiology

Leprosy is considered a rare disease in the United States and Canada, but while the exact number of cases is unknown, it is estimated that there are 15 million lepers in the world. About one half of the cases are in China and India, and cases may be found in most tropical and subtropical countries. In the United States cases are found in the southern coastal states. Present data place the number of cases in the United States at approximately 2,000.

In 1971, the United States Department of Health, Education, and Welfare reported 131 cases of leprosy, while Statistics Canada reported nine cases. In 1972, 130 cases were reported in the United States, and ten cases in Canada. In 1973, the number of cases in the United States was 146, while Canada had a total of fifteen cases reported. During 1974, Canada had a total of eleven cases reported. During the first twenty-five weeks of 1974, the United States reported sixty-eight cases. Between the years 1960 and 1969, the Vital Statistics of the United States reported sixty-two deaths as a result of leprosy. No deaths have been reported in Canada since 1971.

Leprosy is generally present for a number of years before it is diagnosed. Although specific information is lacking, it is believed that there is no natural immunity to the disease. Children of lepers should be separated from the parents at birth because the chances of infection are much greater in infants and young children.

Sex and age factors

The disease affects both male and female with the ratio being about 2:1. However, this ratio has varied in different geographic areas. There is no racial immunity, and the disease makes its appearance at any time of the year. Children and young adults appear to be most susceptible, with the first symptoms appearing around puberty. About 50% of the cases occur in persons before 20 years of age, and about 80% before 35 years of age. The disease is not hereditary, but since children are highly susceptible, the percentage of infection in children associated with leprous parents is very high (30-40%).

Transmission

Leprosy is believed to be transmitted through contact with the degenerating lesions of the skin or the mucous membrane of the upper respiratory tract. Man is the only known reservoir of the infection, and it appears that transmission is directly from person to person. Leprosy is only contracted after prolonged or intimate contact, and even then a person often escapes infection. However, characteristics of the disease contribute to some uncertainty as to the specific mode of transmission. Studies have indicated that socioeconomic factors such as overcrowding and unsanitary conditions, inadequate diet, and sexual promiscuity contribute to its spread. Certain social customs such as eating, sleeping, and smoking together have been cited as possible factors in its spread.[1]

Incubation period

The incubation period is variable, being as short as five and one-half months or as long as fifteen years. The average incubation period is about five years. Because of the long history of the disease and the banishment of lepers during its early existence, many people have a fear of the disease. Leprosy is not considered highly communicable, and no person working in the leprosarium has ever contracted the disease.

Classification

There are two main classes of leprosy, lepromatous (nodular form) and tuberculoid (anesthetic leprosy). The lepromatous form of the disease is considered the most infectious. The skin test (lepromin) is negative, but the skin lesions contain large numbers of Hansen's bacillus. Early symptoms may be unrecognized. There is a gradual thickening of the skin with the development of a granulomatous condition. The lesions frequently appear as macules, becoming nodular in character (leproma). There is a slow involvement of the peripheral nerves, with some degree of anesthesia and loss of sensation and gradual destruction of the nerves. There is atrophy of the skin and muscles and eventual absorption of small bones, primarily the bones in the hands and feet. There is ulceration of the mucous membrane of the nose, and nodules may occur in the mouth, throat, and larynx. Because of the absorption of small bones and ulceration, natural amputation may occur.

In the tuberculoid form the lepromin test is positive, but the organism is rarely isolated from the lesions. The tuberculoid macules are elevated with clearing at the center and are more clearly defined than in the lepromatous form. Anesthesia is present, and involvement of the peripheral nerves occurs more rapidly than in the lepromatous form.

Both forms of the disease are characterized by remissions and exacerbations, and in the tuberculoid form the bacillus may be found in lesions during exacerbations. The course of the disease is prolonged over years, and absolute cure cannot be determined. Mortality usually results from complications and rarely from the disease.

Diagnosis

By the time the patient seeks medical care for the disease it may be well advanced, with destruction of nerves, atrophy of skin and muscles, and ulcerations. The disease is not easily diagnosed, and even in the presence of skin lesions the true diagnosis may be missed. A diagnosis of leprosy is most often made with scrapings from the nasal septum or biopsies of the skin of the ear that have been stained for acid-fast bacilli. A careful clinical history and study of the symptoms with complete physical examination are necessary in making an accurate diagnosis.

Treatment

The understanding and treatment of leprosy has undergone a great change during the past twenty years. The present treatment is sulfone therapy and the drug currently used is dapsone. The drug is administered orally, and dosage varies with the degree of tolerance for the agent. The Expert Committee on Leprosy of the World Health Organization, which met in 1966, recommended beginning with a small dose and gradually increasing it over a period of four to six months until the maximum dose was reached.[3] There is no evidence that cure is obtained, but the disease is arrested, and over a five-year period about a 50% reduction in positive smears is obtained. Present evidence indicates that therapy must be continued for life. The use of physical therapy and particular care to the hands and feet are indicated. Rehabilitation and recreational and occupational therapy are extremely important aspects of the total therapy regimen for the patient with leprosy.

Nursing care

If the patient is admitted to the general hospital, routine isolation and medical asepsis are carried out. The nurse should understand that any personal danger is slight. The nurse should also realize that the patient needs moral support and encouragement, probably more than most patients with other diseases.

Complications

Leprosy is a long debilitating disease, and serious complications frequently arise. Death is usually caused by complications such as tuberculosis or chronic amyloid nephrosis. The patient is highly susceptible to traumatic injury and burns because of loss of sensation, and secondary infections are not infrequent. The patient may have prolonged attacks of lepra fever, or lepra reaction, or repeated attacks of erythema nodosum, accompanied by malaise, painful joints, neuritis, and fever, and orchitis may occur in the male patient.[2]

Prevention and control

Leprosy is best prevented by good living conditions. It should be emphasized that the great majority of people are naturally resistant to leprosy. All cases of leprosy are reportable to the health department. Control measures are frequently difficult. The long incubation period makes it difficult and complicates locating contacts outside the immediate family. Prolonged and intimate contact with lepers is hazardous. All lepers in the United States and Canada found to be discharging *mycobacterium leprae* are sent to a leprosarium. If patients improve and discharge no bacilli for a period of six months, they may be paroled. These patients are subsequently examined twice a year. When the patient returns home no children or young people should live in the house. The patient should remain semisegregated with his own room, linens, and dishes. One of the major problems is to keep patients under regular treatment.

REFERENCES

1. Rogers, Sir Leonard, and Muir, Ernest: Leprosy, ed. 3, Baltimore, 1964, The Williams & Wilkins Co.
2. Doull, James A.: Current status of the therapy of leprosy, J. Am. Med. Assoc. **173**:363-373, May 28, 1960.

10
BACTERIAL MENINGITIS

Etiology

Meningitis may be caused by several kinds of bacteria, including the pneumococcus, staphylococcus, streptococcus, and tubercle bacillus. The species *Neisseria meningitidis* (meningococcus) is the organism causing most epidemics of meningitis. The meningococcus has been classified into four serologic groups, A, B, C, and D. The A strains are generally responsible for most epidemics, whereas B and C strains cause sporadic cases; strain D is rare in North America. The meningococcus is of a coffee-bean shape, is gram negative, is nonmotile, does not form spores, and is aerobic. The organism is sensitive to disinfectants, low humidity, and heat and does not survive long outside the body. The disease is pathogenic only for man. Invasion of the body occurs in three steps:

1. Implantation of the meningococcus in the nasapharynx (most remain localized here)
2. Entrance into the bloodstream with the production of a septicemia
3. Localization in the meninges

Epidemiology

Meningococcal meningitis was first described during an epidemic in Geneva in 1805. Through the years the disease has been known by several names, including cerebrospinal fever, spotted fever, brain fever, and sinking typhus. The disease is worldwide in scope. In 1974 an epidemic occurred in Brazil. One hospital in San Paulo reported receiving one hundred persons a day suffering with the disease. In 1971, the United States Department of Health, Education, and Welfare reported 5176 cases. In Canada during this same period the Public Health Section, Health and Welfare Division, Statistics Canada reported 209 cases with a death rate of 6.9%. In 1972, 4634 cases were reported in the United States, and 361 cases in Canada. In 1973, the number of cases in the United States was 2510, while in Canada a total of 436 cases were reported. During 1974, 1297 cases were reported by the U. S. Communicable Disease Center, and in Canada, 352 cases were reported by Statistics Canada. In the 10-year period between 1960 and 1969 there was an annual average death rate in the United States of 725 persons per year. In 1971, Statistics Canada reported forty-seven deaths.

Age and seasonal factors

The disease may occur among all age groups and among all races, with the exception of epidemics that occur among military personnel. Most cases occur in the age group from 8 to 12 years, with mortality greatest among very young and elderly persons.

While sporadic cases may occur at any time of the year, the disease tends to be seasonal, occurring primarily from spring to fall. There appears to be some evidence of a cyclic occurrence of the disease.

Transmission

The infectious organism enters the upper respiratory tract, and it is spread by direct contact with droplet infection from the nose and mouth and by indirect contact with articles contaminated by secretions from the upper respiratory tract. Direct person-to-person contact is usually necessary for infection to result. It has been demonstrated that many healthy persons carry the organism in the nose and throat, but apparently have a high degree of resistance to clinical infection. However, it is also probable that most persons are susceptible to recognized clinical disease. Meningococcal infections are not highly communicable, and there seems to be a high degree of natural immunity to them. Under ordinary conditions probably 2 to 5% of the general population are carriers.

Incubation period

There is no well-defined incubation period, since the meningococcus may be present in the nasopharynx and the reaction be so mild that it is not observed. The best estimates place the probable incubation period between two and seven days. It is generally considered that the causative organism reaches the central nervous system by the bloodstream, although it may reach the meninges directly from the nasopharynx.

Communicability period

The communicability period lasts until the meningococci are no longer present in mouth and nasal discharges.

Clinical manifestations

The onset of meningitis may vary from a slowly developing syndrome to an acute, rapidly developing or a fulminating form. In general, the early symptoms include severe headache, nausea, vomiting, and photophobia. Forward flexion of the head causes pain and resistance in the posterior neck. Later the head is retracted, and opisthotonos spasm occurs. The patient may be comatose or irrational. There is muscular spasm, the reflexes are exaggerated, the neck is stiff, and the Kernig and Brudzinski signs are positive. The temperature ranges between 100° and 103° F., but it is irregular, the pulse is rapid, and the respirations are irregular. Hemorrhagic manifestations are common in the disease, with petechiae occurring because of vascular damage from endotoxic material.

In infants convulsions may indicate the onset of the disease. Infants in whom the fontanelles have not closed usually display bulging as a common symptom.

Types of meningitis

Meningitis is divided into two main types: bacterial (pyogenic) and aseptic.

Bacterial meningitis (pyogenic). The incidence of bacterial meningitis has been significantly reduced since the introduction of antibiotics.

Meningococcal meningitis. This type is commonest in children, but no age is exempt. The reservoir is man, and human carriers spread the infection by droplets. Overcrowded living conditions play an important role in the spread of this disease. Onset is usually rapid followed by the usual clinical manifestations. Petechial rash is quite frequent. Sometimes the petechiae coalesce producing large patches called "ecchymoses." There are often associated signs of septicemia.

Hemophilus influenza meningitis. This is the second most common type of meningitis in children. The onset is relatively slower than that of meningococcal meningitis. The majority of the children have a preceding infection of the upper respiratory tract. Rash is not a feature of this disease.

Pneumococcal meningitis. This type of meningitis is common in infants under 1 year of age and in patients over 50 years of age. It may develop either as a complication of an ear infection or pneumonia. The onset is difficult to differentiate from that of meningococcal meningitis except that a rash is not present. Response to antibiotic therapy is slower, and the mortality rate is high.

Meningitis due to gram-negative bacilli. This type is also called "neonatal meningitis" because it is frequently seen in newborn babies. Signs of meningitis in the newborn are quite different from those seen in adults—ir-

Table 5. Bacteria causing meningitis

Common	*Uncommon*	*Rare*
Meningococcus	*Mycobacterium tuberculosis*	Salmonella
Pneumococcus	Streptococci	Brucella
Haemophilus influenzae	Staphylococci	
Gram-negative bacilli (*E. coli*, *Pseudomonas*, and *Proteus*)	*Listeria monocytogenis*	

ritability, refusal to suck, fever, convulsions, and bulging fontanelle. Very often these infants have severe gastroenteritis. Management of this type of meningitis with antibiotics is very difficult. Very often this type of meningitis may follow a neurosurgical procedure.

Diagnosis

The diagnosis of meningitis is made by laboratory examination of blood, spinal fluid, and nasopharyngeal material. In severe septic infection the organism may be identified in blood smears, and it may be possible to isolate the organism in specimens taken from hemorrhagic lesions. Examination of specimens must be made quickly because of the rapid disintegration of the cells. Examination of spinal fluid reveals an increase in polymorphonuclear leukocytes, which alone is of diagnostic significance. There is an increase in protein, and sugar level is reduced in relation to the number of organisms present. Usually the same organism can be isolated from the nasopharynx, blood, and spinal fluid. A colloidal gold test may be performed on the spinal fluid, and in the presence of central nervous system involvement, colloidal gold will be precipitated.

Differential diagnosis

The most frequent diseases in which differential diagnosis is encountered are poliomyelitis, tuberculous meningitis, and epidemic encephalitis.

Treatment

The polyvalent serum, although therapeutic, has been replaced by chemotherapeutic agents. There is no unanimity among physicians concerning the specific drug of choice, but it appears that several of the sulfonamides have been found effective. Among these agents are sulfadiazine, sulfisoxazole, sulfadimetine, and the tetracyclines. In most cases crystalline penicillin G is administered in combination with sulfonamide therapy. There is also a variation in the preferred route of administration and in the dosage. Sedatives may be needed for restlessness. The specific chemotherapeutic agent, route of administration, and dose will be determined by the physician for each individual patient. For severe brain edema intravenous urea or mannitol may be used. Lumbar punctures are done to reduce intracranial pressure, for diagnosis, and for intrathecal administration of medications.

Nursing care (symptomatic)

Patients with meningococcal meningitis are isolated until cultures fail to show meningococci in the nasopharynx. All discharges from the nose and mouth, and articles soiled therewith should be disinfected. Patients who have received adequate therapy for a period of not less than twenty-four hours may be released from isolation. The nurse assisting the physician in securing specimens of spinal fluid, blood, and nose and throat smears should record the character and pressure of spinal fluid, label specimens, and see that they are sent to the laboratory immediately. All specimens should be marked "contaminated."

The patient should be placed in a quiet, well-ventilated, slightly darkened room, and noise of any kind should be avoided, especially as convulsions are quite frequent, especially in children. Protection from injury must be assured. The headaches experienced are very severe and require strong analgesics for relief. Side rails on the bed or restraints may be necessary for an irrational patient, and the patient should not be left unattended until fully conscious and oriented. If restraints are used, they must be released frequently, the position changed, and skin care given.

During the acute phase of the disease a rectal temperature should be taken every two hours, and pulse and respiration should be taken frequently. Antipyretic drugs and tepid or alcohol sponges are given according to the physician's orders. The patient must be turned frequently and good skin care provided to prevent decubiti. Cold water mattress may be used to help reduce elevated temperature. Hydration of the patient is very important, and if possible the patient should be encouraged to drink sufficient fluid. Eye care is provided to prevent drying of the conjunctiva. If sufficient fluids are not taken orally, parenteral fluids will be ordered. It is important that accurate records of intake and output be maintained. The patient should be watched for urinary retention or incontinence. Intravenous fluids should be administered carefully if vomiting is a problem and the patient observed for signs of intracranial pressure. Plasma, plasma expanders, or blood may also be used to offset shock.

It should be remembered that meningitis is a debilitating disease and that nutrition and body tissues suffer. The mouth, lips, and nares need frequent care to avoid sordes about the teeth and gums and herpes simplex of the lips. A mild, nonoily lubricant such as petroleum jelly may be used on the lips, and a solution of lemon juice, glycerin, and peroxide used to clean around the teeth and gums.

If the patient is conscious, the diet during the acute stage should be liquids that are high in carbohydrates. As the patient convalesces, a full diet may be offered. Throughout care the doctor and nurse should use every precaution to avoid infection or development of the carrier state. Observations must be made of return of functions to the extremities, of any changes in behaviour, or signs or symptoms indicating the occurrence of otitis media, pneumonia, obstruction, hydrocephalus, subdural collection of fluid, paralysis, spasticity, or contractures.

Complications

Complications may arise from involvement of the cranial nerves. Severe herpes simplex is frequently encountered, and pneumonia may occur. In meningococcemia acute congestive heart failure caused by interstitial myocarditis may complicate the disease and results in a high mortality rate. Otitis media and ophthalmia may occur. Infection may enter the ventricles and cause obstructing hydrocephalus. Headache may persist. Intellectual faculties may be impaired. Children may have paralysis, spasticity, or contractures.

Prevention and control

All cases of meningococcal meningitis should be reported to the health department. No quarantine is required, and there is no preventive immunization available at the present time. However, research is being done on a vaccine. The incidence of secondary cases among contacts is low, and no follow-up of contacts is considered necessary. When epidemics of meningitis occur in institutions or military barracks, chemoprophylaxis with one of the effective chemotherapeutic agents may be administered to limit spread of the disease. However, if control is to be effective, the entire community must be considered.[1]

REFERENCE

1. Gordon, John E.: Control of communicable diseases in man, ed. 10, New York, 1965, American Public Health Assn., Inc.

11

PERTUSSIS (WHOOPING COUGH)

Etiology

The genus *Bordetella* includes *B. pertussis, B. parapertussis,* and *B. bronchiseptica.*

Whooping cough, one of the most highly communicable of all diseases, is caused by *B. pertussis.* It affects the respiratory tract and is especially serious in infants and young children. The *B. pertussis* organism is a gram-negative, nonmotile, nonspore-forming coccobacillus that may form capsules. It is generally aerobic, but under certain conditions it may be anaerobic. The organism survives for only a short time outside the body and for only a few hours in dried sputum. It is easily destroyed by disinfectants, ultraviolet light, and heat.

Epidemiology

Pertussis is both endemic and epidemic on a worldwide basis. The disease was unknown prior to the sixteenth century, and the first epidemic recorded occurred in Paris in 1578. The disease was first called "chin-cough," and was called "pertussis" in 1679. Although the incidence of pertussis has been declining, thousands of cases are still occurring. Pertussis is one of the major causes of death in young children—90% in children under 5 years of age. The United States Department of Health, Education, and Welfare reported 3036 cases in 1971. In Canada during the same period, Statistics Canada reported 3002 cases. In 1972, 3287 cases were reported in the United States, and 1297 in Canada. In 1973 the number of cases in the United States was 1759, while Canada had a total of 969 cases. During 1974, 1555 cases were reported in Canada; during the first twenty-five weeks of 1974, 850 cases were reported in the United States. In the 10 years between 1960 and 1969, 675 deaths were reported in the U. S. In 1971, Canada reported nine deaths from whooping cough.

Age and seasonal factors

Pertussis, a communicable disease of one or two month's duration, may occur at any age, but it is primarily a disease of young children. Dubos reports that in the United States 64% of the deaths occur in children under 1 year of age but that 40% are under 5 months of age.[1] Unimmunized children may contract the disease outside the home and expose infants and preschool children in the home. The case rate for children in the same family is very high, and both case rates and fatality rates are higher among females than among males.

Although the disease may occur at any time of the year, the greatest incidence is during the winter and spring months. There is some evidence of cyclic epidemics occurring every two to four years.

Transmission

The portal of entry is the mucous membranes of the respiratory system. Transmission is by droplet infection and direct contact from infected persons. Carriers do not exist. While exposure is possible by contact with articles freshly soiled by respiratory secretions, most cases are probably the result of direct contact with a case.

Incubation period

The incubation period is considered to be from five to twenty-one days.

Communicability period

The disease is communicable during any stage and often during convalescence.

Prodromal period

Pertussis is characterized by three distinct stages: (1) the catarrhal stage, (2) the paroxysmal stage, and (3) the convalescent stage. The onset of the catarrhal stage is insidious with coryza, sneezing, lacrimation, and a dry bronchial cough—symptoms of an ordinary cold. The cough becomes nocturnal and gradually more severe. During this stage it is difficult to distinguish pertussis from acute bronchitis, and it is during this stage that the disease is most communicable and probably the greatest transmission occurs. In ten to fourteen days the disease enters the paroxysmal stage, during which the coughing occurs in paroxysms. These are repeated series of violent sharp coughs in one expiration terminating in a high-pitched inspiration of air (whoop) caused by the spasmodic closure of the glottis. The "whoop" may be absent in adults and very young children. Depending upon the severity of the disease, the number of paroxysms will vary from about ten to as many as forty or fifty during a twenty-four-hour period. During the paroxysm the face becomes cyanotic, veins in the face and neck are distended, the eyes are red, and there is vomiting of copious amounts of mucus. In severe cases epistaxis or even hemorrhage may occur. The convalescent stage is marked by a gradual decrease in the paroxysms of coughing, the vomiting ceases, and after about six weeks from the onset the attack subsides.

During severe paroxysms parents frequently become alarmed, and unnecessary attention is given to the child. After recovery it is not unusual for such children to prolong coughing and vomiting to gain attention and special favors.

The white blood cell count increases and by the end of the catarrhal stage may reach as high as 15,000 to 30,000 leukocytes with a greatly increased number of lymphocytes.

Complications

Pertussis is a very serious disease during infancy. There are numerous possible complications with pertussis. In infants and very young children the tissues around the bronchioles become inflamed, and interstitial pneumonia occurs. The air passages may become obstructed by mucous plugs and result in atelectasis. Convulsions due to lack of oxygen to the tissues may occur in pneumonia and atelectasis. Severe paroxysms of coughing may give rise to umbilical hernia and hemorrhage. Central nervous system involvement and otitis media are always possible complications. In the 25% of the children who have whooping cough before they are one year old, death is usually from bronchopneumonia.

Diagnosis

During the catarrhal stage, bacteriologic diagnosis may be made by the cough plate and nasal swab technic. The uncovered cough plate is held about 6 inches from the mouth during an attack of coughing. The nasal swab is introduced through the nose to the posterior pharyngeal wall. After incubation for forty-eight to seventy-two hours the *B. pertussis* organism may be identified.

A history of exposure and the characteristic paroxysms of coughing with the whoop and vomiting are usually diagnostic of pertussis.

Treatment (symptomatic)

A number of chemotherapeutic agents have been tried in the treatment of pertussis with varying degrees of success. Drugs in current use include tetracycline, chloramphenicol, streptomycin, sulfadiazine, and sulfisoxazole. Hyperimmune convalescent serum or gamma globulin produced from it has been found to give good results. Penicillin and sulfonamides protect children from secondary infections. Sedative drugs may be used to lessen the severity and frequency of paroxysms; however, caution should be exercised so that the patient does not become too heavily sedated, which may interfere with the removal of mucus.

Infants and very young children should be hospitalized if possible. The room should be cool and well-ventilated, and humidity may be supplied by the use of a humidifier. Because of vomiting, a feeding or meal may be lost. After twenty minutes, the child should be fed again. Numerous small feedings are indicated rather than larger, less frequent meals. Adequate hydration is necessary, and unless adequate fluids are taken by the oral route, parenteral fluids may be necessary.

Nursing care (symptomatic)

A major objective of good nursing care is to prevent complications. The nurse must remember that the bacilli enter the body by the nose and mouth, and are thrown off from the patient in the buccal and nasal secretions, and in the sticky sputum that is coughed up. The patient should be isolated and medical asepsis carried out. During paroxysms the patient should not be left alone, and suctioning equipment should be available for emergency use in preventing obstruction of the airway. A small child may be wrapped and held with the head forward while mucus is being removed from the mouth. Sunshine and fresh air are important, but the child should be protected from drafts. The child should be kept as quiet as possible since excitement and activity may precipitate a paroxysm. Giving warm baths, keeping the bed dry and free of soiled linen, and paying attention to bowel elimination are nursing responsibilities. Fluid intake and the amount of food eaten, or if an infant, the amount of formula taken and retained, should be recorded. The nurse should offer small frequent feedings to maintain the nutritional status. If the child vomits, another feeding should be given. Small amounts of sedatives may be given to quiet the child. Children may receive active immunization. The vaccine may be given as part of the diphtheria-pertussis-tetanus immunization. The vaccine is not a curative measure. Four to six weeks must be allowed for immunity to develop after injection.

Prevention and control

Man possesses no natural immunity. Pertussis should be reported to the health department. Nonimmune children should be excluded from school for fourteen days from the last known exposure. Previously immunized children should be given a reinforcing injection of vaccine, and infants not immunized may be given gamma globulin to provide passive immunity. Patients should be isolated for four to six weeks from the onset of the disease. When possible, recovery should be determined by negative bacteriologic cultures.

Effective control measures should include efforts to locate subclinical or unreported cases and the encouragement of immunization. Public education in active immunization and early diagnosis, together with reporting of all cases should be encouraged.

REFERENCE

1. Dubos, Rene J., and Hirsch, James G., editors: Bacterial and mycotic infections of man, ed. 4, Philadelphia, 1965, J. B. Lippincott Co.

12

PNEUMOCOCCAL PNEUMONIA (BACTERIAL)

Etiology

Bacterial pneumonia is the prototype of all bacterial pneumonias. It may be caused by any of several etiologic agents, including pneumococcus, *Staphylococcus aureus, Streptococcus pyogenes* (group A hemolytic streptococci), *Klebsiella pneumoniae* (Friedländer bacillus), and *Haemophilus influenzae.* Bacterial pneumonia may be primary or secondary, complicating another disease.

Pneumococcal pneumonia is caused by a gram-positive, nonmotile, nonspore-forming, encapsulated, lancet-shaped coccus. The organism is usually arranged in pairs or in short chains. It is classified into more than seventy-five immunologic types based on the chemical differences in the polysaccharide substances that compose the capsule surrounding the cell. Although any of the types may cause infection, only about eight types are responsible for more than three fourths of the infections in man. The pneumococcus and *Streptococcus viridans* have many biologic characteristics in common. Because of this, there has been some attempt to classify pneumococcus as a species of streptococcus. Therefore, pneumococcus pneumonia and streptococcus pneumonia or diplococcus pneumonia may be considered the same disease.[1]

Epidemiology

Infected persons and healthy carriers are the reservoir and source of the pneumococcus organism. Since the carrier rate may be as high as 70% in well persons, the nonimmune person who may carry the pneumococcus in his throat has a good chance of developing pneumococcal pneumonia secondary to viral infections of the upper respiratory tract. Pneumococcal pneumonia occurs sporadically in the United States and Canada, but an increased incidence generally occurs during epidemics of respiratory disease such as influenza.

Age, race, and seasonal factors

Pneumococcal pneumonia may occur at any age, but it occurs most frequently in infants and aged persons. Urban areas where crowding exists or institutions such as mental hospitals, barracks, and prisons appear to favor transmission of the pathogenic types. The incidence is greater among the Negro race and Indians than among the Caucasian race. It is also more common among men than women.

The disease may occur at any time of the year, but peaks are usually reached during the winter months in northern latitudes. Certain occupational groups that are exposed to extremes of temperature such as in steel mills or in shipbuilding have a greater incidence of pneumonia than the general population.

Transmission

The reservoir of infection is man. The infectious agent is transmitted by direct contact with the patient and carrier, and by indirect contact through droplet spread and fomites.

Incubation period

The incubation period is relatively short and may be from one to three days.

Clinical manifestations

The onset of bacterial pneumonia is generally acute, being ushered in by a severe chill, acute pleural pain, and profuse diaphoresis. There is a rapid rise in temperature from about 102° to 106° F. The pulse rate becomes rapid and full, and respirations become rapid, with dilation of the nostrils and a short grunt on expiration. The patient becomes dyspneic, cyanosis appears about the lips, and an anxious expression may be noted. He may become confused and even delerious. The skin is hot, dry, and flushed. The dry cough becomes productive, with the characteristic "rusty" sputum caused by the red blood cells that are mixed with the other constituents. The patient tends to lie on the affected side, when one or more lobes of a lung are involved. However, in some cases both lungs may be affected. Leukocytosis is present at the onset and may reach as high as 50,000 per cubic millimeter of blood in some cases, but generally the range is between 15,000 and 30,000 per cubic millimeter of blood.

Complications

When the patients are untreated, complications may occur in one fifth of the cases. Pleurisy with effusion is the most common complication, but it may be missed and cause no major problem. If it is diagnosed, aspiration of fluid may be necessary.

Empyema, an accumulation of pus in the thoracic cavity, is rarely seen today because of the use of chemotherapeutic agents. Bacteremia with meningeal or cardiac involvement is rare. Preexisting chronic pulmonary disorders may delay clearing of the pneumonic lung areas.

Diagnosis

The diagnosis of pneumococcal pneumonia may be made on clinical evidence and confirmed by radiologic and bacteriologic examination. Early in the disease breath sounds may be inconclusive, but by the second or third day they are of diagnostic significance. A roentgenogram of the chest should be made on every patient with suspected pneumonia. Sputum specimens should be collected for laboratory examination and identification of the pneumococcus. Blood cultures are made from which the organism can be identified. Routine laboratory examinations of blood and urine are carried out. In some patients an electrocardiogram may be ordered.

Treatment

Pneumococci are highly susceptible to the action of antimicrobial drugs, and resistance to the drugs is rarely encountered. In some cases resistance to sulfonamides has occurred. The drug of choice is penicillin G, which is bactericidal. If complications are present, larger doses than normal may be given. Maintenance doses may be administered orally or parenterally. The tetracycline drugs are considered as effective as penicillin. The sulfonamide drugs are bacteriostatic and retard growth of the causative organism. In some cases their use has been found helpful in assuring phagocytosis of the pneumococci.

In the presence of dyspnea, cyanosis, and very rapid pulse rate, oxygen may be administered with the exception of an emphysematous patient, when extreme caution must be exercised.

The use of narcotics or barbiturates is rarely necessary, but chloral hydrate may be necessary for restlessness and insomnia.

Nursing care

The patient with bacterial pneumonia should be hospitalized if possible, and whether in the home or in the hospital, he should be on complete bed rest. Isolation is generally recommended for twenty-four hours after initiating antibiotic therapy. Concurrent disinfection should be carefully adhered to, and reasonable cleaning and airing of the room should be done after recovery of the patient.

Specific nursing care of the patient includes positioning the patient to provide the greatest amount of comfort. Depending on the amount of dyspnea present, the head of the bed may be elevated to any height that will lessen respiratory difficulty. The patient may be comfortable if positioned on the affected side and supported by pillows. Skin care with attention to pressure areas and warm baths will help to refresh the patient and relieve restlessness. Care of the mouth is extremely important and should be given at frequent intervals because of the purulent sputum. Herpes simplex about the lips and mouth is common, and a mild lubricant may relieve irritation caused by the condition.

The problem of abdominal distention arises in many patients with pneumonia. It can often be prevented by small low enemas administered daily. A well-lubricated rectal tube inserted for twenty minutes may also give relief, or drugs such as neostigmine bromide (Prostigmin bromide) or surgical pituitrin may be ordered. Hydration of the patient is important but should not exceed 3000 ml. in twenty-four hours. Excessive amounts of fluid may lead to pulmonary edema, and fluids may be restricted in elderly patients because of congestive heart failure.

During the acute phase of the disease, diet should be liquid or semisolid, but it should be nourishing and of high caloric value. Liquids or foods known to be gas forming should be avoided.

The temperature should be taken every four hours and pulse and respiratory rates determined frequently. Antipyretic drugs such as aspirin and tepid or alcohol sponges may be employed for patients with a severely elevated temperature. Since the use of the chemotherapeutic drugs in the treatment of pneumonia, the temperature falls by lysis. Nearly 75% of the patients will have an elevated temperature for only about five days, while less than 10% will have fever for longer than three weeks.

Immunity

Recovery from a pneumococcal infection offers the individual immunity to that specific type of pneumococcus causing the infection—an immunity of six to twelve months. However, there is no immunity to other types. Man appears to have a comparatively high natural resistance to the pneumococcus, and he usually never contracts pneumonia unless his resistance has been lowered.

Prevention and control

Bacterial pneumonia is reportable to the health department only in the case of epidemics. Since pneumococcal pneumonia usually follows injury to the respiratory system, efforts should be directed toward preventing common colds, influenza, or other upper respiratory infections. It has been established that immunization with influenza vaccine reduces the incidence of influenza, and it seems certain that the incidence of pneumococcal pneumonia occurring secondarily to influenza will also be reduced. Efforts should be made to protect the very young and elderly persons or those with chronic pulmonary disorders against respiratory infections. Environmental factors such as exposure to cold and dampness and physical conditions of fatigue or alcoholism may be contributory factors in lowering resistance to pneumonia.

Because of the antibiotic resistance encountered in pneumococci, vaccine therapy is coming back. The vaccine is new. It is now in the design of a polyvalent vaccine given in a single injection. It incorporates polysaccharides from the twelve types of pneumococci most likely to cause disease.

REFERENCE

1. Dubos, Rene J., and Hirsch, James G., editors: Bacterial and mycotic infections of man, ed. 4, Philadelphia, 1965, J. B. Lippincott Co.

13

SCARLET FEVER (SCARLATINA) AND SEPTIC SORE THROAT

Etiology

Scarlet fever is caused by *Streptococcus pyogenes,* group A hemolytic streptococcus that produce erythrogenic toxin. Although scarlet fever has been recognized as a separate disease entity for centuries the present opinion is that scarlet fever and streptococcal sore throat are different manifestations of the same basic disease. If the streptococci causing the sore throat produces erythrogenic toxin, and the recipient of the infection is not immune to it, then scarlet fever with its characteristic rash results. If the streptococci do not produce erythrogenic toxin, or if the recipient is immune to the toxin, then only the sore throat results.

Epidemiology

Scarlet fever is endemic and epidemic in many parts of the world. The mortality is generally low, about 1% in the United States.[1] In 1860 England and Wales reported that in every million children under 15 years of age, 2500 died from scarlet fever.[2] In 1971 Statistics Canada reported 10,814 cases; in 1972, 12,224 cases; in 1973, 15,694 cases, and in 1974, 20,114 cases. Scarlet fever and streptococcal sore throat are not Specified Notifiable Diseases in the U. S.; they are classified as *Acute Diseases Optionally Reported.* In 1972, forty-six states reported a total number of 421,517 cases; while in 1973, forty-six states reported a total of 474,212 cases.

Age, race, and seasonal factors

Scarlet fever is an acute infection of childhood, although persons of any age may contract it. It occurs primarily in children between 3 and 10 years of age. Why infants and children under 3 years of age are not affected by the disease is not clearly understood. Since these children have negative Dick tests, it is believed that prior exposure and sensitization to the erythrogenic toxin is necessary before the organism can cause manifestation of scarlet fever.[3]

Top reports that the disease is more common among members of the Caucasian race than among the Negroid races and that there is a slight tendency for a greater frequency among males than among females.[4]

The disease tends to appear in cycles, with only sporadic cases in some years followed by a year during which it reaches an epidemic state. The disease may occur at any time of the year but is primarily seasonal, occurring between the late fall and spring months.

Transmission

Sources of infection are the oral and nasal secretions of patients or carriers; and purulent discharges from lymph nodes, ears, and other lesions. Fomites may also transmit the disease. The prevalence of carriers of streptococcal bacteria has been authenticated through surveys in which large numbers of persons have been found to carry group A streptococcus. The organisms are present throughout the illness, and may persist in the nose and throat or in their secretions for weeks or months after the illness. As long as the person harbors the organisms, the person is a dangerous source of infection. At various times the organism has been transmitted through food, especially milk.

Incubation period

The incubation period is short compared to that of many diseases. It may be as short as twenty-four hours or as long as ten days, but the first clinical signs generally appear between two and five days.

Communicability period

The disease is communicable from onset to recovery.

Prodromal period

The period between the onset of the symptoms and the appearance of the characteristic rash is twelve to forty-eight hours. The rash lasts twenty-four hours to ten days.

Clinical manifestations

The disease may have an abrupt onset with fever ranging from 101° to 104° F., sore throat, enlarged lymph nodes, vomiting, and headache. The infection may or may not be ushered in with a chill. There is a great increase in the pulse rate, and the skin feels hot and dry. The skin rash appears at about twenty-four hours after the onset of the disease. It forms a distinct skin eruption with massive exfoliation. The rash results from an acute hyperemia of the skin with petechial hemorrhages. The rash varies in its manifestations, usually beginning on the face and extending downward. It may appear quickly or take several days, and it may be very light or extremely heavy. The rash consists of a diffuse general erythema and a punctate rash superimposed on the erythema. The punctate spots do not appear on the face, and the erythema on the face fades, leaving a distinct pallor around the mouth (circumoral pallor). The tonsils are enlarged and give the appearance of follicular tonsillitis. In severe forms there is severe swelling of the uvula and posterior pharyngeal wall. The tongue is heavily coated and with the appearance of the skin rash, the papillae on the tongue become swollen and the tongue assumes a reddish gray appearance. When the white coating desquamates, the red "strawberry" tongue results. With convalescence it assumes its normal appearance.

Scarlet fever may be very mild or very severe. Mild cases are frequently completely missed. Most cases are considered moderately severe, and while recovery is usually uneventful, a few patients may develop complications.

Desquamation of the skin begins in about ten days, or it may be much later. Flaking of the skin is generally first observed around the neck, chest, and back. Rather large scales may be shed from the palms of the hands and the soles of the feet. Desquamation at the ends of the fingers and toes and under the edge of the nails may be noted. The rash is the only symptom that differentiates scarlet fever from "strep throat."

Complications

Numerous complications may arise from scarlet fever. Among the commonest are suppurative otitis media, mastoiditis, cervical adenitis, pneumonia, peritonsillar abscess, rheumatic fever, and acute nephritis. In more severe cases a septic form of the disease occurs in which the hemolytic streptococci invade the bloodstream. The temperature may be elevated as high as 108° F., with a very rapid pulse rate. All symptoms are intensified, and respiratory problems may develop because of posterior pharyngeal occlusion. Middle ear and mastoid involvement frequently occur in this form of the disease.

A septic form of arthritis caused by an accumulation of infected exudate in the joint cavity may occur. Streptococci are not isolated from the joint, and recovery is expected without permanent damage to the joint.

Streptococcal meningitis may develop and is believed to result from bloodstream involvement.

Diagnosis

The clinical manifestations of scarlet fever are frequently sufficient to provide a diagnosis. Cultures may be taken from the throat to identify the type, serologic group, and strain. Tests that have been used include the Schulz-Charlton and the Dick tests. These tests have not proven reliable in the diagnosis of scarlet fever. The Schelling hemogram has been shown to have some diagnostic value.

One of the primary difficulties in the diagnosis of scarlet fever is that of differential diagnosis. Diseases with a rash give the most problems and include measles and German measles. Certain drugs may cause a rash, and dermatitis caused by hypersensitivity to certain plants. Acute follicular tonsillitis may be easily confused, although there is no rash. Because of severe throat symptoms in scarlet fever, diphtheria may be suspected.

Treatment

Treatment of the patient with scarlet fever depends in part on the severity of the disease and the existence of complications. The general treatment is aimed at the prevention of complications, and bed rest is mandatory for one week. The patient is isolated and concurrent disinfection carried out. Diet may be offered as tolerated, but adequate fluid intake is important. If sufficient fluids are not taken by mouth, parenteral fluids may be ordered. Comfort measures such as an ice collar to the throat or warm saline throat gargle may be ordered. Drug therapy includes penicillin, which is the drug of choice. The suggested unit dose will vary among physicians. The initial dose is generally given by intramuscular injection, after which the maintenance doses may be given by the oral route. Patients unable to take penicillin may be given tetracycline. In general the sulfonamide drugs are not recommended. Drug therapy is continued for about ten days, and is effective in preventing complications such as rheumatic fever.

Complications are rare since the use of antibiotic therapy, but their occurrence is treated according to the condition and symptoms presented.

Nursing care

Isolation and medical asepsis should be carried out. The patient should be protected from drafts and chilling, but the room should be comfortable and well ventilated. For severe infections of the upper respiratory tract the room should have increased humidity. Pruritus may be relieved by warm cleansing baths followed by gentle rubbing with warm olive oil. The nose should be kept free of mucus and a mild lubricant such as petroleum jelly applied to the external nares and the lips. Frequent use of a warm gargle will help to keep the throat free from the accumulation of mucus. Hot or cold applications may be applied to painful cervical lymph nodes. Liquids should be offered freely and the patient encouraged to drink an adequate amount. Intake and output records should be maintained to determine adequate fluid balance. Slightly elevating the head of the bed will facilitate nasal drainage and aid in preventing sinus involvement. The nurse should be constantly alert for symptoms that may indicate complications. Small children who are unable to talk may roll their heads and pull at their ears when pain in the ear is present. Any unusual elevation of temperature, decrease in urinary output, pain in joints, headache, or vomiting should be reported to the physician immediately.

Immunity

Immunity relates to scarlet fever antitoxin in the blood. Infants inherit an immunity from their mother, but it is lost within one year. From that point on, susceptibility increases until 6 years of age. From 6 years of age until adult life susceptibility decreases. The majority of adults are immune. An attack of scarlet fever is usually followed by permanent immunity. Immune persons may harbor the microorganisms for a long time and spread the disease.

Tests for immunity. The Dick test consists of an intradermal injection of streptococcal toxin. In susceptible persons erythema occurs at the site of injection within twenty-four hours. In immune persons no reaction occurs. The Schulz-Charlton test is a skin test that is made by injecting into the skin of a patient with a rash a small dose of scarlet fever antitoxin. If the rash is due to scarlet fever, it immediately fades or is blanched.

Prevention and control

Most countries require that scarlet fever be reported to the health department. Family contacts should be examined and kept under observation for the duration of the incubation period. No follow-up of extrafamily contacts is indicated in sporadic cases. In epidemic situations the source of the infection should be determined, and food and milk should be investigated as possible sources.

Active immunization with scarlet fever toxin is not in general use. When indicated passive immunity may be provided by hyperimmune human gamma globulin, and prophylactic doses of penicillin may be effective. Currently, a highly purified vaccine designed to prevent childhood streptococcal infections is being tested. However, its efficacy will not be known for some time.

REFERENCES

1. Gordon, John E.: Control of communicable diseases in man, ed. 10, New York, 1965, American Public Health Assn., Inc.
2. Paul, Hugh: The control of communicable diseases (social and communicable), Baltimore, 1964, The Williams & Wilkins Co.
3. Samter, M.: Immunological diseases, Boston, 1965, Little, Brown & Co.
4. Top, Franklin H., and Wehrle, Paul F.: Communicable and infectious diseases, ed. 7, St. Louis, 1972, The C. V. Mosby Co.

14

TUBERCULOSIS

History

The history of tuberculosis antedates that of most other communicable diseases. Examination of Egyptian mummies shows evidence of extrapulmonary tuberculosis of the bones. The disease was known in Greece in 429 B.C. and was described by Hippocrates. Because of the clinical characteristics of the disease, Aristotle and Hippocrates gave it the name "phthisis," meaning a "wasting away of the body." Later phthisis was translated to mean "consumption." The disease was commonly referred to as consumption until well into the twentieth century, and when the course of the disease was rapid, it was called "galloping consumption."

Sylvius (1614-1672), a French anatomist, gave the name "tubercle" to nodular lesions discovered during autopsies, and the present name "tuberculosis" was derived from tubercle. In 1865 Jean Antoine Villemin (1827-1892), a French surgeon, expounded the belief that tuberculosis was an infectious disease, but it was not until 1882 that Robert Koch identified the etiologic agent as the tubercle bacillus.

Etiology

The primary and only essential cause of tuberculosis is the tubercule bacillus. Pulmonary tuberculosis is caused by the *Mycobacterium tuberculosis* (tubercle bacilli), which is only one of several mycobacteria known to be pathogenic for man or animals. Among these mycobacteria are the following:

1. Classified mycobacteria
   a. *Mycobacterium tuberculosis.* The cause of pulmonary tuberculosis in humans.
   b. *Mycobacterium bovis.* The cause of tuberculosis in cattle and may be transmitted to humans through unpasteurized milk from infected cattle. It causes extrapulmonary tuberculosis. This type has practically been eliminated as a cause of tuberculosis in Canada and the United States.

c. *Mycobacterium avium.* The cause of tuberculosis in birds; it is very rare in humans.
d. *Mycobacterium leprae.* The cause of leprosy.
e. *Mycobacterium paratuberculosis* (John's bacilli). The cause of enteritis in cattle; not pathogenic for man.
f. *Mycobacterium microti* (vole bacillus). This is not pathogenic for man. It has been used for vaccines to immunize cattle against tuberculosis and has sometimes been used in place of BCG vaccine to immunize humans.

2. Unclassified mycobacteria (tentatively classified)
   a. *Mycobacterium kansasii.* The cause of pulmonary lesions in humans.
   b. Orange bacillus. This has been implicated in disease of cervical lymph nodes in children.
   c. Battey bacillus. The cause of atypical tuberculosis in humans.
   d. *Mycobacterium fortuitum.* The pathogenicity for man is not established.

In this chapter we are concerned with human pulmonary tuberculosis and the increasing significance of atypical tuberculosis caused by the Battey bacillus.

The mycobacteria are strongly acid-fast, strictly aerobic, nonspore-forming, and nonmotile rod-shaped organisms. In staining properties they differ from other organisms in that they cannot be considered gram-negative or gram-positive, and discoloration cannot be accomplished with alcohol once they have been stained with a basic dye. There has been some unconfirmed evidence that during the life cycle of the tubercle bacilli, minute living forms exist that will pass through a filter.[6]

Chemically the tubercle bacillus differs from any other bacterial cells, since about one third of the cell consists of fats. These lipid substances have been separated into several groups, some of which seem to have an effect on the tuberculous process. The activity of these lipid substances is related to the inflammatory process of the granulomatous lesions, the multiplication of reticuloendothelial cells, the changing of macrophages to epithelioid cells, and the virulence of the organism.[13]

The tubercle bacillus is known to remain alive for long periods outside the human body. It offers considerable resistance to ordinary disinfectants such as ammonium compounds, mineral acids, and alkaline agents. On the contrary the organisms are readily killed when exposed to sunlight and heat as in boiling, autoclaving, and pasteurization processes.

Epidemiology

Tuberculosis is one of the most widespread communicable diseases, and unlike most other diseases it has a very long period of infectivity in addition to being the most chronic and the most persistent.[15] In 1971 Statistics Canada reported 3943 cases, while the U. S. Department of Health, Education, and Welfare reported 35,217 active cases. In 1972 32,932 cases were reported in the United States. During the same period of time Canada had 3909 active cases reported. In 1973, the United States had a total of 31,015 cases, while Canada had 1875 cases reported. In the 10 years between 1960 and 1969, 8224 deaths occurred in the United States on a yearly average. In Canada during 1971, 447 deaths occurred. Aldelman points out that the national tuberculosis rate does not reflect the incidence of tuberculosis in many large metropolitan cities, where the rate may be twice that of the national rate.[1]

When chemotherapeutic drugs became available, eradication of tuberculosis appeared to be in sight; however, reduction has been slow, and most authorities believe that it is going to take decades, if not centuries, to achieve. About 35 million persons in the United States harbor latent tubercle bacilli in their bodies, and about 75% of the new cases reported each year are believed to be the result of a breakdown of these latent infections.

Age, sex, and race

Tuberculosis affects all ages, sexes, and races. Tuberculosis is a health hazard of lower socioeconomic groups, densely populated areas, persons over 50 years of age and under 5 years of age, and the chronically ill.

At the present time in the United States there are well over 250,000 cases under medical supervision, and thousands of persons have had the active disease in the past who now make up a high-risk group. It is a disease of civilization and cities. It has been greatly reduced in prevalence in many countries of the West, but it still flourishes in great numbers in the Orient and in the tropics. In our cities there is also estimated to be a substantial number of persons with active disease who have not been diagnosed, and who pose a threat of infection to others.

In the world today about 25 million persons are thought to be infected with the bacillus; between 1 and 2 million of these break down with active disease during their lifetime. Every year 2 or 3 million new infectious cases occur, and about 3 million die of the disease annually.

Pulmonary tuberculosis is becoming an uncommon disease among the young in Canada and the United States, and is a rare cause of death among Caucasians. White males over 40 years of age are the chief victims of pulmonary tuberculosis—for some unknown reason. Mexicans, Negroes, and Indians are very susceptible and contract it at an early age.

Predisposing factors

Factors known to be closely related to the incidence of tuberculosis may be categorized as environmental, socioeconomic, familial, habits and attitudes, defense mechanisms, and immunologic factors.

Tuberculosis is primarily a disease of the urban environment. As the population shifts from a rural to an urban community, there is an increased incidence of tuberculosis. Today tuberculosis is a serious problem in many of the large cities. However, in some underdeveloped countries of the world tuberculosis is a problem in the rural as well as the urban areas.

It is a known fact that a positive correlation exists between tuberculosis and social stratification. Poverty has always been associated with tuberculosis. Masses of people crowded into substandard housing, with their slums and ghettos, reduced financial resources, and insufficient medical care provide the milieu for increase of the disease. The social factors involved are usually a community problem, and the facilities of the health department are unable to resolve them. In the developing countries of the world public health is frequently a luxury, and community facilities cannot cope with the problem. After both world wars the incidence of tuberculosis increased. Famine and serious economic depressions that result in lowering nutritional standards may also lower the body's resistance to infection.

Certain occuptional groups including doctors, nurses, and other health service personnel are at risk because of their constant association with known or unknown cases of infection. Among other high-risk occupations are those in which dust, silicone, asbestos, and coal create an environmental hazard. Occupations in which strenuous physical exertion is required, where there is low earning power, or there is total unemployment are all related to the social level of population most frequently infected with tuberculosis.

There is no evidence that tuberculosis is inherited, although the belief exists among some lay persons. However, there is some element of heredity in reactions to infections that make certain persons either more or less susceptible than others. It is known that tuberculosis frequently is a family disease. Studies have indicated that close family members of a patient with tuberculosis are from three to four times more likely to die from the disease than an equated group of unrelated persons.

Unfortunately some persons think of tuberculosis as a social stigma and delay examination and diagnosis. The development of attitudes toward the existence of infection may lead to delay in examination or to neglect in following the prescribed therapy. The efforts of the nurse to teach the patient or family how to prevent the spread of infection may be regarded lightly or ignored. Efforts to develop new habit patterns and attitudes may prove a difficult task, and delay may carry the person beyond the point when cure may be achieved.

A breakdown of the body's defense mechanisms may predispose the individual to tuberculosis. Nutritional inadequacy from insufficient food, failure of the body to utilize food, or lack of necessary nutritional requirements may lead to lowered resistance to infection. The general health of an individual may be affected by loss of sleep, dissipation, harassing strain, emotional stress, or lack of medical care for remedial defects. Exposure to respiratory infections, overwork, and fatigue may also be contributing factors. Teenage motherhood or frequent pregnancies, debilitating disease, and mental stress or mental illness may result in improper functioning of the normal defense mechanisms of the body. The presence of chronic diseases such as diabetes, alcoholism, other chronic lung diseases, and silicosis may predispose the individual to tuberculosis.

The question of immunity to tuberculosis has not been completely determined. There is some evidence that a healed primary lesion may confer some immunity against reinfection tuberculosis; however, evidence has not been conclusive. There is no natural immunity. The best evidence so far concerns the use of Calmette Guérin (BCG) vaccine to produce an active immunity.

Transmission

Tuberculosis is usually transmitted by inhaling tubercle bacilli expelled from persons with active disease by coughing or sneezing. Droplets expelled from the respiratory tract during coughing, sneezing, or laughing remain suspended in the air as tiny droplet nuclei. These nuclei may be carried about by air currents, and a single nuclei containing a tubercle may be inhaled and deposited deeply in an alveoli of the lungs, where it becomes implanted and begins multiplication. The belief that droplet infection may transmit tuberculosis is now questioned because droplets tend to settle too quickly to be inhaled (Fig. 9).

When the tubercle bacillus gains entrance to the body, it may involve every tissue and organ of the body. There are primarily three ways by which it spreads within the body: (1) by lymphatic spread in which the or-

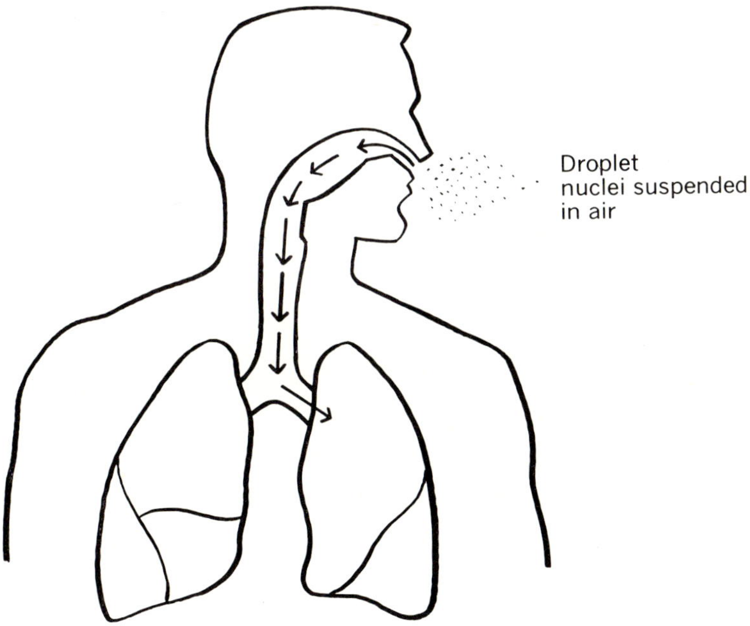

Fig. 9. Droplet nuclei containing the tubercle bacillus are inhaled and deposited in the lungs.

ganism may be disseminated from a nearby lymph node to involve an entire chain of nodes; occasionally it may be carried along the lymph channels and enter the bloodstream by way of the thoracic duct (see primary infection); (2) by the blood if a vessel in the mediastinum is penetrated by an infected lymph node or growing tubercle; and (3) by the sloughing of a necrotic discharging cavity, allowing the organism to reach the bronchi and initiate new lesions in the parenchyma of the same or the other lung.

Pathogenic patterns

Mycobacterium bovis (bovine tuberculosis) affects cattle and is pathogenic for man. It is transmitted through unpasteurized milk and milk products from infected cattle. Infection may also result from inhaling droplet nuclei, which may be present in barns where infected cattle are housed, or by handling contaminated animal products. The incidence of this type of tuberculosis in the United States and Canada has declined because of tuberculosis control of cattle and the emphasis on pasteurization of milk.

Primary tuberculosis. Primary tuberculosis has also been known as "childhood tuberculosis" or "first infection tuberculosis." Until recently it was seen almost exclusively in infants and children. Because of the declining incidence of tuberculosis, infants and young children are more often escaping exposure, and first encounter with the organism may be delayed until adolescence or even adult life. Therefore "primary infection" is the accepted clinical classification regardless of the age when it occurs. With the first infection "primary tuberculosis" begins. The primary infection results from respiratory inhalation of the tubercle bacilli. The organism may be deposited in any part of the lung parenchyma and almost always involves the hilus and mediastinal lymph nodes. Primary tuberculosis is an acute disease, and its course may be rapid and progressive. There may be fever and malaise. However, the vast majority of persons go through this stage without any apparent illness. When progressive, the type of lesions are exudative, resulting from the inflammatory process and necrotic debris. These lesions may slough, causing bronchogenic spread to other lung areas. The tubercle bacilli may be disseminated throughout the body by the lymph channels or by bloodstream invasion resulting in generalized infection. Depending on the number of organisms involved, death may occur rather quickly, or miliary tuberculosis or tuberculous meningitis may occur. The progressive form of primary tuberculosis appears to be more common among young adult Negroes than among young white adults.

Primary tuberculosis may heal with no recognized symptoms. A "latent phase" follows, which usually lasts for the rest of the person's life. In fact roentgenography in later life may show only minute calcifications to indicate an earlier infection, or a reactive tuberculin test may be the only evidence of previous infection. Before the decline in tuberculosis it was estimated that from 70% to 80% of all adults had a reactive tuberculin test but no evidence of disease. Even today it is estimated that about 75% of persons with reactive tuberculin tests show no evidence of disease on roentgenographic examination[16]; the evidence indicates that most primary tuberculosis heals without causing disease. It is also known that 5% of these persons will develop tuberculosis some time during their lives. The exact reason is not clearly understood, but it is believed that stress situations may be a contributing factor. It is now recommended that these persons be kept under surveillance by the health department.

Primary tuberculosis heals by one of two ways: by resolution, in which the caseous exudate is absorbed, or by calcification, in which calcium and lime salts are deposited in the lymph node lesion.

Postprimary tuberculosis. Reinfection tuberculosis is also known as postprimary tuberculosis or adult-type tuberculosis and is the most common form of the disease. As the term would imply, reinfection tuberculosis is a new infection (exogenous), however, the term may be misleading since the origin of the infection may be "endogenous," resulting from a breakdown of primary tuberculosis. An endogenous infection may be caused by a caseous lymph node rupturing into a bronchus or by lymphatic or bloodstream transportation of the tubercle from a lymph node focus of infection. Also reinfection tuberculosis may be the result of exacerbation of a healed postprimary lesion. Such infections may occur months or many years after an initial primary infection. This gives rise to the question of resistance (immunity) from the first infection and its possible duration. An exogenous infection may imply that a new infection from without has been superimposed in a patient with an active lesion.[5] Whatever the cause may be, a primary infection may give rise to a progressive infection regardless of the age at which it occurs, whereas the reinfection type may be from a primary infection or superimposed infection from without.

Primary and reinfection tuberculosis exhibit quite different characteristics. The lesions of postprimary tuberculosis are most frequently in the upper parts of the lung although lesions may occur anywhere in the parenchyma. It starts as a small patch of tubercular pneumonia below the apex of one lung, more often on the right side than on the left. Lesions in the mediastinal lymph nodes rarely occur, and fibrosis with cavity formation that progresses downward from the apex characterizes postprimary tuberculosis. Productivity is usual, and lesions rarely heal by resolution. The disease is chronic and progresses by contiguous spread, forming cavities whose contents are discharged into the bronchi producing lesions in the tracheobronchial tree and larynx.

Healing of postprimary tuberculosis cavities may be from fibrosis (scarring) that completely or partially fills the cavity, or the cavity may become filled with caseous debris. This occurs if the body is relieved of the stresses that precipitated the onset of the disease. Some cavities remain open but are clean without evidence of disease. It is possible for cavitation to exhibit all of the various characteristics at the same time, that is, new cavities in the stage of formation, healed cavities, and progression of the present cavities.

Extrapulmonary tuberculosis. The incidence of extrapulmonary tuberculosis has shown a remarkable decrease in the United States and Canada because of the control of tuberculosis in dairy herds and through the use of chemotherapeutic drugs.

Generalized hematogenous tuberculosis is caused by a dissemination of the tubercle bacilli to every organ and tissue of the body by way of the bloodstream. The organism is liberated into the bloodstream by erosion of a caseous lesion or into the thoracic duct from the lymphatic system.

Miliary tuberculosis resulting from generalized bloodstream infection may be acute, subacute, and rarely chronic. Miliary tuberculosis occurs more frequently in infants and young children after a primary infection. The miliary lesions may involve organs other than the lungs, including the spleen, kidneys, bones, or other organs. Tuberculous meningitis may be a complication of miliary tuberculosis.

Tuberculosis involving bones and joints may result from hematogenous dissemination or from primary infection by the *Mycobacterium bovis* organism. While persons of any age may be affected, it is commonest in children. The infection may attack synovial membranes, progress slowly with few symptoms, and continue for years before the bone is involved. The knee is a frequent site of infection. When the bone is affected first, the infection progresses rapidly with destruction of the bone and abscess formation. In this type of abscess the usual signs of inflammation are lacking. The greater trochanter is a common site for the lesions, and the shaft of the long bones are rarely affected. The spine, hip, and knee are frequent sites for tuberculosis of bones, but ankles, wrists, shoulders, and elbows may be involved.

Atypical tuberculosis. In recent years the role of certain acid-fast bacilli, presently unclassified, has received intensive study. It is now definitely known that some of these bacilli produce pulmonary and extrapulmonary disease in man. Atypical tuberculosis may be caused by the Battey bacillus,* and, clinically, tuberculosis caused by the Battey bacillus and that caused by *Mycobacterium tuberculosis* are indistinguishable. Atypical tuberculosis is a chronic pulmonary disease with cavitation, and it has been found most commonly in men past 45 years of age. It has frequently been associated with emphysematous conditions. At the present time there is no evidence that the disease is transmitted from person to person; therefore, it does not constitute a public health problem.[4] Evidence at the present time suggests that the organism may be present without causing progressive disease. There is a great deal still unknown about the unclassified mycobacteria and their role in causing disease in man.

Clinical manifestations of pulmonary tuberculosis

The onset of pulmonary tuberculosis is usually insidious.

Primary tuberculosis. Most individuals with primary tuberculosis have no symptoms. However, if present, they are no more than those of a slight

---

*The Battey bacillus was discovered at Battey Tuberculosis Hospital, Rome, Ga.

cold. In case of progressive disease resulting from hematogenous dissemination, symptoms will be characteristic of extrapulmonary lesions and symptoms.

Postprimary tuberculosis. In uncomplicated postprimary tuberculosis the onset is insidious. Frequently by the time the individual seeks medical attention the disease is well advanced. There may be loss of weight, malaise, feeling of fatigue, loss of strength, night sweats, and unexplained low-grade temperature, all of which may be present in other disease conditions. As the infection progresses, a cough develops, which becomes productive; however, the cough may also be unproductive. There may be anorexia and nausea, and in women amenorrhea may occur. The patient may become anemic, nervous, depressed, and irritable. Sputum may be bloodstreaked, or frank hemorrhage may occur. Chest pain may vary from only an occasional ache to acute pain if pleurisy is present. Fever generally remains low grade and is present only in the afternoon. In acute onset there may be considerable elevation of temperature; otherwise, fever is regarded as less significant than it was some years ago. Dyspnea does not occur until the lungs are extensively involved, unless there is a pleural effusion, which may occur early. The extent of symptoms and their severity will vary with the individual and whether the disease remains confined to the lungs or becomes a generalized infection.

Complications

The complications of tuberculosis may fall into several categories: those resulting from hematogenous dissemination of the tubercle bacillus, the presence of preexisting or superimposed chronic nontuberculous disease, and the emotional factors related to the reactivation or diagnosis of the disease.

Some of the complications resulting from bloodstream involvement have been reviewed previously, that is miliary tuberculosis, bone and joint involvement, and tubercular meningitis as complicating miliary tuberculosis. The spread of the disease through the body may not always be considered as a true complication. True complications usually arise from active progressive pulmonary tuberculosis. Hemoptysis must always be considered a possibility in pulmonary tuberculosis. It may occur at any stage of the disease and usually indicates the presence of a cavity or tracheobronchial ulceration. Bleeding may be only blood-streaked sputum or a massive hemorrhage resulting in death. The condition must always be regarded as an emergency requiring prompt action on the part of the nurse.

Spontaneous pneumothorax may result from air seeping into the pleural cavity. It occurs suddenly with an acute pain. The affected lobe or lung may reexpand normally, or the condition may cause immediate death. Tuberculous empyema may follow spontaneous pneumothorax. Prior to the use of chemotherapeutic drugs, artificial pneumothorax was a common procedure in treatment of the disease. At the present time it is used to a very limited extent.

Pleurisy may occur at any stage of the disease, frequently with effusion.

It may occur in primary tuberculosis as well as in postprimary infection. Pleurisy with effusion in any person with a reactive tuberculin test, although other clinical signs of the disease are lacking, is considered to be tuberculous until proved otherwise.

Other complications that may arise include tuberculous laryngitis, a fairly common complication. Ulcerations may occur in the bronchi, trachea, pharynx, tongue, soft palate, and oral mucosa. These involvements occur most frequently in patients with far-advanced disease.

There are various nontuberculous pulmonary conditions that are thought to have a close relationship to tuberculosis. Some of these conditions may be superimposed on an already-existing tuberculosis infection, or their presence may be identified when diagnosis of tuberculosis is confirmed. The question of which came first may not be possible to determine, nor the extent to which one affects the other.

Silicosis has long been identified with tuberculosis. It is thought to predispose to tuberculosis, and its presence may tend to aggravate the infection. The coexistence of the two diseases is called silicotuberculosis.

Emphysema is characteristically a disease of older persons, especially of men. It may not be a coincidence that more tuberculosis is being found among the older male population. Existence of the two conditions often presents problems of diagnosis, although their relationship to each other is unknown.

Chronic bronchitis or bronchiectasis may exist in the patient with tuberculosis. Symptoms of chronic bronchitis and tuberculosis are very similar, and coughing in bronchitis may facilitate the spread of the tubercle bacilli.

Carcinoma of the lung gives rise to symptoms similar to those of tuberculosis; however, the two diseases may exist simultaneously. A diagnosis of tuberculosis may require extensive examination before it is confirmed. If the tuberculous lesion is inactive, the carcinomatous lesion may cause reactivation of the tuberculous infection.

A number of other diseases including those caused by fungus such as histoplasmosis, cardiovascular disease, certain gastrointestinal disorders such as peptic ulcer, and diabetes may exist together with tuberculosis in the same individual. Tuberculosis case rates for persons with diabetes are several times higher than those for the general population because of their increased susceptibility to infection.

A previous reference to mental stress as a predisposing factor in tuberculosis was made. It is not completely understood, but psychic trauma is believed to play a part in the activation of the disease.[5] The nurse must also consider the emotional factor when a person learns for the first time that he has tuberculosis. The need for understanding and for someone who cares is very important, and frequently the nurse is the one person who can provide this kind of emotional support.

Today, pregnancy during pulmonary tuberculosis is no longer feared or considered an indication for therapeutic abortion. Under chemotherapy the mother can have a healthy baby without added risk to herself or to the child.

Classification

There are numerous ways in which tuberculosis may be classified, and proper classification depends on proper and sound diagnosis. Throughout the course of the disease reexamination may result in reclassification of the infection. Those aspects of classification that are important to the nurse are extent of the disease, clinical activity, and bacteriologic status.

The extent of the disease may indicate a "minimal" infection, usually without cavitation. Lesions may be present in one or both lungs, but there is limited involvement. "Moderately advanced" may indicate infection in one or both lungs, with or without cavitation. The total area involved in one or both lungs does not exceed the area of one lung. If cavitation is present, the diameter is limited to less than 4 cm. "Far-advanced" tuberculosis indicates that the lesions and cavitation have progressed beyond the moderately advanced stage.

The activity of the infection is described as "active, quiescent, or inactive," or it may not be possible to determine the exact state of activity. Active tuberculosis is generally based on roentgenographic examination and may show progression of disease as in new lesions or extension of cavitation. The patient casts off bacilli in sputum or in other excreta. Although active, examination may also indicate improvement. Quiescent means quiet or still. Therefore, a quiescent tuberculosis may not be actively progressing but may not be considered as inactive. Cavities may be present, but examination indicates improvement. In order to be classified as quiescent, the bacteriologic findings must be negative. Tuberculosis may be considered as inactive when all lesions show definite healing, all bacteriologic findings are negative, and cavities show no extension. For positive inactive classification, status of the disease must show improvement at regular intervals for at least a period of six months. When tuberculosis is suspected but diagnosis has not been completed, the status of "activity undetermined" may be made.[5] The status may be especially hazardous to nurses caring for such patients, since on completion of the examination the disease may be found to be infectious.

Bacteriologic status is determined by the examination of sputum or gastric washings. The culture technic has been proved as the most reliable method for identifying the acid-fast tubercle bacilli. In case of generalized tuberculosis, bacteriologic examination may include examination of spinal fluid, pleural fluid, urine, and biopsy materials. In the past, serology tests have not been found satisfactory for general use; however, several new types of serologic tests are being investigated at the present time.

Diagnosis

Tuberculosis cannot be recognized by casual observation. The demonstration of tubercle bacilli is necessary to prove the diagnosis of tuberculosis.

The diagnosis of tuberculosis is also based on personal and family history, clinical examination, sputum examination, tuberculin testing, and roentgenologic studies.

Examination of the patient includes a total evaluation of all of the findings. No one aspect of the examination may be considered diagnostic. The tuberculin test is a valuable tool when a differential diagnosis is involved, and skin tests for fungal infections may be performed.

Although clinical examination is considered less important than formerly, it may be significant when related to the total examination. Laboratory and bacteriologic examinations of body fluids are of primary importance, since no diagnosis of tuberculosis can be made without specific identification of the tubercle bacillus. A failure to find the organism does not always rule out the possibility of the disease, and repeated examinations may be required. The diagnosis of atypical tuberculosis can be made only by culture methods.[14]

Roentgenologic studies are valuable when done by a competent radiologist. The interpretation is of prime importance, since findings may indicate pulmonary disease other than tuberculosis or coexisting with tuberculosis.

Treatment

The treatment of tuberculosis has undergone many changes since the discovery of chemotherapeutic drugs. Lives have been saved and many more prolonged. Collapse procedures have almost been eliminated, more success has been achieved in resectional surgery, the number of hospital beds has been reduced, and hospital stay has been shortened with post-hospital ambulatory care programs.

The classification of chemotherapeutic agents used in the treatment of *Mycobacterium* tuberculosis and atypical tuberculosis is as follows:

1. Primary drugs
   a. Streptomycin (SM) — The first effective medication against tuberculosis, it was introduced in 1945. It is taken by injection and may cause dizziness in some patients.
   b. Para-aminosalicylic acid (PAS) — Introduced in 1949, PAS increases the effectiveness of other medications. It is taken orally. In some patients it may produce a skin rash.
   c. Isonicotinic acid hydrazide (Isoniazid [INH]) — Introduced in 1952, it is the most effective medication against tuberculosis. It is taken orally. Serious side effects are uncommon, and it is well suited to long-term use in the home treatment of patients after discharge.
2. Secondary drugs
   a. Pyrazinamide (PZA)
   b. Viomycin (VM)
   c. Cycloserine (CS)
   d. Kanamycin (Kantrex) (KM)

e. Ethionamide (Trecator) (ETHA)

f. Ethambutol (EMB) — Introduced in 1967, it is a very effective drug along with other medicines.

g. Rifampin (RFN) — Newest of the medicines, it is very effective taken orally and in combination with other drugs.

All these drugs produce toxic reactions, and although their use has been a major contribution in the treatment and control of tuberculosis, it should be pointed out that the ideal drug is yet to be discovered.

The primary toxic effect of streptomycin is damage to the eighth nerve, resulting in incoordination and vertigo. Allergic reactions including nauea, vomiting, diarrhea, and skin rash may occur. Para-aminosalicylic acid may cause nausea and vomiting, gastric irritation, and reduced prothrombin time in the blood. Isoniazid appears to be less toxic than the other drugs; however, peripheral nervous system disturbances may occur. Allergic manifestations involving the central nervous system, nausea, vomiting, delirium, and convulsions are possible in the hypersensitive person.

Not all patients respond to the same drugs, and drug-susceptibility tests should be done for all patients to ensure the agent that will be most effective. This is particularly important in diseases caused by the unclassified mycobacteria. Most patients with atypical tuberculosis respond poorly, if at all, to the primary drugs, and drug-sensitivity tests become exceedingly important for this group of patients.

There is some variation in methods of drug therapy, but, in general, a combination of drugs is given. Factors that may affect the treatment plan include the pathology and type of lesion, the growth of the bacilli, and the degree of patient resistance. In moderately or far-advanced cases of pulmonary tuberculosis, therapy is initiated with all of the drugs. Isoniazid, 3 to 5 mg. per kilogram of body weight, is given daily in divided doses by the oral route. Para-aminosalicylic acid, 10 to 15 gm. daily in divided doses, is administered orally before meals, and streptomycin, 1 Gm. daily is administered intramuscularly and reduced to 1 Gm. biweekly after a few weeks.[8] When a regimen using two drugs is used, streptomycin and isoniazid are generally the drugs used.

Chemotherapy should begin when the diagnosis is made and continued for at least two years. In some situations it may be continued longer. When therapy is inadequate or discontinued too soon, relapse may occur. Some types of lesions may respond quickly, others slowly, and in fibrotic or fibrocavernous lesions it may be ineffective, but it will render sputum negative and help to prevent further spread of the disease.[17]

Prognosis

With present day chemotherapy prognosis has greatly improved. A fully cooperative, intelligent patient under competent medical treatment has odds in his favor to recover without becoming chronically ill. The goal of modern treatment has become nothing less than 100% recovery rate.

Factors influencing recovery are cooperation of the patient; heriditary temperament and constitution; virulence of the organism; intensity, continuity, and duration of treatment; and development of complications.

Resectional surgery

The success of resectional surgery has been facilitated through the use of chemotherapeutic drugs. It is now possible to remove all evidence of disease by wedge or segmental resections, or in selected cases a lobectomy or pneumonectomy may be advisable. Some physicians believe that the need for resectional surgery has almost been eliminated. However, there is a small proportion of patients who choose not to remain on therapy, whose lesions do not respond to therapy, or who develop new active lesions after chemotherapy treatment. The need for and the type of surgery is determined on an individual basis after consideration of all of the factors involved. Resectional surgery is often necessary and appears to offer the best chance for cure in pulmonary cavitation caused by the *Mycobacterium kansasii.* Other procedures such as artificial pneumothorax, pneumoperitoneum, and thoracoplasty are rarely used today.

Case finding

Present-day methods of case finding have changed from those of a decade ago. The older method of mass survey was centered on the general population and was costly and largely unfruitful in finding new active cases of tuberculosis. The present emphasis is centered on specific groups of people in whom tuberculosis is most likely to be found. Among these groups are family contacts to infectious tuberculosis patients, and there is increased emphasis on tuberculin testing of preschool children and those beginning high school. A reactive tuberculin test in the preschool child increases the possibility of finding an infected adult in the home. The World Health Organization has stated that children who are tuberculin reactors represent the best index of the current transmission of disease in the community.[18] Tuberculin testing and x-ray examination of reactors should in-

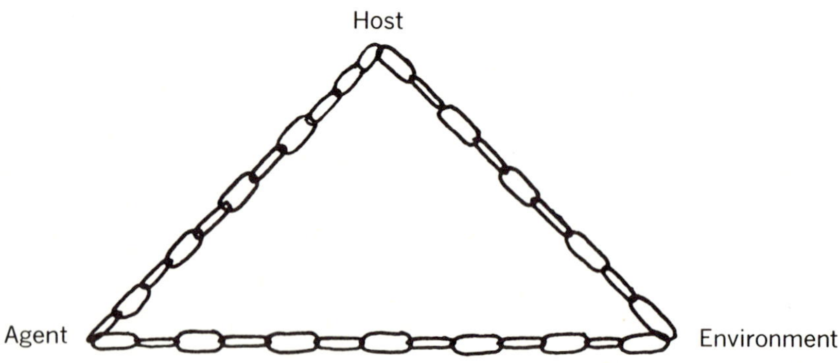

Fig. 10. Epidemiologic chain of infection. (Courtesy National Medical Audiovisual Center, Chamblee, Ga.)

clude adults such as teachers in public schools, nursery schools, day care centers, bus drivers, custodians, and lunchroom personnel (Fig. 10).

Examination of long-term institutionalized persons in mental hospitals, nursing homes, and prisons should be included in a case-finding program. The increase in the number of elderly persons and the incidence of tuberculosis in this age group, together with the increased population in nursing homes, should provide a fertile field for finding new cases.

Some general hospitals secure roentgenologic examination of all hospital admissions.

Persons receiving public relief represent a segment of the population in which the incidence may be high. Persons in slum areas and the nonwhite male population, persons with diabetes, persons with silicosis, persons receiving steroid therapy, hospital personnel, or economic and racial groups where the incidence of tuberculosis is high represent high-risk groups.

While there are gaps in our present knowledge about tuberculosis, we do have sufficient information to reduce the present tuberculosis rates if emphasis is placed on segments of the population where tuberculosis is known to exist.

Tuberculin skin testing

These tests are specific for tuberculosis infection, except those that occur from cross reactions with infection by the atypical mycobacterium. Principles underlying the tuberculin test involve a delayed hypersensitivity to the proteins of the *Mycobacterium tuberculosis* organism. As is characteristic in other diseases, antibodies are not involved in reactivity to the tuberculin test but, rather, cells. Following the primary infection a delay of about six weeks occurs, after which the defense mechanisms of the body become extremely sensitive to the bacillus proteins. At this time a minute amount of these proteins injected into the body will elicit a reaction involving swelling and discoloration, the extent of which depends on the degree of hypersensitivity and the size of the injected dose.

The use of the tuberculin test as a case-finding technic has given new emphasis when it is used among high-risk groups and in areas where the incidence of tuberculosis is high. It has great value in locating early infections, when treatment is most effective.

The tuberculin test is carried out with old tuberculin (OT), a heat-killed concentrated filtrate of the *Mycobacterium tuberculosis* organism, or with purified protein derivative (PPD), which contains the active protein or fraction made from the filtrates of the tubercle bacilli. Solutions of these preparations deteriorate very quickly, and for accurate results only fresh preparations should be used. Diluted solutions should not be allowed to stand at room temperature but should be refrigerated.

Multiple-puncture skin tests such as the Heaf, the Tine, the jet injector, and the Mono-Vacc are useful in the physician's office or in mass screening. Equivocal results should always be checked by repeating with a standard Mantoux test.

Mantoux test. The Mantoux test is the most commonly used method of tuberculin testing and is the standard with which all other methods must be compared. The dermal test is performed by injecting 0.1 ml. of a 1:100 dilution of old tuberculin into the skin of the forearm. Some prefer to begin testing with a weaker dilution and if no reaction is noted, to retest with a stronger dilution. The present trend is away from using the weaker dilution. A tuberculin syringe and a one-quarter-inch, 25-gauge needle should be used. The needle should be sharply beveled, and needles and syringes used for tuberculin testing should not be used for any other purpose. The test should be read after forty-eight to seventy-two hours, and familiarity and skill are required for accurate reading. It is presently considered that reactions of 8 to 10 mm. or more in diameter represent a high risk of developing tuberculosis. The intracutaneous test using purified protein derivative is the same as that using old tuberculin (Fig. 11).

Sterneedle. The Sterneedle is a multiple-puncture device for intradermal tuberculin testing. The device consists of six needles within the Sterneedle cartridge that automatically penetrate the skin to a controlled depth through a film of concentrated tuberculin purified protein derivative solution. The Sterneedle cartridge tip is dipped into the solution, after which it is placed on the flexor surface of the upper third of the forearm and rotated 90 degrees to spread the tuberculin. The handle of the device is then pressed, releasing the six points to carry the tuberculin into the skin. The cartridge

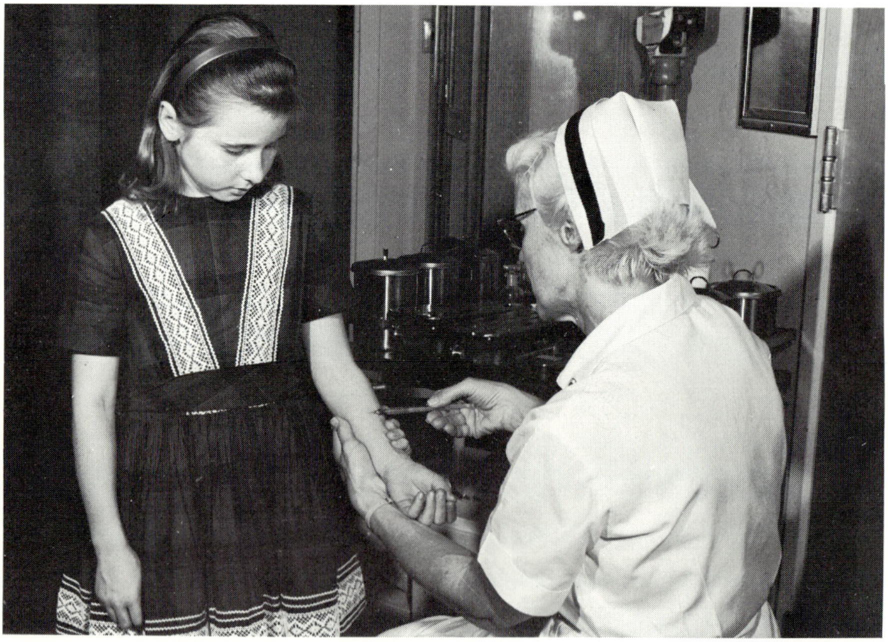

Fig. 11. Nurse performing Mantoux tuberculin test on a young girl. (Courtesy National Medical Audiovisual Center, Chamblee, Ga.)

is then discarded; cartridges may be autoclaved and reused. The test is read three to seven days after its administration. A positive test is indicated if four or more puncture points are endurated with erythema (Figs. 12 and 13).

Tine test. The Tine test is an intradermal test and consists of a stainless steel disc attached to a plastic handle. Each disc has four triangular-shaped prongs or tines, which are 2 mm. long and are spaced about 4 mm. apart. The tines have been dip-dried into four times concentrated U. S. Standard old tuberculin. The total unit is disposable. The test is performed on the

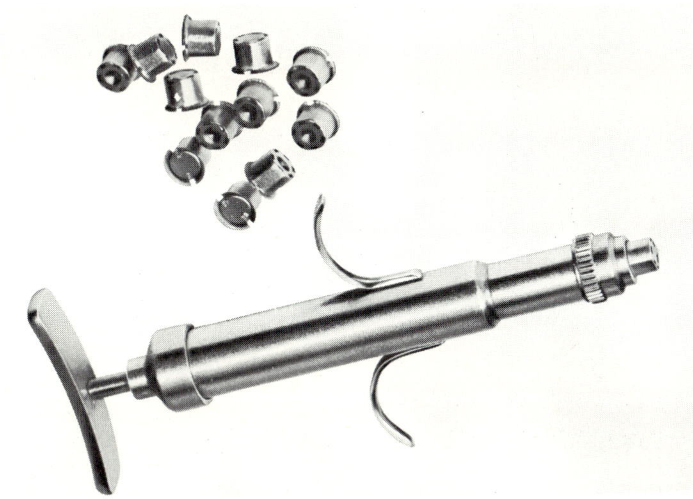

Fig. 12. Sterneedle for tuberculin testing. (Courtesy Panray Division, Ormont Drug & Chemical Co., Inc., Englewood, N. J.)

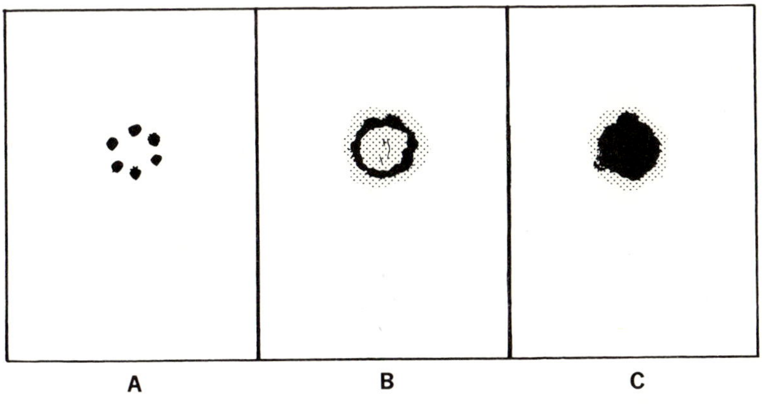

Fig. 13. Reading the Sterneedle tuberculin test. **A,** Positive reaction if four or more puncture points show induration. **B,** Grade 2 reaction. **C,** Grade 3 reaction.

A

B

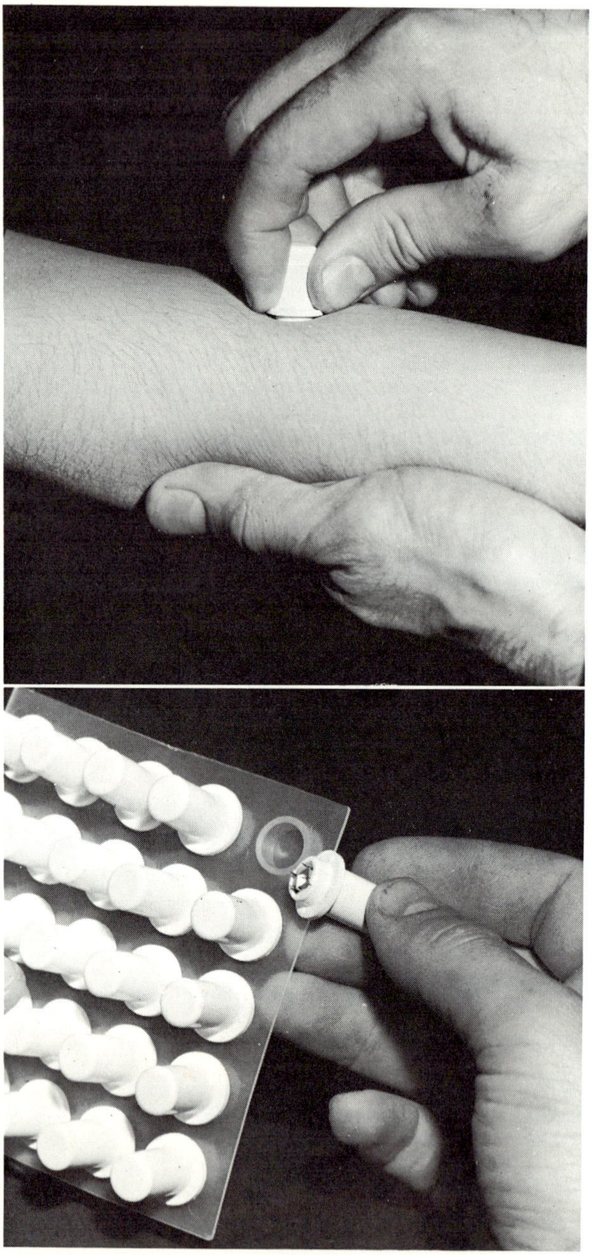

Fig. 14. Tuberculin Tine test. **A,** Administering the Tine tuberculin test. **B,** Disposable sterile plastic unit holding disposable tines coated with tuberculin. (Courtesy Lederle Laboratories, Division of American Cyanamid Co., Pearl River, N. Y.)

inner surface of the midforearm after cleaning with acetone, ether, or soap and water. The skin is slightly stretched, and the Tine test pressed into the skin and held for one second. When the unit is removed, the four puncture sites should be visible. The test is read in forty-eight to seventy-two hours. Each unit is sterile and should not be reused. Research using the Tine test indicates that results are comparable to the intradermal test using the injected technic. The test is reported to have the advantages of (1) eliminating the problem of syringes and needles; (2) being sterile and disposable and eliminating the danger of cross-infection; (3) being inexpensive and well suited for mass testing in remote and underdeveloped areas of the world; and (4) being performed by trained technical personnel, conserving the time of nurses and physicians. (See Fig. 14.)

Jet injector. The jet injector is a new method of administering the tuberculin test. The technic uses a jet gun and permits rapid testing of large numbers of persons quickly. Considerable skill and special training in its use are required. However, it has the advantage of eliminating the fear of needles when testing young children. Morse and co-workers found that by comparison, agreement between tests administered with the jet gun and those using the intradermal technic was 97.4% (Fig. 15).[3]

Other tests. The patch test uses dried tuberculin, which is placed on gauze and held in place with adhesive tape. The test is used to a very limited extent, since it is not considered as reliable as the Mantoux test. A

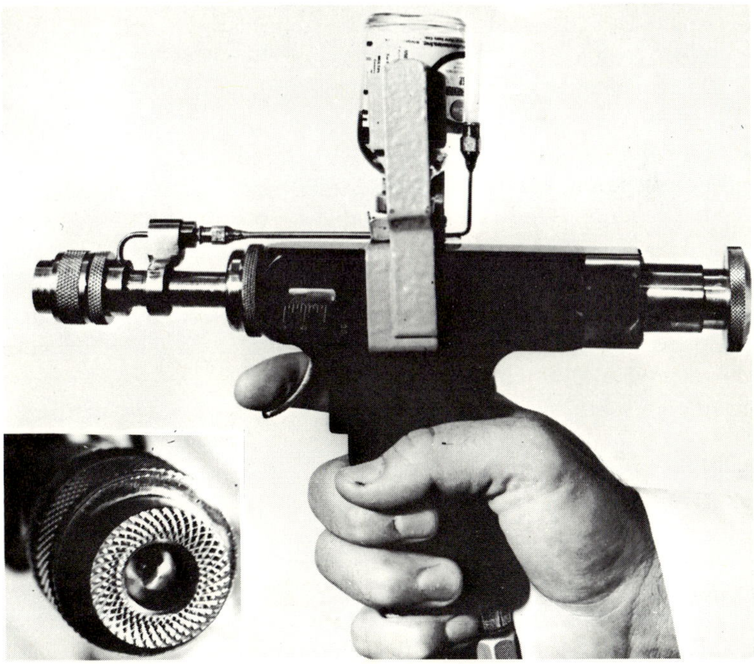

Fig. 15. Jet injector. (Courtesy National Medical Audiovisual Center, Chamblee, Ga.)

similar technic, the jelly patch test, uses tuberculin jelly, which is squeezed onto the cleansed skin and covered for forty-eight hours. The dressing is then removed, and the test is read seventy-two to ninety-six hours after it was performed.

The von Pirquet test is a scratch test and is no longer being used.

Calmette Guérin vaccine (BCG)

The BCG vaccine is prepared from living strains of attenuated tubercle bacillus, and it is used to immunize persons for tuberculosis. The vaccine has had wide use throughout many countries, where good results have been reported in reducing tuberculosis rates. The use of BCG vaccine in the United States and Canada is a controversial issue. In 1962 the Tuberculosis Control Advisory Committee on BCG vaccine reported to the Surgeon General of the United States Public Health Service that in most instances BCG vaccination is not needed and that its widespread use would interfere with the use of the tuberculin test as a diagnostic tool. Therefore, its use is not indicated. However, the committee stated exceptions in which its use on an individual basis might be justified.[2]

The National Tuberculosis Association has approved BCG vaccination for tuberculin-negative persons; however, in keeping with newer trends in case finding, they do not recommend mass vaccination. They advise BCG vaccination of the following: (1) children in areas where the incidence of tuberculosis is high, (2) hospital personnel who are in danger from undetected tuberculosis, (3) tuberculin-negative persons in homes where they are exposed to tuberculosis, and (4) inmates and personnel in prisons and mental hospitals where the incidence of the disease is high.[9]

The vaccine is administered intracutaneously over the deltoid muscle, and a multiple-puncture method quite similar to that used for smallpox vaccination is employed. It may also be administered by a scarification technic similar to the von Pirquet technic of tuberculin testing.

The vaccine is administered only to persons with negative tuberculin tests. Age is not a factor if the individual is tuberculin negative. Two tuberculin tests are administered six weeks apart to allow for any prior exposure that may have sensitized the individual. Vaccinated persons should be protected from known tuberculosis patients for periods varying from six weeks in adults to eight to twelve weeks in infants. After this period a tuberculin test is done that should be reactive if the immunization has been successful. The protection afforded by BCG vaccination wanes slowly. A good level of protection is maintained for ten years.

The vaccine is not administered to persons during attacks of communicable disease and is not given simultaneously with inoculations for other diseases.[10]

Nursing care in the general hospital

The nursing care of tuberculosis patients in the communicable disease hospital follows a technic prescribed by the institution. Procedures are adhered to through a planned continuous program of teaching all hospital personnel and patients, with sufficient supervision and counseling to ensure compliance.

Physicians, nurses, paramedical personnel, as well as other employees in most general hospitals are at a distinct disadvantage because of possible exposure from unknown cases of tuberculosis.

The patient with tuberculosis or suspected tuberculosis who is admitted to the general hospital may fall into one of several categories. He may be admitted (1) to evaluate the status of the infection after chemotherapy, (2) to provide relief and treatment for allergic manifestation resulting from chemotherapy, (3) to establish differential diagnosis, (4) for diagnosis of probable symptomatic tuberculosis, or (5) to await transfer to a tuberculosis facility.

There is no need for patients to wait for transfer to a tuberculosis hospital today. Because of the shortened hospitalization and ambulatory and home care programs, hospital beds for new admissions are available immediately.

Some hospitals may have a communicable disease unit, but in most cases the patient will be admitted to a private room, cubicle, or ward bed on a regular medical unit. Since chemotherapy renders most patients noninfectious very quickly, many changes have been made in their care. In many cases a patient who is noninfectious may occupy a cubicle or ward bed with unit precautions. Any patient with a positive sputum and who is coughing or otherwise infectious must be placed in a private room and isolation technic carried out. It should be pointed out here that the use of gowns in airborne infections such as tuberculosis are ineffective and not necessary. Gowns are used only for prolonged personal care or while changing the bed. Neither are masks indicated for personnel except in instances of intimate face to face contact. If anyone is to be masked, it should be the patient. Masking of the patient is indicated only if his condition is such that he is unable to control or unwilling to cover his cough, when visitors are in the room, or when the patient is taken out of the room for any reason. Patients with tuberculosis or suspected tuberculosis should not be placed in halls with the bed screened.

Although most hospitals have communicable disease procedures, frequently they overemphasize factors of least importance, while underestimating important ones. It should be kept in mind that tuberculosis is not a highly communicable disease and that most persons have a high degree of resistance to it; however, any person discharging tubercle bacilli is in a communicable disease state, and certain precautions should be taken.

A prime factor in nursing care is the proper care and handling of sputum to prevent the organism being disseminated by air currents. This begins by teaching the patient to cover the nose and mouth completely when coughing. The patient should be taught how to place several layers of tissue in the cupped hand to receive sputum. The tissue is then carefully folded over the sputum and placed in a cuffed paper bag pinned to the side of the bed. The nurse may remove the bag by placing the hands under the cuff to avoid soiling them, and the entire contents should be burned at once. In pulmonary tuberculosis the urine and feces are not infectious and may be placed in the public sewage system without prior disinfection.

Ventilation is one of the most important factors to be considered in patient care. Good ventilation in the room dilutes the number of nuclei and moves them out into the air currents, where they are readily killed by sunlight. Ultraviolet light placed in a room will kill nuclei in a few seconds.

Handwashing facilities are a requirement. Washing of one's hands is quite efficient in removing organisms that have been picked up from direct contact with infected sputum. While automatic knee or foot controls and automatic soap dispensers are ideal, ordinary methods may be safely used. Special care of the nails should be given after patient contact.

In the case of hemoptysis or emesis the bed should be changed immediately and linens cared for according to the policies of the institution.

Specimens of sputum for bacteriologic examination are collected in containers designed for that purpose. The specimen should consist of the first sputum raised in the morning and should be collected before the patient has brushed his teeth. No mouthwash or antiseptic gargles should precede collection of the specimen. The specimen should be properly labeled, marked contaminated, and sent to the laboratory.

The tuberculosis patient needs rest and should be provided with a quiet environment to afford the maximum amount of rest. Visitors are permitted, but they should not be allowed to cause the patient to become fatigued.

Patients with tuberculosis need a well-balanced diet, but it is generally agreed that a diet high in calories and supplements of vitamins and minerals is unnecessary.

Patients need a great deal of emotional support and understanding when they learn for the first time that they have tuberculosis, as do their families. Newly diagnosed patients should not be left alone for long periods. Frequent short trips to the room will indicate to the patient that the nurse is interested in his welfare.

Prevention and control

The prevention and control of tuberculosis is now being centered on the long-term follow-up and surveillance by health departments and private physicians of high-risk groups. According to Soper, if eradication of tuberculosis is to be achieved, emphasis must be placed on the complete elimination of the disease, not merely reducing the incidence through control measures.[15] Thus, the new philosophy is centered about preventing the occurrence of disease and rendering the infectious patient noninfectious as quickly as possible.

It is believed that prophylactic isoniaizd is a practical tool to use in preventing tuberculosis in contact groups.

At this time prophylactic isoniaizd therapy is recommended for: (1) all children under 3 years of age who are tuberculin reactive; (2) all adolescents with recent infections; (3) all age groups who convert from negative to positive tuberculin reactions; (4) persons whose disease appears healed, but in whom reactivation is possible; and (5) all individuals with conditions that may predispose them to tuberculosis. This group includes tuberculin-reactive persons receiving corticosteroid agents, diabetic patients, patients with inactive tuberculosis who become pregnant.[11]

It is recommended that student nurses and medical students who have negative tuberculin tests be retested every three months. If the test converts to positive, x-ray examination should follow, and in the absence of tuberculosis they should be placed on isoniazid prophylaxis. Some schools of nursing and some medical schools are presently following this regimen.

Sufficient evidence has been collected during the past few years to indicate that tuberculin tests, x-ray examination when indicated, and prophylactic therapy should be required of all school personnel including teachers, custodians, bus drivers, practice teachers, nursery school teachers, baby sitters, and all other persons who have contact with young children.

All cases of pulmonary and extrapulmonary tuberculosis should be reported to the health department, and this is mandatory in most countries. This is the basic method of control along with chemoprophylaxis. Patients who are infectious should be hospitalized, if possible, until noninfectious. Concurrent disinfection, including care of sputum and isolation in a well-ventilated room until the patient is noninfectious, is indicated. All general measures to improve economic conditions, working conditions, housing, nutrition, sanitation, and health hazards also serve to reduce the incidence of tuberculosis.

As effective chemotherapy shortens the infectious period and the hospital stay, the clinic or physician's office becomes very important in the control program. These are now the centers both for diagnosis and for prolonged treatment.

Note: It is not possible to review all aspects of tuberculosis in this chapter. The nurse may consult other references and the fine articles that appear in nursing journals.

REFERENCES

1. Aldelman, Samuel L.: Tuberculosis in large urban centers. Am. J. Public Health **56**:1546-1553, Sept., 1966.
2. Chamberlain, W. Edward, Davey, Winthrop N., Farnsworth, Stanford F., Gray, A. L., Hutcheson, R. H., Long, Esmond R., and Perkins, James E.: Use of BCG vaccine, Public Health Reports **77**:680, Aug., 1962.
3. Morse, Dan, Hall, Clifton, Kaluzny, Alex, and Runde, R. H.: Comparative tuberculosis testing, intradermal gun versus intradermal needle, Am. Rev. Respir. Dis- **96**:107-110, Jan., 1967.
4. Corpe, Raymond F., Runyon, Ernest H., and Lester, William: Status of disease due to unclassified mycobacteria, Am. Rev. Respir. Dis. **87**:459-461, March, 1963.
5. Diagnostic standards and classification of tuberculosis, American Thoracic Society Committee on Revision of Diagnostic Standards, New York, 1961, National Tuberculosis Association.
6. Dubos, Rene J., and Hirsch, James G., editors: Bacterial and mycotic infections of man, ed. 4, Philadelphia, 1965, J. B. Lippincott Co.
7. Ferebee, Shirley H., and Mount, Frank W.: Tuberculosis morbidity in a controlled trial of the prophylactic use of isoniazid among household contacts, Am.

Rev. Respir. Dis. **85**:490-510, April, 1962.
8. Modell, Walter, editor: Drugs of choice 1974-1975, St. Louis, 1974, The C. V. Mosby Co.
9. NTA issues statement on BCG vaccine, Am. J. Nurs. **65**:24, Feb., 1965.
10. Paul, Hugh: The control of diseases (social and communicable), Baltimore, 1964, The Williams & Wilkins Co.
11. Planning eradication of tuberculosis, Currents in Public Health, vol. 7, no. 6, Columbus, Ohio, 1967, Ross Laboratories.
12. Riley, Richard L.: Air-borne infection, Am. J. Nurs. **60**:1246-1248, Sept., 1960.
13. Samter, Max, editor: Immunological diseases, Boston, 1965, Little, Brown & Co.
14. Schaffer, W. B.: Serologic identification of the atypical mycobacteria and its value in epidemiologic studies, Am. Rev. Respir. Dis. **96**:115-118, Jan., 1967.
15. Soper, Fred L.: Problems to be solved if the eradication of tuberculosis is to be realized, Am. J. Public Health **52**:734-745, May, 1962.
16. Top, Franklin H. and Wehrle, Paul F.: Communicable and infectious diseases, ed. 7, St. Louis, 1972, The C. V. Mosby Co.
17. Weiss, Moe: Chemotherapy and tuberculosis, Am. J. Nurs. **59**:1711-1714, Dec., 1959.
18. World Health Organization Expert Committee on Tuberculosis, eighth report, Technical Report Series, Geneva, 1964, World Health Organization.

15

STAPHYLOCOCCUS AUREUS INFECTION

Characteristics of staphylococcus

The staphylococcus bacteria belong to the family Micrococcaceae, and *Staphylococcus aureus* is the pathogenic species of the family that causes severe infections. Together with a nonpathogenic species *Staphylococcus epidermis* (formerly *Staphylococcus albus*) which is sometimes responsible for very mild, limited infections, they are a part of the resident population of bacteria that inhabit the normal skin and mucous membrane.

The *Staphylococcus aureus* is a gram-positive, nonmotile, nonsporulating organism that grows in irregular clusters resembling a bunch of grapes. However, they may grow in various formations, including pairs or chains. They do not have flagellae, and some strains that may show capsules have not been found to be pathogenic. Cultures of staphylococci produce a pigment varying in color from golden orange to yellow or white. A few strains of the organism produce a heat-stable toxin called enterotoxin resulting in food intoxication.

Exactly how long the organism may remain alive outside the body is unknown. Various estimates range from weeks to months. Staphylococci are the most resistant of all nonspore-forming organisms to the action of heat, drying, and chemicals. In dried pus they may live for weeks and even months. The staphylococcus has adapted quickly and easily to sulfonamides and antibiotics, with the result that they may have become resistant. As much as 80% are resistant to penicillin.

Staphylococcus is an optionally reported disease in the U. S. However, in 1972 four states reported a total of 718 cases. New Hampshire reported 165 cases; Delaware 127 cases; Arkansas forty-nine cases; and Oregon 377 cases. In 1973, five states reported a total of 574 cases. No statistics are available for Canada as it is not a notifiable disease.

Epidemiology

Staphylococcus bacteria are not newcomers to the field of communicable disease, but their importance has been highlighted by the increasing number of nosocomial infections in recent years. There seems little doubt that the organism may have been man's companion through the ages. However, its recognition as a specific microorganism did not occur until the nineteenth century. Studies by Pasteur and Ogston as early as 1880 established its pathogenicity, and in 1882 Ogston named the organism staphylococcus from a Greek word meaning "a bunch of grapes."

The natural habitat of the staphylococcus is the human anterior nares, skin, and throat. In a study of ambulatory patients made at Massachusetts General Hospital by the Harvard Medical School, 79% of the patients were found to carry staphylococcus. The organism was isolated from all three areas, nose, skin, and throat, in 30% of the patients studied.[1]

There is wide variation in the carrier state. Some persons carry the organism intermittently with change in the phage type at intervals. Others may carry the same phage type for long intervals, whereas some may carry more than one phage type at the same time, and others never carry the organism at any time. The carrier rate varies from infancy to adulthood, with the adult rate between 30% and 50%. However, it is not unusual for the rate to be lower in nonepidemic situations and to increase during epidemics. Roodyn conducted a study over a period of seven years in which he found 11% of eighty-one patients had recurrent infections with the same phage type of staphylococcus.[10]

The small number of serious infections seem to indicate that most normal persons are not affected by the presence of the organism. However, in nosocomial infections certain groups seem to be at risk. Surgical patients, newborn infants in nurseries, maternity patients, and elderly debilitated patients comprise the high-risk group.

Pathogenicity

Staphylococci cause boils, pustules, pimples, furuncles, abscesses, carbuncles, paronychias, and infections of accidental or surgical wounds. Staphylococci also produce systemic diseases, and all organs in the body may be affected. They may cause empyema, endocarditis, brain abscesses, cystitis, pneumonia, meningitis, pyelonephritis, otitis media, food poisoning, osteomyelitis, and arthritis. They may also be involved in mixed infections, and associated with other pathogenic organisms.

Transmission

Staphylococci are normal inhabitants of the skin, mouth, throat, and nose of man. Ordinarily, they live in these areas with no effects, but once they penetrate the body's defences of the skin and mucous membrane, they cause extensive serious disease if the organism is highly virulent or the body resistance is low. Staphylococci penetrate the skin through the hair follicles and ducts of the sweat glands. Staphylococci are spread by direct person-to-person contact. Nasal carriers can also transmit the organisms. Prevention of the spread of the organisms requires rigid precautions as to handwashing, disposal of infected dressings, disinfection of bedding, dishes, and thermometers. All the details of barrier isolation technique should be used. One of the most important measures in controlling their spread is the maintenance of good housekeeping standards.

During the period when the staphylococcus is in the normal process of drying, in the dust or in the lint from bedding, there is a reduction in the number of organisms released into the environment. As the drying process continues, injury to the cell occurs that results in a reduced capacity to cause infection.[8] Although the viable organism is reported to dry and live in dust for weeks or months, its infective potential appears to be greatly reduced.

The prime source of infection however, is the infected patient, and when he is placed in a ward with noninfected patients, he contaminates the immediate environment. It is possible to culture the same phage type from the nose and throat of other patients in the ward. The organism disappears from the environment but remains in the noses and throats of the patients, and as a new patient is admitted to the ward, he becomes infected with the same phage type.[1] Thus, it may be concluded that environment may play some part. Staphylococcus disseminated from an infected lesion finds occupancy in the noses and throats of closely associated patients, where it remains to infect new patients. Farrer found the highest incidence of infection in patients in wards where cross-infection occurred and the lowest attack rate in patients in private rooms.[5]

The newborn infant who acquires an infection while in the nursery, either impetigo or as a carrier, has been found to carry the organism for many months and disseminates it to family members. In a study made by Hurst and Grossman concerning staphylococcus infection among families of newborn infants, they found that 44% of infants infected in the hospital continued to carry the organism, which was transmitted to 27% of mothers, 2% of fathers, and 12% of siblings. The study indicated that forty-three infants and fifty-one family members developed staphylococcal infection.[7] Studies made by Roodyn over a seven-year period showed that eleven of seventeen infections occurring in the home were caused by person-to-person spread.[9]

Age, sex, racial, and seasonal factors

There are no known predisposing factors for staphylococcal infection. Investigations as to sex, age, and seasonal variations are limited and varied. An effort to study seasonal variation was made at Johns Hopkins University, where the greatest number of infections occurred in January of each year, suggesting some relationship to season. Two thirds of the infections occurred on the surgical service, but no other significant factor developed during the study.[11]

Farrer and MacLeod studied age, sex, and racial factors at the University of Pennsylvania Hospital in Philadelphia and found the largest number of infections among persons from 50 to 59 years of age. The smallest number of infections occurred in infants between 1 month and 1 year of age. The incidence was highest in males and twice as high in white than in nonwhite persons. Farrer and MacLeod did not find any seasonal variation. Most investigations showed increased incidence among persons with chronic diseases.[5]

Elderly persons from underprivileged socioeconomic environments and having one or more attendant diseases have a greater incidence of staphylococcal infections. There may be a relationship between socioeconomic status and infection rate among ward patients. Most hospitals tend to place patients who are economically depressed in wards where rates are usually less than in private or semiprivate rooms, and the incidence of infection has been shown to be greater among ward patients.

Clinical manifestations

Staphylococcus aureus is probably the most frequent cause of pyrogenic infections in man. The clinical example of staphylococcus disease is the abscess. Cutaneous pustular diseases include pustules, furuncles (boils), and the carbuncle. Although these infections are usually self-limiting, some individuals may have recurring episodes over an extended period of time. Family members have a risk rate that is four times greater than exists among the general population.[3] The cutaneous lesions are usually treated in the physician's office or in an outpatient clinic. Although they are generally considered minor, hematogenous spread of *Staphylococcus aureus* may cause abscess formation in any tissue of the body.

Staphylococcal bacteremia results from the constant presence of the organism in the blood. The mortality rate is high, varying from 30% to 50% in some areas to as high as 80% to 90% in other areas. Staphylococcal bacteremia may also be caused by the *Staphylococcus epidermidis* strain and if not treated, runs a rapid and highly fatal course. All patients with bacteremia are gravely ill with fever, malaise, chills, and anorexia.

Staphylococcal endocarditis results from bloodstream infection and is most likely to affect hearts already damaged from rheumatic fever or when congenital malformations are present. The patient is acutely ill with symptoms of fever, chills, loss of weight, and petechiae.

Acute hematogenous osteomyelitis is most frequent in young persons, and neonatal osteomyelitis is most frequent in infants under 1 month of age. In children and young adults the long bones of the lower extremities near the knee are most commonly involved, but other bones including the spine may be affected. As the disease progresses, the periosteum and soft tissues become involved with abscess formation. The disease is accompanied by chills, elevation of temperature, malaise, and increased pulse rate. The involved areas become painful, tender, and swollen, and a toxic condition may be present.

Staphylococcal pneumonia is a frequent complication of viral influenza and may follow measles and pertussis. It may also occur as a primary disease with accompanying complications including lung abscess or empyema. Pneumonia caused by *Staphylococcus aureus* differs very little from pneumonia caused by the pneumococcus, except that a greater lung area may be involved. The patient may be acutely ill with considerable elevation of temperature, dyspnea, cyanosis, and retrosternal pain. Staphylococcal pneumonia in young infants is likely to be acute and highly fatal.

Meningitis may be caused by the staphylococcus and results from dissemination of the organism in bacteremia. It may also occur from cutaneous staphylococcal lesions.

Staphylococcus food intoxication results from the ingestion of food containing enterotoxin produced by certain strains of the organism. About two to four hours following ingestion of the contaminated food the disease occurs with an abrupt onset. There is nausea, vomiting, diarrhea, abdominal cramping, and prostration. In severe cases there may be fever, muscular cramps, and headache with severe dehydration. Recovery is usually rapid; however, in young infants or debilitated persons who are excessively dehydrated, death may occur.

Bacteriologic diagnosis

Infections caused by *Staphylococcus aureus* are pyogenic, and diagnosis is readily established by the examination of exudate from the lesion using a smear technic or by cultures. An easily performed "slide test" can be done very quickly and is frequently used as a screening technic.

When bacteriologic examination implicates the staphylococcus as the etiologic agent in serious infections, antibiotic sensitivity tests are usually done. This enables the physician to select the most effective therapeutic agent.

Epidemiologic identification

Bacteriophage typing is not diagnostic but is used to differentiate between the various strains of staphylococcus. Bacteriophages are bacterial viruses that attack bacteria and, in certain cases, dissolve the bacterial cell. Each phage is specific in its capacity to cause lysis of a specific strain of bacteria. Because of the numerous strains of staphylococcus, some of which are not pathogenic, each phage is identified by a number. The specific strain of staphylococcus that is lysed by the phage is designated by the same number as the phage.

For the process of routine typing, phages are placed in four groups identified by Roman numerals, I, II, III, IV, and a miscellaneous group. Each group contains several phage types, and each phage in the group may cause lysis of the same strain, whereas it is possible for a specific strain to be lysed by a phage in more than one group. Bacteriophage typing also provides certain information concerning antibiotic resistance. There are still a large number of staphylococcus strains that are not typable.

Antibiotic resistance and hospital-acquired (nosocomial) infection

With the discovery of penicillin it appeared that the problem of staphylococcus infection had been solved. It had been known before the antibiotic era that certain strains of staphylococcus produced a number of enzymes, including penicillinase. In time it was discovered that penicillinase inactivated penicillin. More recent investigations indicate that the presence of the enzyme under certain conditions may reduce the effectiveness of penicillin on other kinds of pathogenic organisms.[3]

Systemic staphylococcal disease is often acquired in a hospital, especially in patients who have had surgery or who are already ill with a serious disease. In one regard the problem is related to modern antibiotic therapy. Antibiotics are usually bacteriostatic in nature, not bactericidal. Since they have been administered so freely, and the staphylococci are well equipped for survival, antibiotic-resistant strains have developed. Other factors adding to this problem of hospital-acquired staphylococcus infection is that more people are coming to the hospitals and surgical techniques have expanded, thus involving more persons.

Treatment

The treatment of staphylococcal infections includes the application of warm moist compresses for minor cutaneous lesions such as pustules and boils. The skin about a draining lesion should be kept clean with a germicidal agent to prevent infecting other areas. Surgical incision may be necessary in some cases, but therapeutic drugs rarely are necessary. Patients should be cautioned against pinching, squeezing, or other manual manipulation to prevent hematogenous spread of the organism. Carbuncles cover a wide area in subcutaneous fatty tissue and frequently require incision and drainage. A frequent site of this lesion is the back of the neck, but their occurrence about the nose and lips is not uncommon. Because of the rich blood supply about the face, any damage to the protective wall around the lesion may cause hematogenous spread with very serious complications. The appropriate antibiotic is frequently administered and if given early, may prevent the need for surgical intervention.

Staphylococcal pneumonia is considered a medical emergency. It often affects the very young and debilitated elderly persons. Antibiotic therapy must be based on antibiotic sensitivity tests. Penicillin is the drug of choice, but the widespread penicillin resistance may limit its use. Alternative semisynthetic penicillin drugs such as methicillin, oxacillin, and nafcillin, may be effective. In addition to the problem of drug resistance, patient sensitivity may be encountered. Vancomycin may be administered to these patients. Other drugs that may be used for the penicillin-sensitive patient include cephalothin, lincomycin, and novobiocin. Other treatment for the patient with staphylococcal pneumonia is the same as that for patients with pneumococcal pneumonia.

Osteomyelitis usually results from hematogenous spread of staphylococcus from some focal point. In the early stages of the disease the appropriate antibiotic is administered. The patient is placed on complete bed rest, and intravenous fluids are administered to relieve dehydration. The anemic patient may be transfused with whole blood. Efforts are directed toward building up the patient's general resistance. The diet is high protein, with vitamin supplements if needed.[2] After relief of the acute condition, surgery may be necessary to remove areas of necrotic bone (sequestrectomy).

Bacteremia may result from many different kinds of bacteria. When the physician is faced with a life-threatening situation, antibiotic therapy is usually initiated promptly. On the basis of signs and symptoms and clinical examination, the physician selects the antibiotic believed to be most effective. As a rule, drugs known to be bactericidal are preferred. Large doses of the antibiotic are administered intravenously, and treatment must be continued over a period of time. As soon as possible a complete bacteriologic diagnosis is established. If the causative organism is staphylococcus, sensitivity tests may be done.

It is important to reduce the number of organisms in the body as quickly as possible, and to do this any abscess or other focus of infection is incised and drained if possible.

Staphylococcal food intoxication is generally treated on the basis of symptoms. Diarrhea is treated with an antidiarrheic given after each stool. Drugs such as codeine or meperidine (Demerol) may be given to decrease bowel motility and relieve muscular aching. If diarrhea and vomiting are prolonged with important electrolytes being lost, intravenous replacement may be indicated. Most cases recover with no specific treatment.

Although synthetic penicillins have not been affected by penicillinase and have been lifesaving in many situations, there has been some evidence that methicillin-resistant strains are occurring.

Nursing care

It is important for the nurse to appreciate fully the significance of nosocomial infections—what it means to the patient, his family, the community, and hospital personnel. Strict isolation and medical asepsis with careful handwashing are requirements that cannot be minimized. In addition to the gown an effective mask should be worn, and gloves should be worn when the nurse is dressing contaminated wounds. All soiled dressings should be wrapped securely and burned immediately. They should not be deposited in trash containers to be disposed of at a later time. The greatest care must be taken not to let the pus come into contact with anything that will spread it. Hands should be thoroughly washed following any care given, even though gloves may be worn. Sputum from patients with staphylococcal pneumonia should be cared for in the same way as dressings, collected in tissues, placed in a paper bag, and burned immediately. The use of disposable equipment may help in preventing spread of the infection. Nondisposable equipment must be thoroughly disinfected, and individual thermometers properly disinfected after use. Disposable thermometers are preferable.

Specific nursing care of the patient depends on the clinical diagnosis. Some patients may require the administration of intravenous fluids, and intake and output records should be maintained. Many patients may be debilitated, and there is need to improve their overall condition and resistance. A diet high in protein, vitamins, and calories is frequently recommended.

The patient with a staphylococcal infection may need considerable emotional support. He may have entered the hospital for clean surgery, and through no fault of his own he is required to spend additional days in the hospital. The increased cost, threat of transmitting the infection to his family, and restriction of his personal liberty creates a situation that may be difficult for him to accept. An understanding nurse who appreciates the total problem may do much to relieve the tension and anxiety felt by the patient.

Immunity

A considerable degree of immunity is possessed by healthy man. Patients with debilitating diseases are much more susceptible. Having had a staphylococcal infection seems to produce no detectable immunity to the organism.

Prevention and control

In Chapter 2 it was stated that man is the cause of his own illness and death. In the case of staphylococcal infections this seems to apply. If man is the cause, it is inherent in man to find the solution to the problem.

There is no specific solution to the problem at this time or to the prevention and control of nosocomial infections. However, it seems the most important measures of controlling staphylococcal infections are the maintenance of good housekeeping and the adherence to strict aseptic technic. A variety of studies made in the United States and abroad indicate that *Staphylococcus aureus* behaves differently in different situations. Many earlier studies were devoted to the role of the carrier, whereas more recent studies tend to show that carriers play a minor part in transmitting infection. The part played by dust, air currents, and contaminated fomites has not been proved to be the specific source of infection. It appears that the most likely source is the person with a lesion, the patient, physician, nurse, or other hospital personnel.

There are numerous factors in most hospitals that deserve careful consideration. Because of the shortage of professional nursing personnel, many hospitals are making wide use of volunteer untrained persons. These persons are permitted in and out of patients' rooms and the nursery, and they frequently participate in some aspects of patient care. From the literature it appears that little attention has been given to the potential hazard involved by the indiscriminate use of such persons.

On the basis of current information there are certain guiding principles that bear consideration:

1. Provide maximum protection to high-risk groups, including all surgical patients, infants, postpartum mothers, elderly and debilitated patients, and patients with agranulocytosis.
2. Isolate all patients with draining wounds positive for staphylococcus and maintain isolation until the wound is clean and cultures are negative.
3. Encourage all personnel to report any lesion of pustular type and remove such persons from all nursing duties until they are free of the organism.
4. Limit the use of antibiotics that are likely to result in resistant strains of staphylococci, with the possibility that such resistant strains might be disseminated to other patients in the hospital.
5. Establish an infection committee to investigate and evaluate risks and to have a planned attack if an epidemic should occur.
6. Provide a special examining room for physicians to examine infants. Require the physician to wear a gown and mask and to wash the hands before entering the nursery or handling an infant. Allow no person in the nursery except those assigned to care for the infants unless absolutely necessary.[4]
7. Supervise closely food handling and refrigeration facilities for foods in which enterotoxinogenic strains of staphylococcus may multiply.
8. Provide abundant handwashing facilities throughout the hospital and stress washing hands between patients.
9. Place greater emphasis on aseptic technic in operating rooms and delivery rooms and when changing dressings.
10. Provide convenient and proper facilities for immediate disposal of contaminated dressings and sterilization of equipment.

Public health control includes the reporting of epidemics to the local health officer (no individual case report required). Two or more cases may be considered an epidemic. In case of an epidemic an effort should be made to locate the source of the infection.[6]

REFERENCES

1. Burke, John F., and Corrigan, E. A.: Staphylococcal epidemiology on a surgical ward, N. Eng. J. Med. **264**:321-326, Feb. 16, 1961.
2. Conn, H. E., editor: Current therapy 1968, Philadelphia, 1968, W. B. Saunders Co.
3. Dubos, Rene J., and Hirsch, James G., editors: Bacterial and mycotic infections of man, ed. 4, Philadelphia, 1965, J. B. Lippincott Co.
4. Edgeworth, Dorotha: Nursing and asepsis in the modern hospital, Nurs. Outlook **13**:54-56, June, 1965.
5. Farrer, Sanford, M., and MacLeod, Calvin M.: Staphylococcal infections in a general hospital, Am. J. Hygiene **72**:38-58, Jan., 1960.
6. Gordon, John E.: Control of communicable diseases in man, ed. 10, New York, 1965, American Public Health Assn., Inc.
7. Hurst, Valeri, and Grossman, Moses: The hospital nursery as a source of staphylococcal disease among families of newborn infants, N. Eng. J. Med. **262**:951-956, May 12, 1960.
8. Mattman, J. R., Orr, J. H., and Hinton, Norman A.: The effect of desiccation of

staphylococcus pyogenes with special reference to implications concerning virulence, Am. J. Hygiene **72**:335-342, March, 1960.
9. Roodyn, Leonard: Epidemiology of staphylococcal infections, J. Hygiene **58**: 1-10, March, 1960.
10. Roodyn, Leonard: Recurrent staphylococcal infections and duration of the carrier state, J. Hygiene **58**:11-19, March, 1960.
11. Thornton, George F., Fekety, F. Robert, and Cluff, Leighton E.: Studies on the epidemiology of staphylococcal infections, seasonal variation, N. Eng. J. Med. **271**:1333-1337, Dec. 26, 1964.

16
TETANUS

Tetanus was known and the symptoms described centuries ago. It was first described as an infectious disease in 1884, and in 1889 Shibasaburo Kitasato, a Japanese bacteriologist, isolated the tetanus organism and identified it as the cause of tetanus. In 1890, Kitasato and Von Behring were able to prove the role of antitoxin in the disease.

Etiology

Tetanus is a toxemia resulting from a powerful exotoxin produced by the *Clostridium tetani* (tetanus bacillus). The organism is a gram-positive, anaerobic, nonmotile, spore-forming bacterium. Next to *Clostridium botulinum,* the *Clostridium tetani* produces the most lethal poison known. The neurotoxin produced has a special affinity for central nervous system tissue. Present evidence supports the belief that the toxin formed at the site of injury reaches the central nervous system by way of the motor nerve trunks and the spinal cord rather than by the blood as formerly believed.[4]

The natural habitat of the organism is in the intestines of certain herbivorous animals and man. Here it does no harm. It is found widely distributed in the soil especially in manured farmlands. The spore-forming organism has almost no power to invade tissue, but when deposited in a wound where anaerobic conditions exist, there is rapid production of toxin. Once the toxin is absorbed by nervous tissue, it becomes fixed and cannot be neutralized by antitoxin.

The spores formed by the organism are extremely resistant and may remain dormant for months or even years, but they are still capable of causing infection if deposited in a wound.

Epidemiology

Tetanus is endemic throughout the world, although it is a preventable disease. In the United States about 500 cases occur annually.[2] The United States Department of Health, Education, and Welfare reported 116 cases in 1971. In Canada during this same period Statistics Canada reported six cases. In 1972, 128 cases were reported in the United States and three in Canada. In 1973 the number of cases in the U. S. was 101, while Canada had a total of three cases. During 1974, ninety-three cases were reported by the U. S. Communicable Disease Center, while in Canada for this same period six cases were reported. Between 1960 and 1969 Vital Statistics of the U. S. reported 1735 deaths. No statistics on death rates are available for Canada. The incidence of tetanus in many countries remains high. Colombia, South America, reported 7842 cases from 1958 to 1962, with the annual incidence remaining stable. In the Philippines, where the incidence has been increasing, 15,400 cases were reported between 1958 and 1963. Mexico reported 2000 cases in 1958, 2500 in 1959, and 2600 cases in 1961.

Tetanus occurs in infants from infection of an unhealed umbilicus (tetanus neonatorum) with soil or feces during the neonatal period. Most deaths occur in infants under 28 days of age, and there is an average of seventy-seven deaths per 100 cases, two thirds of which are nonwhite. Of 319 cases occurring in Bombay, India, all were between 3 and 30 days of age with 73% mortality. The younger the infant the greater the mortality.[1] The incidence of tetanus after surgery has been greatly reduced, the greatest danger now being from surgery of old ulcers and scars. There is a high incidence among drug addicts, particularly those who use heroin. In addition to using contaminated syringes and needles, the heroin itself is frequently contaminated. Burns and criminal abortions are also responsible for a few cases.

The incidence is much higher among the nonwhite population, with more cases among males. Nonwhite females have a rate three times higher than that for the white male. Case reports show a seasonal pattern with more cases occurring during the warm months.

Communicability period

This disease is not communicable from person to person.

Incubation period

There is a positive relationship between the length of the incubation period, the rapidity with which the disease develops, and the fatality rate. If the incubation period is less than seven days, two thirds of the cases end fatally, and if severe spasms occur within the first twenty-four hours, the mortality may be 90%.[2] The average incubation period is ten days, but it may vary from three to twenty-one days.

Clinical manifestations

The onset of tetanus may be insidious or it may be acute. The bacillus produces a powerful toxin having an affinity for the nervous system. There is restlessness, hyperirritability, stiffness of the jaw and neck muscles, stiffness of the extremities, headache, fever, and convulsions. Pain and tingling sensation may be present at the site of the wound. Tonic spasms of muscles develop, with the extensor muscles predominating. The stronger muscle groups are affected; that is, muscles closing the mouth are stronger than those opening it; therefore, spasms of the muscles keep the mouth closed, leading to the name "lockjaw." A later condition, trismus spasm of the facial muscles, causes a grinning expression called risus sardonicus (sardonic grin). Spasms frequently involve the respiratory muscles, predisposing the patient to hypoxia and pulmonary infection. The spasms are exceedingly painful and may be so severe as to cause compression fractures or muscle rupture. A state called "opisthotonos" may develop. In this position there is backward arching of the back, while the feet and head remain on the bed. This position develops due to the dominance of the extensor muscles of the spine.

Spasms may be precipitated by exteroceptive stimuli such as noise or bright lights, by proprioceptive stimuli resulting from moving or turning the patient, and interoceptive stimuli from flatus in the intestinal tract, distention of the bladder, or mucous plugs in the bronchi.

The patient is apprehensive and may have difficulty swallowing. Consciousness is not lost. Laboratory examination of the blood, urine, and spinal fluid shows that they are normal. The temperature is elevated to 101° to 104° F., and there is profuse diaphoresis. Urine may be retained due to spasms of the urethral muscles. Cyanosis and asphyxia may occur due to muscle spasms of the larynx and chest. The rate of metabolism is increased because of the intense muscle hyperirritability. Death may result from aspirative pneumonia or exhaustion.

Treatment

The treatment of tetanus takes into consideration three factors: (1) the neutralization of toxin in the circulation, (2) destruction of the *Clostridium tetani* spores, and (3) supportive therapy.[3]

There is no uniformity in the treatment of tetanus, and although tetanus antitoxin has been used for years in treatment, there are widely divergent views concerning its use and the amount that should be given. Tests for sensitivity to serum must be done before the antitoxin is administered. Although foreign objects in a wound should be removed, opinions differ concerning debridement and injection of antitoxin into the wound. Homologous (human) serum antitoxin has become available, and it is reported that some hospitals are no longer stocking equine antitoxin.[6] Long-acting penicillin over a period of time is effective against spores. Antibiotics should be given to prevent wound infection.

A combination of muscle relaxant, sedative, and tranquillizing medications will help to control tetanospasm. The combination relaxes the patient without them being heavily sedated.

Agreement seems fairly uniform that a tracheotomy should be done early, before the patient's condition becomes critical, necessitating the procedure.[3]

Supportive therapy includes the maintenance of fluid and electrolyte balance and nutrition. An indwelling catheter may be inserted to prevent bladder distention, and small enemas may be used to relieve constipation and prevent formation of flatus. Parenteral fluid therapy, oxygen, a respirator, suctioning apparatus, and gavage feeding may be necessary. After the patient recovers, roentgenograms should be taken to detect fractures or aversion of muscle insertions.

Nursing care

Caring for the patient with tetanus requires a closely coordinated program, which includes the surgeon, medical internist, anesthesiologist, and nurse. The patient should be attended at all times, and nursing care is exacting. The patient must be kept free from all external stimuli that will initiate spasms. Therefore, he should be placed in a darkened, quiet room. All unnecessary movement of the patient should be eliminated as far as possible. Vital signs and muscle tone must be closely monitored. Secretions must be suctioned and the tracheotomy cannula kept free of mucus to prevent aspiration. An automatic cycling respirator may be used. Nasogastric feedings of a formula or puréed diet to maintain nutrition may be given and oral care given to prevent sordes.

The nurse must be alert for signs that may indicate worsening of the patient's condition, that is, rise in temperature, respiratory difficulty, twitching of muscles, convulsions, cyanosis, and urine retention, which must be reported at once to the physician. An accurate intake and output must be kept.

Isolation, concurrent disinfection, and quarantine are not considered necessary.[5] In case of open wounds, dressings should be wrapped in paper and burned.

Prognosis

Death from tetanus usually occurs in two to five days and results from respiratory spasm, exhaustion, shock, or aspiration pneumonia. Death occurring later is frequently caused by acidosis, alkalosis, disturbances of electrolytes or enzymes, or cardiorespiratory arrhythmias. If the patient survives for one week after the onset, the prognosis is usually favorable. A long incubation period generally favors a good prognosis. If treatment is delayed, the fatality rate is increased. After the tetanus toxin has affected the nerve tissue, the antitoxin cannot effectively neutralize it, hence the great importance of giving the antitoxin as soon after injury as possible.

Prevention and control

Universal immunization for tetanus would completely eliminate the disease. Tetanus toxoid should be administered early in life. At the present time it is given in combination with dipththeria toxoid and pertussis vaccine to infants with periodic booster doses. Adults should receive three injections of tetanus toxoid; since it is long acting, there is no regular schedule for recall doses. When a wound occurs that is likely to cause tetanus, a "booster dose" should be given immediately.

All wounds should be thoroughly cleaned and foreign bodies removed. There is no uniform agreement concerning the administration of prophylactic tetanus antitoxin. The present trend seems to favor the administration of a reinforcing dose of tetanus toxoid if more than one year has elapsed since the last dose of toxoid. In persons with no previous tetanus immunization, human tetanus immune globulin or homologous human serum antitoxin may be given.

Tetanus neonatorum should be prevented by education of mothers concerning the care of the unhealed umbilicus and through education and supervision of midwives.

All cases of tetanus should be reported to the health department, and persons traveling abroad are advised to secure active immunization for the disease.

REFERENCES

1. Athavale, V. B., and Pai, P. N.: Tetanus neonatorum, J. Pediatr. **67**: 649-657, Oct., 1965.
2. Cirksena, William J.: Tetanus, Am. J. Nurs. **62**:65-69, April, 1962.
3. Conn, Howard F., editor: Current therapy 1968, Philadelphia, 1968, W. B. Saunders Co.
4. Dubos, Rene J., and Hirsch, James C., editors: Bacterial and mycotic infections of man, ed. 4, Philadelphia, 1965, J. B. Lippincott Co.
5. Gordon, John E.: Control of communicable diseases in man, ed. 10, New York, 1965, American Public Health Assn., Inc.
6. Shirkey, Harry C.: Tetanus immune globulin (human) in prophylaxis against tetanus, J. Pediatr. **67**:643-645, Oct., 1965.

17

TULAREMIA (RABBIT FEVER)

Etiology

The bacillus causing tularemia is presently named *Pasteurella Francisella) tularensis*. It is a gram-negative, nonmotile, nonspore-forming bacterium, coccoid in form, or it may appear as very small rods. The variation in shape is believed to be related to its virulence and immunologic characteristics. The organism does not have flagella, and it is believed that capsules may form in the tissues. The organism is not highly resistant to heat but has been known to survive freezing and drying. It may be rendered inactive by 0.1% formalin or in 1 part per million (ppm).

Epidemiology

Tuleremia is an acute infectious disease of wild animals. It is believed to be a very old disease, but it was first described in 1911 in Tulare County, California. The disease was found in rodents and appeared similar to plague. In 1912 the causative agent was identified and named *Bacterium tularense*. The disease was later identified in man and given the name tularemia. Tularemia is a plaguelike disease affecting rodents, some arthropods, and wild animals, especially rabbits. Since discovery of the disease in man there has been a gradual decrease in the number of cases reported. If untreated, about 5% of cases will end fatally. The organism is extremely sensitive to streptomycin, and since its introduction into therapy the death rate has declined.

The disease exists in many countries of the world, including the United States and Canada, as well as most of Europe, Russia, Mexico, Japan, and Turkey. In 1971 an outbreak of tularemia occurred in Sweden. All data collected indicated that the infection was generally transmitted through inhalation of dust from hay contaminated with animal feces.

Any person, regardless of age or sex, may contract the disease. Immunity follows one attack of the disease, although laboratory workers have been known to be reinfected. In areas where the disease has occurred, there is evidence of subclinical infection based on positive skin tests. In 1971 Statistics Canada reported one case, while the U. S. Department of Health, Education, and Welfare reported 187 cases. In 1972, 152 cases were reported in the United States. During this same period of time Canada reported no cases. In 1973, the United States had a total of 171 cases reported, while Canada reported one case. During 1974, seven cases were reported by the Public Health Section, Health and Welfare Division, Statistics Canada; while in the United States, the U. S. Communicable Disease Center

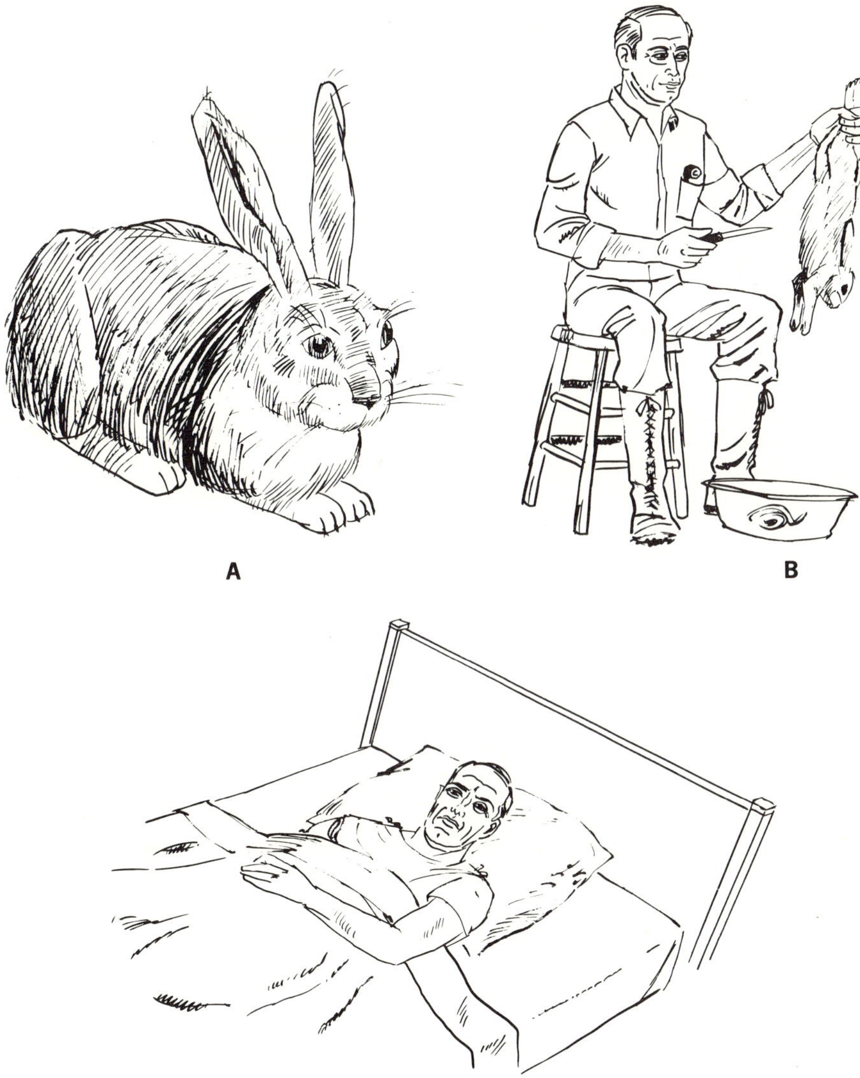

Fig. 16. Tularemia. **A,** Infected rabbit. **B,** Man is infected by inoculation while dressing a rabbit. **C,** Illness occurs in about three days after inoculation.

reported 135 cases. In the 10-year period between 1960 and 1969, twenty-five deaths were recorded in the U. S. No deaths were reported in Canada.

Tularemia is seasonal and is related to the rabbit-hunting seasons in various sections of the country and to the peak incidence of vector activity (Fig. 16).

Transmission

The principal reservoir is wild animals such as rabbits, squirrels, and rodents. It is transferred from animal to animal by the bite of a tick (wood tick, dog tick, and Lone Star tick) and certain species of the deer fly, the squirrel flea, and the ordinary bedbug. Transmission to man occurs by mechanical inoculation through the skin resulting from the bite of the infected vector, by inoculation while handling infected animals, by ingestion of inadequately cooked rabbit meat, and by drinking water that has been contaminated by rodents and animals. Accidental inoculation is a frequent occurrence among laboratory workers. As far as is known at this time the disease is not transmitted from man to man.

The greatest source of infection in the United States and Canada results from handling infected rabbits. Inoculation occurs while skinning and dressing the animal, and butchers handling the infected meat are frequently infected. An infected rabbit held in cold storage may remain infectious for two to three weeks; if it is kept frozen it may be a source of infection for up to three years or more.

Incubation period

The incubation period varies from one to ten days, with an average of three days.

Clinical manifestations

Tularemia in man is an acute febrile and prostrating infectious disease. Several types of the disease are recognized, and each is closely related to the portal of entry of the organism. The commonest type is cutaneous, in which an ulcer develops at the site of inoculation. The oculoglandular type usually occurs from rubbing the eye with the contaminated hand. The conjunctiva is the site of primary infection. An enteric or typhoidal form is caused by the ingestion of infected rabbit meat that has been insufficiently cooked and a pneumonic form in which pneumonia is secondary to the disease. A glandular type may occur with no evidence of a primary lesion. The lymph nodes are involved, but ulceration is absent.

The onset of the disease is usually abrupt, with influenza-like symptoms, headache, fever, vomiting, generalized aching, diaphoresis, chills, and prostration. The regional lymph nodes become tender and enlarged. A papular lesion develops at the site of inoculation, usually on the hands, arms, or face. The lesion eventually ulcerates and breaks down with necrotic debris in the center. The patient remains febrile for two to three weeks, with his temperature elevated from 102° to 104° F.

In the ocular type of the disease a similar papule that becomes ulcerated forms on the upper or lower eyelid. The entire conjunctiva becomes inflamed and congested, with lacrimation and involvement of the regional lymph nodes. If untreated, serious damage to the eye may result.

The enteric infection is characteristic of typhoid fever in many respects. Necrotic ulcers occur throughout the gastrointestinal tract, beginning with lesions and abscess formation in the mouth and pharynx. Gastrointestinal lesions may become hemorrhagic. Lymph nodes are enlarged and toxemia and death may occur quickly unless the infection is diagnosed and properly treated.

Tularemia commonly causes a pneumonic complication and may occur in the absence of enlarged lymph nodes. The condition may resemble caseous tuberculous lesions. There is evidence that this form of the disease may result from inhalation of the organism.

Although few cases of tularemia are reported, and the fatality rate is as low as 5%, persons who contract the disease are sick people, and convalescence is slow, varying with the virulence of the organism and the severity of the disease. The patient may be incapacitated for weeks or months. Clinically, tularemia may be confused with cat-scratch fever.

Diagnosis

Tularemia should be suspected if there is a history of handling rabbits or if the person has been bitten by vectors of the disease. Diagnosis may be made on the basis of clinical findings but should be confirmed by bacteriologic and serologic findings. Examination of sputum and gastric washings may recover the causative organism. The newer method of fluorescent antibody technic has aided in identifying the organism.

The agglutination test may provide a specific diagnosis; however, the agglutinins do not appear in the blood until sometime between seven and twenty-one days after the onset of the disease and may be as long as five weeks. The need for a test that will aid in an earlier diagnosis has led to work with the hemagglutination test, which uses human red blood cells. Results indicate that the hemagglutinins appear by eleven days after the beginning of illness.

There are three intracutaneous skin tests that are of diagnostic value: (1) the polysaccharide antigen test will produce an erythematous area and wheal during the second week of the disease; (2) the *Pasteurella tularensis* antibody test will produce a wheal in five days; and (3) the protein antigen test is a delayed sensitivity test similar to the tuberculin test and will give results in seven to ten days after infection.[3]

Immunity

One attack of tularemia results in permanent immunity.

Treatment

Streptomycin is the antibiotic of choice and is given for five to eight days. Some strains of the organism have been found to be resistant to streptomycin. Other antibiotics that have been used successfully include chloramphenicol and tetracycline. Other treatment is symptomatic and supportive.

Nursing care

There is no isolation of the patient, but concurrent disinfection should be practiced where there are suppurating ulcers or lymph nodes.[1] The febrile condition of the patient requires intensive nursing care not unlike that given to any patient with a febrile disease, such as typhoid fever. Because of the prolonged convalescence, the patient should be in a pleasant environment. A high-calorie diet of easily digested foods should be offered.

Prevention and control

The widespread infection among rodents makes control difficult. There should be interstate control and supervision of the shipment of rabbits and the sale of rabbit food. Rabbit meat should be thoroughly cooked, and rubber gloves should be worn when dressing or handling wild rabbits. In areas where an infected reservoir is known to exist, care should be taken to avoid bites of ticks, fleas, and rodents. In addition there should be no drinking of water from streams in endemic areas.

In parts of the world where the disease is endemic, cases should be reported to the health department, and efforts should be made to locate the source of the infection.

Antitularemia vaccination with living strains of the organism is available and has been widely used in Russia. An aerogenic tularemia vaccine developed at Fort Detrick, Maryland, is administered by inhalation. It is reported to be more effective than the injected vaccine.[2]

REFERENCES

1. Gordon, John E.: Control of communicable diseases in man, ed. 10, New York, 1965, American Public Health Assn., Inc.
2. Rogers, Fred B.: Epidemiology and communicable disease control, New York, 1963, Grune & Stratton, Inc.
3. Samter, Max, and Alexander, Harry L.: Immunological diseases, Boston, 1965, Little, Brown & Co.

18

VENEREAL DISEASES

There are five diseases classified as venereal. Syphilis and gonorrhea are the most important because of their prevalence and the serious complications that they may cause. Chancroid, lymphogranuloma venereum, and granuloma inguinale are considered minor venereal diseases, since they occur much less frequently and their incidence has been declining. There are differing opinions as to whether granuloma inguinale is a true venereal disease. Because of the lack of more specific information about the disease and since the lesions are primarily genital, it has been classed with venereal diseases.

"Venereal" is derived from a Latin word *veneris,* meaning love. It has come to be applied to a group of diseases associated with venery or sexual contact. Because of the very personal nature of these relationships, it was considered improper to mention or discuss them. Early in the 1930s Thomas Parran, Surgeon General of the United States Public Health Service, spoke openly and broadly about the problem of syphilis and its control. Today syphilis and other venereal diseases are considered and spoken of the same as any other communicable disease. However, the lack of knowledge and understanding about these diseases is appalling. Unfortunately it must be stated that nurses are very little better informed than the general public.

Today syphilis is a plague on North American society, and the rate of increase in infectious syphilis is alarming. Nurses must be knowledgeable concerning the total problem and be able to assist actively in its prevention and control.

Between the years of July 1, 1941 and June 30, 1947, the case rate for infectious syphilis rose from 51.7 to 75.6 per 100,000 population.[9] Nevertheless, control forces were at work, and in 1947, 107,000 cases of infectious syphilis were reported treated. Penicillin, the most potent weapon in the treatment and control of syphilis, had come into use. Between July 1, 1956 and June 30, 1957, the rate for infectious syphilis had dropped to an all-time low of 3.8 per 100,000 population. The country settled back into a state of apathy and self-satisfaction, believing that the job was completed. But the year ending June 30, 1958, disclosed that the task was far from completion and that infectious syphilis was again on the increase.

The outbreak of venereal diseases across the United States and Canada appears to be ebbing for the first time in 1974 in a decade. According to statistics, the number of reported cases of infectious syphilis shows a 2% decline in the first few months of 1974, compared with the same period the preceding year. For gonorrhea, by far the most widespread of the venereal diseases, the rate of increase for 1973 was less than 1%.

However, despite apparent inroads, venereal diseases continue to be a major public health problem in the United States and Canada. In the United States in 1973 there were 309,681 new, unreported cases of gonorrhea, a 12.7% rise from the preceeding year. The 25,080 new unreported cases of syphilis represented a 4.5% increase.

Because many cases of venereal diseases are not reported, public health sources estimate that the actual figures are much higher. In the United States in 1973 it was estimated that there were 2.5 million new cases of gonorrhea, and 85,000 to 90,000 new cases of syphilis. In Canada venereal diseases extract a toll of approximately 425,000 Canadians per year. Of the half million cases of gonorrhea in Canada in 1973, only 10% were reported.

Today syphilis is killing 3000 persons annually, crippling thousands, and costing millions annually for institutional care of the syphilitic insane.

Sociological factors

The very marked increase in incidence of venereal and sexually-transmitted diseases during the past twenty years is a matter of anxiety to health authorities in all countries of the world. These diseases are now among the commonest conditions affecting mankind during the prime of life.

In 1969, more than half of the cases of venereal disease were reported in persons under 25 years of age. The greatest increase of infection has occurred among boys and girls between 10 and 14 years of age, and among teenagers 15 to 19 years of age. In 1972, the 15- to 24-year-old age group accounted for 50% to 80% of all venereal diseases (Tables 6 and 7). Similar increases have been reported all over the world and there has been much speculation as to the cause. A World Health Organization study concluded in 1970 confirms that the spread of venereal infections can be mainly attributed to the rapid environmental, social, and behavioral changes that the world has undergone in the last decades. The following factors may have some bearing on the matter.

Modern means of communication and travel are two reasons for the rapid spread of syphilis and gonorrhea. In some countries more than one half of all the new cases are held to be imported from other countries.

The majority of workers moving into industrial and urban areas are young people separated from their families and traditions. They have many casual encounters, increasing their risk of contracting venereal disease.

The stresses of economics have resulted in later marriages and in earlier and more widespread sexual experience before marriage. This new set of behavioral patterns extends to both heterosexual and homosexual behavior, and into all classes of society.

Because homosexual behavior is still not fully accepted, such relationships are subject to the pressure that arise from subterfuge. Homosexuals often have difficulty in maintaining stable relationships, so they may seek promiscuous companions. The social and psychological milieu of the homosexual provides a situation in which venereal disease can thrive.

The decline in conventional religious standards may contribute to the increase of venereal disease, since clear standards of right and wrong, which previously inhibited sexual behavior, have now become weakened.

A widely held belief that since biological urges are pleasurable they are good may, along with a more permissive attitude toward sex, contribute to increased sexual activity and, hence, increased venereal disease.

Increases in the use of oral contraceptives and intrauterine devices have also contributed toward the spread of venereal diseases, because they have largely eliminated the man's need to use the condom, an effective guard against venereal diseases. They have eliminated the fear of pregnancy and allowed more casual relationships to occur. Many women have stated that they thought "the pill" would protect them against venereal diseases. On the contrary, it makes them more susceptible to gonorrhea, since its ingredients affect the flora of the vagina, providing an ideal alkaline environment for the growth of gonococci.

Venereal diseases can be treated, controlled, and prevented only if all contacts of the infected person are treated and if all cases are reported by physicians. Social and psychological attitudes dictate the extent to which contacts are named and traced and the accuracy of physicians' reports. People usually withhold information about the identity of their contacts. Many private physicians, who treat about 80% of all venereal disease cases, fail to report them to public health authorities, and so contacts are not traced. Many doctors feel that reporting their patients' condition is a breach of the doctor-patient relationship, even though they are legally required to report all cases.

Health education has not kept pace with the radical social changes of our time. Often young people with venereal disease know nothing about the disease and do not know how to cope with it or where to turn for help.

There are more people in the world today, and many are living to a greater age; as a result, their sexual lives are beginning earlier and are lasting longer. This greater span also increases the chances of spreading infection.

Another reason so many people are infected annually is complacency. With the advent of treatment with penicillin in 1943, new cases of syphilis fell rapidly and gonorrhea decreased. Venereal disease seemed to have been conquered. With the incidence (and therefore apparently with the risk of infection) subsiding, government funds for control and educational programs were curtailed, and the public lost interest. Moreover, in recent years, venereal disease organisms, especially those of gonorrhea, have developed a resistance to many antibiotics. This means that without very careful follow-up, the patient would be treated, symptoms would be masked, and a total cure would not be achieved. Such masking of symptoms and apparent "false" cures occur frequently among persons who obtain antibiotics illegally. As a result they unknowingly remain infectious.

In spite of the continuing effectiveness of penicillin and other drugs, in spite of efforts to educate the public about the seriousness of venereal diseases, in spite of improved medical education at all levels, and in spite of technological advances and more and better health services in many countries, the humanness of people and the increased opportunities for social and sexual encounters in a rapidly changing world have continued to defeat all the efforts to control venereal diseases.

SYPHILIS

Etiology

Syphilis belongs to the Order *Spirochaetales*, and the family *Treponematageae*. *Treponema pallidum* or *Spirochaeta pallida* is the organism responsible for human syphilis. The *Treponema pallidum* is an actively motile organism, and its rapid rotary motion is one of its distinctive diagnostic characteristics. The organism is strictly anaerobic, and efforts to culture it in the laboratory have not been successful. It does not survive drying and is killed in the human body when the temperature is elevated to 41.5° to 42° C. The organism has been described as most fragile, and viability outside the human host is very limited. The organism is sensitive to arsenic compounds, bismuth, mercuric agents, penicillin, and other broad-spectrum antibiotics. It is quickly killed by ordinary disinfectants and soap and water.

Epidemiology

Syphilis is widespread throughout the world, affects all socioeconomic groups, and is present in all climates. The highest incidence occurs at the lower socioeconomic levels among nonwhite persons. It is prevalent in seaport areas and where migration results in a concentration of people. Health departments treat about 61% of the reported primary and secondary cases, but since only about 11% of cases being treated by private physicians are reported and since some cases do not get treated at all, the exact incidence is unknown.

In 1971, the U. S. Department of Health, Education, and Welfare reported 95,997 cases. In 1972 the number of cases in the U. S. dropped to 91,149. In Canada during this same period Statistics Canada reported 2489 cases in 1971 of primary and secondary syphilis and 3064 cases in 1972. In 1973, the number of primary and secondary cases of syphilis numbered 87,469 in the U. S., and 3764 in Canada. During 1974, 24,080 cases of primary and secondary syphilis were reported by the U. S. Communicable Disease Center. In Canada during 1974, 3658 cases of primary and secondary syphilis were reported. Between the years 1960 and 1969 the U. S.

Table 6. Venereal diseases in the United States–1972-1973

Age	*All venereal diseases* 1972	*All venereal diseases* 1973	*Syphilis—primary and secondary** 1972	*Syphilis—primary and secondary** 1973	*Gonococcal* 1972	*Gonococcal* 1973
0-14	10,672	12,076	323	262	10,349	10,814
15-19	206,087	236,863	3930	3869	202,157	232,994
20-24	398,158	353,877	7112	7175	312,075	333,423
25-29	137,614	187,406	4859	5351	132,755	152,055
30-34	56,960	89,897†	3373	5297†	53,587	84,600†
35-39	28,674		1886		26,788	
40-44	15,531	53,011†	1300	2103†	14,231	20,908†
45-49	8303		723		7580	
50+	8616	8595	923	768	7693	7827
Male	589,828	576,709	16,292	16,888	504,575	509,821
Female	270,787	355,016	8137	7937	262,640	332,800
Total	860,615	931,725	24,429	24,825	767,215	842,621

*Total cases in all stages: 1972, 91,149; 1973, 87,469.
†1973 combines the age groups 30-39 and 40-49.

Table 7. Venereal disease in Canada–1972

Age	*All venereal diseases*	*Syphilis*	*Gonococcal*
Under 1 year of age	18	7	11
1-4	20	3	17
5-9	41	No statistics available	41
10-14	204	5	198
15-19	8353	200	8150
20-24	15,085	502	14,557
25-29	8340	502	7838
30-39	5974	597	5377
40-59	2892	639	2253
60+	493	352	40
Age not stated	2116	138	1985
Total cases	45,536	3064	41,467
Male	29,509	1998	28,531
Female	14,027	1066	12,936

reported an average annual death rate of 2612 persons from syphilis. In 1968 the death rate dropped to 586; in 1969 it dropped further to 543; and in 1970 to 461 persons. In Canada during 1971, Statistics Canada reported thirty-one deaths from syphilis (Tables 6 and 7).

Age, sex, race, and other factors

Numerous studies indicate that the highest incidence of infectious syphilis occurs among teenagers and young adults. In 1972, more than half the cases of venereal diseases in Canada and the United States were reported in persons under 25 years of age. The greatest increase in infection has occurred among boys and girls 10 to 14 years of age, and among teenagers 15 to 19 years of age. In 1972, the 15- to 24-year-old age group accounted for 50% to 80% of all venereal diseases. Similar increases and trends have been reported all over the world.

It attacks both sexes, and does not occur in any particular race or geographical center.

Transmission

Man is its only reservoir. The disease is transmitted by intimate sexual contact, including homosexual relationships, with the exception of a small number of cases of congenital syphilis. When infectious lesions are present in the mouth, the disease may be transmitted by kissing. Transmission through contaminated articles is considered rare, if not impossible. Accidental inoculation or transmission through blood transfusion is possible, but in relation to the total number of cases it must be considered rare. The *Treponema pallidum* enters through a minute abrasion in the skin or through intact mucous membrane. Once in the body the organisms are carried by the bloodstream to every organ in the body. Within a few hours after exposure the infection is systemic.

Incubation period

The incubation period is variable between ten and ninety days, with an average of three to four weeks before symptoms appear.

Diagnosis

An accurate history is important, and often essential to the diagnosis and treatment of syphilis. Both bacteriologic and serologic testing must be done. Clinical diagnosis is presumptive and may be made during the infectious phase of the disease, but it should always be confirmed by laboratory examination.

Darkfield examination. The darkfield examination is the earliest diagnostic test made. Serous exudate is obtained from the primary lesion, placed on a clean microscopic slide, and a cover-glass applied. The specimen is examined immediately under a darkfield microscope. It is difficult to see the *Treponema pallidum* with the ordinary microscope. When a special condenser is used on the microscope, the light rays enter the field from the side, and the *Treponema* may be seen as a fine, silver-colored revolving organism against a dark background. Skill is needed in obtaining the specimen, and familiarity with the *Treponema pallidum* is needed to differentiate it from nonpathogenic Spirochaetales.

Serologic testing for syphilis (STS). Serology tests for syphilis have changed notably since the development of the first test by Wassermann in 1906. Contrary to what some persons believe, the *Treponema pallidum* cannot be isolated from the blood. The test developed by Wassermann utilized the technic of complement fixation.* Today the test has been so improved that of the original, only the name and principle remain. Application of the term "Wassermann test" is now obsolete in the United States and Canada, and should no longer be used.

When referring to serology for syphilis it is recommended the STS (serology test for syphilis) be used. The serological testing is involved mainly with the use of complement fixation and flocculation tests. STS is seldom positive during the first few days of the chancre, but usually becomes positive before the appearance of the secondary stage.

Many tests have been developed by bacteriologists, and each test is known by the name of its originator. Some of these modified tests in use today are known as Eagle, Kolmer, Boerner-Luckens. Each test uses the principle of complement fixation. They represent modifications of the original test of 1906.

The flocculation test, a precipitation test, is based on the principle that when the proper combination of an antigen and serum from a person with syphilis is mixed, a precipitate is formed. The flocculation tests have certain advantages over the complement-fixation tests in that they require less time to perform and the results are more easily read. Thus a large number of tests were developed using the flocculation technic, and each was known by the name of the originator of the test. Among these tests are the Meinicke, Sachs-Georgi, Kahn, Kline, Eagle, Hinton, Davies, Müller, Mazzini, the Venereal Disease Research Laboratory test (VDRL), and the rapid plasma reagin test (RPR). The Venereal Disease Research Laboratory Test (VDRL), probably the most widely used of the tests, is used exclusively for testing cerebrospinal fluid.

Very sensitive tests such as the Kahn "presumptive" test and the Kline "exclusion" test have the disadvantage that positive results may be obtained in healthy persons. Therefore, they are more significant when negative and are used for "screening," thus their names.

The first of the treponemal antigen tests was developed in 1949, and from this beginning a long list of treponemal antigen tests were developed. The FTA test, a treponemal antigen test, was developed in 1957, and it uses nonviable *Treponema pallidum* and a fluorescent-tagged antibody. Several modifications of the original test have been developed. The FTA-ABS test, a test in the same category, is reported to be the most important test for the diagnosis of syphilis in all stages that has been developed so far. Another important test in this category is the TPI test (Treponema pallidum immobilization test).

In 1962 the rapid plasma reagin (RPR) card test was introduced. Everything needed for the test is available in a commercial kit, eliminating the need for laboratory equipment except the microscope. In studies that have been made it appears that this test is comparable with the VDRL slide

*Refer to any microbiology textbook for a review of complement fixation.

test.[12] The VDRL test and the RPR test are used as routine diagnostic aids. The TPI, and FTA-ABS tests are usually used as confirmatory tests in cases in which diagnosis has been difficult.

This abbreviated review of serology for syphilis has been presented to help the nurse understand the changes that have taken place in tests for syphilis. Serological tests for syphilis cannot be considered diagnostic of the disease as they may give a false reading. These tests only give immunological information. None of these tests developed up to the present time are absolutely specific.

Spinal fluid examination. A lumbar puncture to secure a specimen of spinal fluid for examination is considered important in many cases of syphilis. The purpose of the examination is to determine if the *Treponema pallidum* has invaded the central nervous system. This test is the only means of diagnosing neurosyphilis accurately, and evaluating its treatment. It is known that invasion occurs early in the course of the disease. Under ordinary conditions the *Treponema* serum antibody is not present in the spinal fluid, but when it is found, it indicates central nervous system involvement. Significant tests made on spinal fluid are cell count, quantitative protein, and antibody titer. Frequently neurosyphilis can be detected months or even years before development of subjective or objective neurologic evidence of the disease.

Cardiovascular examination. All patients with suspected late syphilis should have a periodic cardiovascular examination with roentgenogram of the chest. Particular attention is given to the aortic valves, where leakage or insufficiency may occur, and to any evidence of bulging in the walls above the valves that may indicate an aneurysm.

Classification

Classification of syphilis by stages is artificial and done only to aid in describing its period of pathogenicity. The stages often overlap. Syphilis is classified as primary and secondary, which is infectious syphilis. Latent syphilis is frequently subclassified as early, if less than four years' duration and late, if more than four years' duration. Congenital syphilis is acquired by the fetus in utero. Symptomatic syphilis of over four years' duration is called late or tertiary syphilis, and this may involve any organ in the body, such as the central nervous system, the cardiovascular system, eyes, and bones.

Primary syphilis. Clinical signs appear from ten to ninety days (average of twenty-one days) following infection. The initial lesion of syphilis is the chancre. The most frequent site of the lesion is the genitalia, although it may occur on other parts of the body, that is, at whatever site *Treponemal* invasion occurred, such as the lips, tongue, tonsils, nipples, fingers, or anus. In the female the lesion frequently occurs on the cervix or labia, whereas in the male it is usually on the penis. There has been some question concerning whether some persons fail to develop the chancre; however, syphilologists generally agree that a chancre is always present at the site of inoculation, but it may not be observed. In case of direct bloodstream inoculation there is no chancre.

The chancre is usually a single lesion and in the absence of secondary infection is painless. The lesion is usually an eroded papule that is firm and indurated, the surface being crusted or ulcerated. The border surrounding the lesion is frequently raised and firm. An enlarged lymph node is usually present in the area draining the lesion. The presence of the lesion and the enlarged lymph node are considered significant in diagnosis. The *Treponema pallidum* can usually be isolated from the lesion and identified by darkfield examination. Serology is usually negative for at least one week and sometimes longer after the appearance of the lesion. A serologic test is always made at the same time as the darkfield examination. If the darkfield examination is negative, the serologic examination should be repeated at regular intervals for at least three months. The primary lesion always heals with or without treatment within four to six weeks. It should be noted that no external treatment such as salves or ointments have any therapeutic value in treatment of the disease. Many patients frequently apply local therapy, rendering darkfield examination difficult or impossible. The disease is highly infectious during this phase.

Secondary syphilis. The secondary manifestations of syphilis occur about six weeks to three months after the primary lesion. There may be a generalized reaction, with slight elevation of temperature, sore throat, and malaise. Numerous lesions frequently appear on the skin and mucous membranes. There may be a generalized skin rash with macules, papules, or pustules. The rashes may resemble those of chickenpox, measles, scarlet fever, or smallpox. Sometimes the rash may be too slight to notice. Typical palmar lesions sometimes appear on the palms of the hands and the soles of the feet. Syphilis is one of the few diseases that may cause eruptions on the soles of the feet and palms of the hands. Moist lesions occur on the mucous membrane in the mouth and inside the lips and are known as mucous patches.

Condylomata lata are elevated flat lesions, appearing about the anogenital area. Condylomata lata and mucous patches are usually teeming with *Treponema,* and frequently a darkfield examination can be made from them. These manifestations generally make their appearance late in the secondary stage of the infection. During this period the disease is highly infectious, and the serology is always reactive. Other symptoms that may occur during the secondary phase are syphilitic alopecia, a temporary loss of hair in small patches. The scalp looks "moth-eaten." Alopecia occurs in less than 10% of the cases. The patient may also have loss of parts of the eyebrows. Lymphadenopathy is present in most cases. As with the primary stage, the secondary symptoms will disappear with or without treatment, in two to six weeks, and the patient lapses into the latent stage. From the viewpoint of transmission, the important secondary manifestations are the rash and mucous membrane lesions. Both are teeming with *Treponemata.* The secondary stage, in fact, is considered more infectious than the primary stage since the lesions are multiple, while in the primary stage they are usually single.

Latent syphilis. During the latent period there are no recognizable symptoms, and diagnosis must be made on the basis of serologic findings. However, examination for any clinical evidence should always be made, and a history of any primary or secondary symptoms should be elicited from the patient. After the infection has persisted more than four years, it is rarely communicable, except in the case of a pregnant woman who can pass it on to her fetus.

Late syphilis or tertiary stage. The late manifestations of syphilis begin to make their appearance between fifteen and twenty years after the onset of the infection. In this stage lesions known as "gumma" develop in internal organs and interfere with the functions of these organs. Syphilis seems to have an affinity for the cardiovascular system and the central nervous system. Gumma may also attack the skin and bone. These lesions are not infectious, but they do cause considerable tissue damage. According to Samter, only about 10% to 15% of persons with latent syphilis develop the complications of late syphilis.[10] These are the unfortunate persons. Research has shown that syphilis shortens the life span and causes years of invalidism or confinement in a mental institution.

Complications

The commonest complication of late syphilis is involvement of the central nervous system. Included is meningovascular syphilis, which gives rise to a variety of symptoms such as headache, dizziness, loss of special senses. Tabes dorsalis (locomotor ataxia) is a manifestation in which the sensory nerve roots of the spinal cord are gradually destroyed. The patient becomes incontinent and impotent and has difficulty walking. He may have attacks of severe vomiting and gastric pain (gastric crisis). General paresis is a more common complication of late syphilis. The disease affects the cells of the cerebral cortex, resulting in a progressive change in the total behavior pattern. The mental aberrations usually become so severe that the individual is placed in a mental hospital. Cardiovascular syphilis is also a common complication. The essential signs are aortic insufficiency, or saccular aneurysm of the thoracic aorta.

Late syphilis is not considered infectious; however, if untreated, it may be transmitted from the mother to the fetus in utero.

Congenital syphilis (prenatal syphilis)

Infection of the fetus in utero occurs after the eighteenth week of gestation. The effect on the fetus is closely related to the stage of the disease in the mother. If pregnancy occurs during the infectious stage of syphilis, the fetus is usually unable to withstand the infection. Frequently abortion or miscarriage occurs if the mother is in the primary or secondary stage of syphilis, or if the pregnancy progresses to term, the baby is stillborn. When pregnancy occurs during late syphilis, the fetus may survive and is born alive at term. Adequate treatment of the mother before the eighteenth week of pregnancy prevents infection of the fetus. Because penicillin crosses the placental barrier, treatment of the mother after the eighteenth week will also cure the fetus.

When a live birth occurs, a cord serology is usually done. A reactive cord serology is not diagnostic of congenital syphilis. It may merely indicate the passive transfer of antibodies across the placenta, and it may occur in a mother who has been adequately treated but may be seroresistant. The infant should always be closely followed and an STS made when the infant is 3 months of age.

In a study of 1220 infants, Nelson and co-workers found that no cases of early congenital syphilis occurred in infants after 3 months of age.[12]

After birth the infant should be closely observed for symptoms, which rarely occur before 3 weeks of age. There may be a skin rash, papular in character, which occurs about the anogenital area, on palms of the hands and soles of the feet, about the mouth, or distributed over the entire body. A typical sign is snuffles characterized by stuffiness of the nose and a mucopurulent nasal discharge. Difficulty in breathing may interfere with feeding and lead to malnutrition. The nasal discharge may cause crusting about the nose, and fissures occur around the mouth.

If untreated, congenital syphilis may progress to late syphilis. Manifestations of late congenital syphilis begin to occur in the child between 6 and 9 years of age. The upper central incisors are deformed, being narrowed, thickened, and notched (Hutchinson's teeth). A rough bulging of the tibia called a saber shin may develop. Between 12 and 16 years of age further complications may develop. The commonest condition is interstitial keratitis, a chronic inflammatory condition of the cornea of the eye, progressing to impairment of visual acuity. The deformed teeth, interstitial keratitis, and involvement of the auditory nerve (eighth nerve) have been called the Hutchinson's triad.

Involvement of the central nervous system may occur at an early age and is always serious. However, it develops most often in the older child and may lead to juvenile paresis.

Congenital syphilis is completely preventable by early and adequate treatment of the mother. The American Social Health Association states that the practice by hospitals of routinely performing blood tests on mothers and their newborn infants has diminished the number of cases of syphilis. Society is again becoming complacent. In 1971, the United States Statistics reported a total of 2052 cases; while in 1972, 1758 cases were recorded. In Canada during 1972, Statistics Canada reported forty-one cases. In 1973, the total number of cases in the U. S. was 1527.

Treatment

The present-day treatment of syphilis in all stages is penicillin, which was first used in 1943. But penicillin obviously should not be used with patients who are sensitive to it. A careful history to rule out penicillin sensitivity is indicated with every patient. Alternate therapy may consist of tetracycline, erythromycin, or doxycyclin (vibramycin).

Primary and secondary syphilis. Current treatment of infectious syphilis is 2.4 to 4.8 million units of benzathine penicillin (Bicillin or Permapen). It will render a patient noninfectious in primary syphilis, and probably in early secondary syphilis, although the disease may need more treatment.

Latent syphilis. The treatment for latent syphilis is benzathine penicillin G, 2.4 million units the same as for primary and secondary syphilis, or procaine penicillin G, 600,000 units given in the gluteal muscle daily for ten days.

Late syphilis. There is some variation in the treatment of late syphilis. It is recommended that 7.2 million units of procaine penicillin G be given in biweekly doses or that 2.4 million units of benzathine penicillin be given weekly for three weeks.

Complications of late syphilis. Opinions differ concerning the treatment necessary in the presence of complications of late syphilis. It has been suggested that 600,000 units of procaine penicillin G be administered daily for ten days or 1.2 million units of PAM every third day to a total of 6 million units. Both Top and Modell recommend doses of procaine penicillin varying from 9.6 million units with biweekly doses for four weeks to 1 million units daily for ten to fifteen days.

Syphilis in pregnancy. Penicillin retreatment in subsequent pregnancies is unnecessary if previous adequate treatment can be documented. If there is doubt as to the adequacy of treatment, retreatment is indicated.

If possible, treatment should be given during the first trimester of pregnancy to ensure protection of the fetus. The treatment recommended is 600,000 units of aqueous suspension of procaine penicillin G daily or every second day, or 600,000 units of PAM every third day or biweekly for ten injections, or 2.4 million units of Bicillin weekly for two doses.

Congenital syphilis. The treatment of congenital syphilis in infants is the same as that for early syphilis, with the unit dose proportionate to body weight. Modell recommends a dose of 200,000 units per kilogram of body weight daily for a total of 1.5 million units.[3]

Syphilis prophylaxis

Some physicians approve the administration of penicillin to persons who have a known exposure to infectious syphilis. It is believed that there is some danger in the procedure unless the dose administered is completely adequate. All persons treated prophylactically should be followed for six months for serologic examination, since the treatment may obscure the manifestations of primary or secondary syphilis.

Syphilis and gonorrhea

Syphilis and gonorrhea may exist simultaneously in the same person. The same type of drugs will act against gonorrhea as syphilis, and will cure early gonorrhea unless the strains of *Neisseria gonorrhoeae* are penicillin resistant.

Reinfection and immunity

Natural immunity to syphilis probably does not exist, and it is known that a person who has had primary or secondary syphilis and has had adequate treatment may become reinfected. It is also possible that in case of exposure and reinfection there may not be the usual characteristic symptoms. Although considerable information is lacking, recent evidence suggests that immunity to syphilis after an infection is not unlike immunity to any other infectious disease.

GONORRHEA

Gonorrhea is probably a very old disease and was identified as different from syphilis in 1790. The term *gonorrhea* was first used by Galen in A.D. 130; however, the disease that he called gonorrhea may not be the same disease known by that name today. In 1879 Albert Neisser, a German physician, identified the etiologic agent, which he called gonococcus. Identification of the causative organism was greatly improved when Hans Gram introduced the technic of Gram stain in 1884.

No progress in the treatment of gonorrhea occurred until the sulfonamides came into use in 1936. Sulfanilamide, the first of a long line of sulfonamides, was first used to treat gonorrhea at Johns Hopkins Medical Center. However, it soon became apparent that the gonococcus was becoming resistant to the sulfonamide agents, but nevertheless they remained the treatment of choice until 1943, when penicillin became available. Penicillin has replaced all other drugs in the treatment of gonorrhea. Because of the success of this treatment, there has been a general apathy and attitude of complacency.

Etiology

Gonorrhea is caused by the *Neisseria gonorrhoeae*, or the gonococcus. The organism is pathogenic only for man. It has the appearance of two slightly flattened, concave coffee beans. They are readily stained with Gram stain and are gram-negative. The organism is nonspore-forming and nonmotile, and it does not form capsules or have flagella. It is fragile and does not survive long outside the body. It is readily killed by drying, sunlight, or ultraviolet light, and it may be killed with ordinary disinfectants.

Epidemiology

In 1971, the U. S. Department of Health, Education, and Welfare reported 670,268 new cases of gonorrhea. In 1972, the number of cases in the U. S. rose to 767,215. Statistics Canada reported 34,405 new cases in 1971 and 41,467 in 1972. In 1973, the number of new cases of gonorrhea reported in the U. S. was 842,621; while in Canada there were 45,266 new cases reported. During 1974, 882,590 new cases of gonorrhea were reported by the

U. S. Communicable Disease Center. In Canada during 1974, 46,760 new cases of gonorrhea were reported. Between the years 1960 and 1969, 158 deaths occurred as a result of gonorrhea in the U. S. During 1971, one death occurred in Canada from this disease (Tables 6 and 7).

As with syphilis, gonorrhea is a worldwide problem, in fact it is one of the most widespread of the venereal diseases.

In the United States, for the year 1973 there were 309,681 new unreported cases of gonorrhea, a 12.7% rise from 1972. In Canada in 1973, of the estimated half a million cases of gonorrhea, only 10% were reported.

The Communicable Disease Center (CDC) of the United States Public Health Services conducted a study of 740,446 women in twenty-two states from mid-1969 to mid-1971. Of all these women tested over this three year period, 8.9% were found to have gonorrhea. The tests were done routinely on all patients in many settings. From this study of the women tested it was found that 80% of those with gonorrhea had no symptoms of the disease. From this sampling, the Venereal Disease Branch of C.D.C. estimated that there were at that time 640,000 female carriers of asymptomatic gonorrhea in the United States.

Transmission

Although both sexes carry the disease, the main reservoir of the disease is the woman. This is because in women it usually causes no signs or symptoms and many women go untreated as they do not realize they are infected, 50 to 80% of women are asymptomatic.

Gonorrhea is transmitted through direct sexual contact, including homosexual relationships. Ophthalmia neonatorum in the infant may occur by passage through an infected birth canal of the mother. The possibility of infection by indirect contact in adults is rare. There has been some evidence of asymptomatic male carriers, but the number of such persons is believed to be small.

The infected secretions and discharges from the male urethra are deposited on the proper type of mucous membrane of the female vulva, urethra, and cervix. The chain of infection continues when the female deposits the organism in the male urethra. Thus, the vicious cycle of infection continues. There probably is no other disease in history in which so many misleading opinions have been given by infected individuals to explain the source of their infection.

The infection of children with gonorrhea often takes place in families in which there is an adult case of gonorrhea. The female child may become infected as a result of sleeping in the same bed with the infectious person, or from the common use of toilets, washcloths, bathtubs, and towels.

Incubation period

The incubation period for gonorrhea is variable. It may be as short as two to ten days or as long as twenty-one days; the average is three to five days. During this stage the disease is infectious and may be transmitted before any symptoms are displayed, as long as the organisms are present in secretions and discharges. The disease may become latent and chronic and remain infectious for months or even for years. Almost everyone is susceptible, and the disease produces no significant immunity.

Clinical manifestations

The classic symptoms of gonorrhea are rarely seen at the present time. The male usually seeks treatment early in the course of the disease—one to three days after sexual contact. The early symptoms in the male appear within twenty-four hours and consist of a burning sensation on urination and redness and edema of the urinary meatus. Soon after the initial symptoms a discharge appears that becomes mucopurulent. The discharge may be severe or mild. Without treatment the condition gradually increases in severity and may persist for weeks. The appearance of these symptoms can hardly be neglected even by the most slothful man. Consequently, male gonorrhea is usually treated soon after symptoms begin. If not treated, prostatitis may occur, and the seminal vesicles, vas deferens, and epididymis may become involved with abscess formation.

Gonorrhea in the female is more likely to become chronic because of a failure to secure treatment early. Untreated gonorrhea in women progresses through three stages. The first stage begins a few days after the sexual contact; the woman may develop urethritis or cervicitis and notice a burning sensation on voiding; or she might notice a slight vaginal discharge. These inflammatory responses are usually too mild to cause the woman any undue discomfort and thus they remain untreated. The infection often involves Bartholin's glands and Skene's ducts with abscess formation. The stratified squamous epithelium of the vulva and vaginal canal is not involved, but the infectious organism passes into the cervical canal, where it causes an inflammatory condition and erosions. The infection ascends and may cause endocervicitis and endometritis. It may reach the fallopian tubes and ovaries, resulting in pelvic inflammatory disease. Severe salpingitis or pelvic peritonitis can necessitate immediate surgical removal of the uterus, tubes, and ovaries in order to bring the infection under control. The urethra is generally involved, and a vaginal discharge is present. Since many women experience periodic vaginal discharge, they are likely to overlook the significance of gonorrheal discharge. If gonorrhea makes such an invasion it usually does so during a menstrual period. Invasion beyond the uterus is called second stage gonorrhea. The third stage involves chronic infection.

Diagnosis

Clinical diagnosis of gonorrhea may be easily made in the male, but it should always be confirmed by bacteriologic examination. A clinical diagnosis is rarely possible in the female. There are a number of laboratory tests available for the diagnosis of gonorrhea. Probably the oldest method and one still in use is the smear technic. A small amount of exudate is placed on a clean glass slide, stained, and examined under the microscope for gram-negative intracellular diplococci. In the female, smears should be taken from the urethra, Skene's ducts, Bartholin's glands, and the cervix. Exudate from at least two of these sites should be examined. The culture method is preferred to the smear technic, but it requires several days before results are obtained.

Several new methods have recently been developed, including a fluorescent antibody test (FA), in which the organism may be identified in one hour. The delayed fluorescent antibody test requires a longer period, but has been proved more effective in the asymptomatic female. Another new test requiring only a short time to complete is the cytochrome oxidase test. This is a paper test that gives a color reaction in the presence of certain bacteria.[8]

In all cases of gonorrhea, examination should be made for evidence of infectious syphilis, including a serologic test for syphilis. The individual may be exposed to syphilis at the same time that gonorrhea is contracted, and both diseases may exist simultaneously in the same person. However, the difference in the incubation period of the two diseases requires that the individual be followed for some time.

Medical programs against gonorrhea are hindered by lack of specific, dependable diagnostic tests. Researchers have also been working to produce a vaccine against gonorrhea and syphilis. The Canadian government is now studying a proposal to test a gonorrhea vaccine just developed by the Canadian Communicable Disease Center in Ottawa. But at this writing no proved vaccine is available.

Treatment

Penicillin still remains the drug of choice for the treatment of gonorrhea. Opinions vary as to results obtained from the use of other drugs. Although some concern has been expressed over the resistance of certain strains of the gonococcus to penicillin, it is generally believed that it is not a serious problem at this time. However, the same precautions should be exercised in administering penicillin for gonorrhea or syphilis as for any other disease because of the increasing incidence of patient sensitivity to penicillin.

The recommended treatment for uncomplicated gonorrhea is 4.8 million units of aqueous procaine penicillin G or procaine penicillin G in oil with aluminum monostearate (PAM). In case of severe complications the patient is hospitalized, and treatment with crystalline penicillin G is administered.

Treatment failure may occur in a small number of patients, and retreatment is required. In case of retreatment the dose may be increased and divided with the administration extended over several days. After the patient is treated he should be followed and serologic examination repeated every thirty days for three months. Self-treatment with penicillin or tetracycline purchased illegally, or left over from an old prescription is usually unsuccessful. The dose is only large enough to mask the symptoms and so the patient thinks a cure has been achieved, until later symptoms appear.

Ophthalmia neonatorum (gonorrhea ophthalmia)

Ophthalmia neonatorum is a severe inflammation of the eye, conjunctiva, or both. It is caused by the gonococcus. A woman infected with gonorrhea may infect the baby's eyes during the birth process. Unless the condition is treated immediately the baby's eyes may be destroyed within a few days.

The use of silver nitrate for the prevention of gonorrheal ophthalmia was introduced in 1888 by Karl Credé. Most health departments supply a 1% solution free to physicians and hospitals. Some countries have enacted legislation making the treatment mandatory. When the drug is properly instilled into the eyes a chemical conjunctivitis occurs that is harmless to the infant. The administration of silver nitrate is not absolute protection; therefore, safety can be guaranteed only when there is a non-infected birth canal. Some work has been done in the use of penicillin as a prophylactic agent, but this needs further research. In view of the increased incidence of gonorrhea and the number of cases of gonorrheal ophthalmia reported, it appears that prophylactic treatment of the eyes of the newborn must be continued.

The incubation period for gonorrheal ophthalmia is about three days and is characterized by a heavy purulent discharge. If untreated, ulceration of the cornea occurs, and blindness may result.[5]

Complications

Although most cases of gonorrhea respond readily to treatment when diagnosed early, delay in securing diagnosis and treatment, self-treatment, and insufficient treatment may delay cure and precipitate severe complications in both the male and the female.

Arthritis is the most frequently encountered complication of untreated gonorrhea. It may occur in both men and women, although it is more common in the female. It may affect any joint, but the knee is most commonly involved. The typical inflammatory reaction occurs with redness, heat, pain, swelling, and tenderness. Necrosis with destruction of the cartilage may result from the infection. It is primarily a disease of young people.

Stricture in the male may follow the inflammatory condition involving the urethra and may require surgery. In the female, Bartholin's glands (usually unilateral) become tender and painful with abscess formation. Salpingitis is a frequent complication characterized by abdominal pain, elevation of temperature, and leukocytosis. Systemic bloodstream infection is possible but rare. Untreated gonorrhea is a frequent cause of childless marriages as the infection has destroyed parts of the genital organs.

NURSING CARE IN SYPHILIS AND GONORRHEA

Very few patients with syphilis and/or gonorrhea are admitted to the general hospital. Most patients are treated in a health department clinic, the private physician's office, and outpatient clinics. In these clinics and in the community, the nursing profession is faced with the challenge of meeting the needs of a new kind of public who expect nurses to be able to deal with their problem in an interested, but tolerant fashion. Nurses can do a great deal to help people if they can discuss these matters in understandable, but unemotional tones.

If nurses are going to care for patients with venereal diseases, they must ask themselves: "Am I an emotionally stable person who can have a sympathetic approach towards the problems of others and not moralize and point a finger?" Nurses must work through their own feelings about sex before they can accept sex both intellectually and unemotionally as being a normal and natural part of human life. Again they must ask themselves: "Do I have an honest desire to meet with people from every walk of life with equal impartiality?" If nurses find themselves wanting to save souls, or if they feel that the discussion of sex is vulgar, then this area of nursing is not for them.

Nurses have been accustomed to considering patients as "sick" persons, frequently treated in hospitals. When looking after patients with venereal diseases, the nurse finds the patients in the community and remaining in their own homes where they are free to make their own rules of conduct. In fact they may even consider the treatment they are undergoing as an invasion of their privacy. The nurse's role is to be aware of all this and to meet the patients halfway. Respect must be given to the patients as individuals, and the nurse must not interfere unnecessarily with their normal way of life. Patients must be approached as equals; not in an authoritarian manner. The reason for each piece of advice that is given must be explained carefully. But once the patients understand, the nurse must allow them to make their own decisions. Most young persons prefer the straight, honest, friendly approach, and shy away from the moralizing, mother approach. Once patients have established in their own minds that nurses are human, advice will be sought more readily.

Patients admitted to the general hospital with medical or surgical conditions may be found to have a reactive serology. This does not always mean that the patient has or has ever had syphilis, since various conditions may give rise to a biologic false reactive (positive) serology in the complete absence of syphilis.

Hospital isolation and strict medical asepsis of the patient with syphilis and gonorrhea, including concurrent and terminal disinfection, is considered unnecessary.[1] Isolation of the patient in the community to prevent spread of the disease is generally impractical and unnecessary. In certain isolated cases such as a recalcitrant prostitute who may continue to spread the infection, the health office may order isolation or quarantine.

Thorough handwashing should follow care of the patient with infectious syphilis. In some instances the use of rubber gloves may be recommended, that is, when giving enemas if moist anogenital lesions are present. The usual care to avoid contamination of the hands should be exercised when changing dressings. There is no need for individual thermometers when proper care and cleaning of thermometers is a routine procedure.

Precautions should be taken to avoid puncture wounds or abrasions when cleaning surgical instruments after surgery of a patient with reactive serology caused by syphilis. Nurses are usually responsible for administering penicillin, and the usual precautions and technic are the same for all intramuscular injections.

It is not a usual procedure for nurses to interview hospitalized patients for contact information. However, patients may volunteer such information, and the nurse should be able to accept it and refer it to the health department for investigation.

The professional nurse should have a basic understanding of venereal diseases and be able to interpret and supervise less well-trained personnel who participate in patient care. It should be realized that all information concerning these patients is considered confidential, and there should be no discussion concerning the patient and laboratory reports.

Nurses should be able to answer the following types of questions that patients will ask.

Some questions asked by patients concerning syphilis

1. Is the infection serious?
2. Can you get syphilis from kissing?
3. How long am I infectious?
4. Will my baby have it?
5. Will I lose my baby?
6. If a condom is used, am I safe?
7. Could I have been born with this disease?
8. How would I know if I had syphilis?
9. Will it keep me from becoming pregnant?
10. When the baby is born will it be deformed?
11. Will the disease disfigure me with awful sores?
12. What are the signs of the second stage of syphilis?
13. How long is the treatment?
14. Could I have syphilis and not know it?
15. Can I get it again after I've had it once and been treated?
16. What can syphilis do to me if it is not treated?
17. Can I die from syphilis?
18. What can I do after intercourse to lessen the chances of infection?
19. Can I get syphilis from using public toilets?
20. Can I get the disease from living in the same household with a person who has syphilis?

Some questions asked by patients concerning gonorrhea

1. As a man, how would I know that I had gonorrhea?
2. As a woman, how would I know that I had gonorrhea?
3. How do I get gonorrhea?
4. How long am I infectious?
5. Is gonorrhea serious?
6. Will gonorrhea keep me from having a baby?

7. If I am cured of gonorrhea, could I get it again?
8. What will gonorrhea do to me if I leave it untreated?
9. Could I have been born with this disease?
10. How long does it take gonorrhea to appear after sexual contact?
11. What affect will it have on my baby when the child is born?
12. How long is the treatment?
13. Could I have gonorrhea and not know it?
14. Can I get gonorrhea from kissing?
15. Can I die from this infection?
16. Can I get gonorrhea from using public toilets?
17. If I have gonorrhea what can I do about others who may be infected?

PREVENTION AND CONTROL

Most countries have laws that require reporting of syphilis and gonorrhea to the health department. Concerted efforts are needed to promote better reporting by private physicians and to promote interest among all hospitals for routine serologic tests for syphilis of all admissions, and of all routine physical checkups and during pap smears.

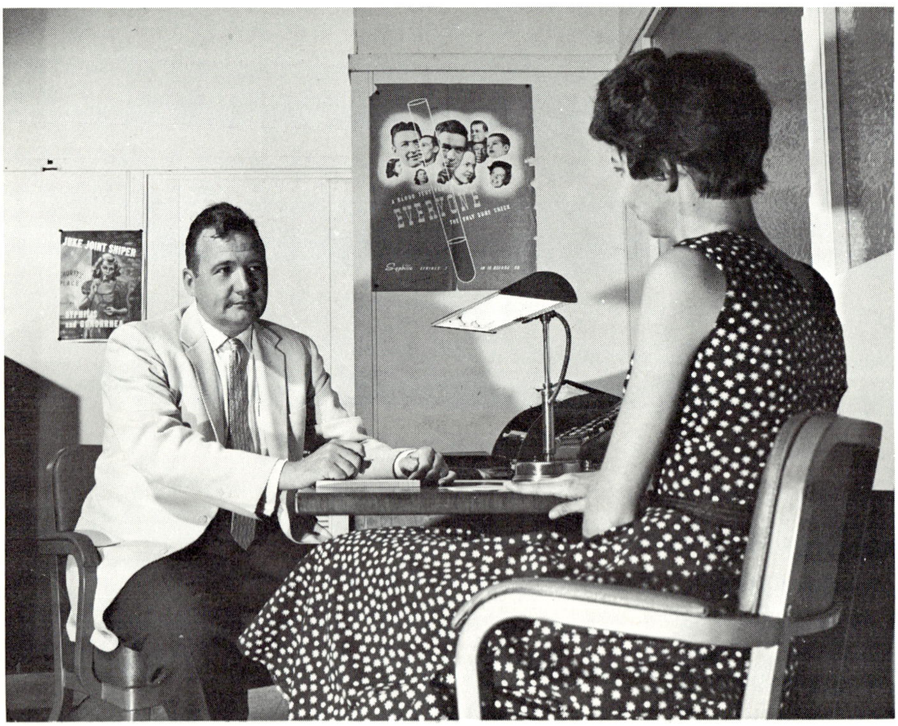

Fig. 17. Contact interviewing. (Courtesy National Medical Audiovisual Center, Chamblee, Ga.)

There should be uniform laws to require a serologic test for syphilis (STS) of all prenatal patients on their first visit to a clinic or physician and to be repeated during the last trimester of pregnancy. Premarital laws have been enacted in many states requiring a physical examination and an STS prior to marriage. Nowhere in Canada are tests for gonorrhea required prior to marriage or during pregnancy. Laws and ordinances requiring STS of food handlers and domestics serve only one purpose—case finding—since venereal disease is not transmitted through food handling.

The control of prostitution is a police function, whereas the prevention of infectious diseases is a function of the health department. In areas where prostitution constitutes a problem in transmitting venereal disease, health departments and police departments need to work closely together.

Laws and ordinances cannot control individual behavior. The sex drive is normal and one of the strongest drives in humans. Efforts to regulate sexual promiscuity through proper sex education should begin early in life, and sex education in the home, in the school, and in public education in the community are important considerations.

Case finding is the most important weapon in the prevention and control of venereal disease. Every case has at least one sexual contact and frequently three or four more. The patient is not only the host, but he also is the vector. Persons trained in the technic of contact interviewing should elicit from the patient sufficient information to investigate and bring to examination and/or treatment every possible source contact and every exposed contact. Wrote Homer: "Fools alone their ulcerated ills conceal."

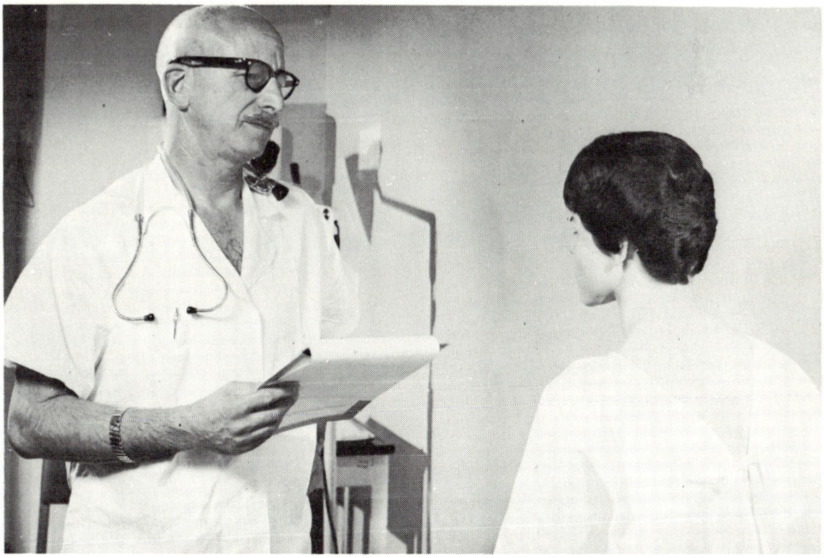

Fig. 18. Physician talking with the patient during the physical examination. (Courtesy National Medical Audiovisual Center, Chamblee, Ga.)

This ancient thought of the Greek poet might well be applied to modern venereal disease's contact (Fig. 17). The contact interviewer does not condemn, moralize, or reproach, but he treats the situation the same as if it were a typhoid fever investigation.

Venereal disease nursing is part and parcel of a family health service. When venereal disease exists, there are other health problems. Treatment in a clinic is not an end in itself. Patients need to be followed long enough to determine the effect of the therapy.

The socioeconomic problems related to increased incidence of venereal disease and its prevention and control are legion, and they must be attacked if eventual eradication is ever to be achieved. However, immediate attack should not be idealistic and philosophic but should be strongly oriented toward case finding and treatment (Fig. 18).

MINOR VENEREAL DISEASES

Chancroid (soft chancre)

Chancroid is the most prevalent of the minor venereal diseases. It was not until 1850 that it was recognized as a separate disease from syphilis. The causative organism, *Hemophilus ducreyi,* was first identified by Ducrey in 1889 and is generally known as Ducrey's bacillus. It is a gram-negative, nonspore-forming, and nonmotile organism that characteristically appears in short oval rods, which may occur in pairs or in chains, and it is easily killed by weak disinfectants.

Chancroid is an acute infectious disease transmitted almost exclusively through close sexual contact but can also be spread indirectly by fingers, towels, clothing, or instruments. It has usually been associated with poor personal hygiene and uncleanliness. The disease occurs worldwide and may affect any age, sex, or race. The incubation period is variable, being as short as twenty-four hours or longer than five days.

The disease begins with a painful anogenital ulcer occurring at the site of inoculation. The period of communicability is usually as long as the disease's duration. Through autoinoculation, numerous small, tender, painful ulcerations appear. The ulcers have a reddened border, and the base exhibits a necrotic purulent exudate with a grayish appearance. The ulcers bleed easily. The patient may have been exposed to syphilis and chancroid at the same time, and both diseases exist simultaneously. Since chancroid has the shorter incubation period, the patient should be observed for syphilis. However, a darkfield examination should be made to avoid overlooking primary syphilis. The main difference between syphilis chancres and lesions of chancroid are the painfulness and softness of the chancroid in contrast with the painlessness and hardness of the typical syphilis lesion. Chancroid is self-limiting. If untreated the disease runs its course in several weeks and then usually disappears with no serious complications. However, an untreated person could die from extensive spread of the ulcers.

Bacteriologic examination including stained smears of exudate taken from the under edges of the lesion will usually give positive identification of the causative organism in about 50% of cases. Cultures of exudate aspirated from a bubo in the inguinal area are more satisfactory, and Ducrey's bacillus can be isolated in about 75% of cases.[6]

Treatment consists of the administration of sulfonamide agents such as sulfadiazine, triple sulfonamides, or sulfisoxazole. Oral administration of 1 Gm. daily for seven to ten days will generally bring about a cure. Several antibiotic drugs are useful, including streptomycin, chlortetracycline hydrochloride (Aureomycin), and oxytetracycline (Terramycin), and may be used if failure of the sulfonamides occurs. However, it is pointed out that antibiotics may mask a syphilitic infection.

Lymphogranuloma venereum

Lymphogranuloma venereum, also known as lymphopathia venereum, lymphogranuloma inguinale, climatic bubo, and tropical bubo, has probably existed for hundreds of years. Symptoms of the disease were described in the eighteenth century. In about 1912 it was recognized as a venereal disease that was transmitted through sexual contact. The causative agent is a virus-like microorganism called a "bedsonia." It is an infectious disease of the lymphatic system.

The disease is most prevalent in tropical and semitropical countries but exists on a worldwide basis.

The incubation period is variable, being from five to twenty-one days; the average is usually seven to twelve days.

The primary lesion appears about the anogenital region or in the vaginal wall in the female. The lesion, which resembles herpes, ruptures, leaving a shallow ulcer with a slightly erythematous area around it. The lesion is painless and may not be noticed. There may be slight constitutional symptoms such as malaise, slight elevation of temperature, and aching of muscles. Spontaneous recovery may occur at this stage, or the disease may progress to a secondary stage.

During the secondary stage regional lymph nodes become painful and swollen. The involved lymph glands are called "buboes." In the male the inguinal nodes are usually the first affected. From slight tenderness they gradually adhere to underlying tissues, forming a large tender mass. Resolution may occur, or suppuration may develop. The infection is generally confined to the lymph nodes, but a generalized infection may result with chills, fever, nausea, vomiting, anorexia, bronchitis, and skin rash. If a generalized infection occurs, all lymph nodes become involved, and there may be enlargement of the liver and splenomegaly.[2]

A third stage of the disease is recognized, during which complications occur. Among the most serious sequelae is rectal stricture, which may lead to proctitis, perirectal abscess, and chronic rectal fistula. Elephantiasis of the male penis and of the vulva and anus in the female may occur.

The disease must be differentiated from syphilis, chancroid, granuloma inguinale, and tuberculous lymphomas. In 1925 Frei developed the skin test for lymphogranuloma venereum, and modifications of the original test are in use today. A complement-fixation test is available, and studies of its use indicate that it may be more valuable in diagnosis of the disease than the Frei test. The organism may also be isolated from biopsy material from the bubo.

The treatment of lymphogranuloma venereum includes the use of chlortetracycline or oxytetracycline for a three-week period, or triple sulfonamides for five to fifteen days. Late manifestations of the disease may require surgical intervention. If untreated, the disease can run a long and debilitating course, but is seldom fatal. No immunity results from an attack.

Granuloma inguinale

The etiologic agent in granuloma inguinale is *Donovania granulomatis* (Donovan body), named after Charles Donovan, an Irish physician who discovered the causative organism in 1905. The Donovan body is a gram-negative, nonmobile, encapsulated organism pathogenic for man.

The exact status of the disease has never been specifically determined. The clinical characteristics of the disease are primarily genital; therefore, it has been classified with venereal diseases, but whether it is a true venereal disease is unknown, and no one is exactly certain if it is communicable or how it is spread.

The disease is endemic in tropical and semitropical countries, and the incidence is predominantly among the Negro race. Among 1387 cases reported 92% were nonwhite persons, but the incidence is about equally divided between males and females. Granuloma inguinale is considered a disease of the poor and the unclean.

The exact incubation period is unknown but is believed to be from one to twelve weeks, or possibly from three to forty days. The disease begins with a bubo in the groin that ruptures, leaving a velvety red lesion that resembles proud flesh in appearance. Soon other lesions develop and coalesce, gradually extending over the entire anogenital area, thighs, and buttocks. The lesions give rise to a very fetid odor, and the patient becomes unemployable and is essentially a social outcast.

Diagnosis is confirmed by finding the Donovan bodies. The organism is deep in the tissue and the exudate and debris are removed. Clean granulation tissue is placed between clean glass slides, dried, stained, and examined under the microscope for the causative organism. Biopsy of clean tissue is regarded as a more desirable diagnostic procedure.

Until antibiotics became available, there was no cure for the disease. Treatment for seven days with tetracycline or streptomycin is usually curative. In addition, oxytetracycline, chloramphenicol, erythromycin, and chlortetracycline have been found equally effective. Treatment with the broad-spectrum antibiotics is continued for from four to six weeks, depending on the severity of the disease.

Serologic examinations should be made of all patients treated for granuloma inguinale, and the patient should be kept under observation for one year.

REFERENCES

1. Gordon, John E., editor: Control of communicable diseases in man, ed. 10, New York, 1965, American Public Health Assn., Inc.
2. Horsfall, Frank L., and Tamm, Igor, editors: Viral and rickettsial infections of man, ed. 4, Philadelphia, 1965, J. B. Lippincott Co.
3. Modell, Walter, editor: Drugs of choice, 1974-1975, St. Louis, 1974, The C. V. Mosby Co.
4. Nelson, Nels A., and Struve, Virginia R.: Prevention of congenital syphilis by treatment of syphilis in pregnancy, J. Am. Med. Assoc. **161**:869-872, June 30, 1956.
5. Ormsby, Hugh L.: Prophylaxis of ophthalmia neonatorum, Am. J. Nurs. **57**: 1174-1175, Sept., 1957.
6. Packer, Henry: Minor venereal diseases in the United States, Public Health Reports **72**:363-366, April, 1957.
7. Paul, Hugh: The control of diseases (social and communicable), Baltimore, 1964, The Williams & Wilkins Co.
8. Pedersen, A. H. B., and Kelly, R. E.: Rapid biochemical presumptive test for gonorrheal urethritis in the male, Public Health Reports **81**:318-322, April, 1966.
9. Proceedings of the World Forum on Syphilis and Other Treponematoses, Public Health Service Publication no. 997, Washington, D. C., 1964, U. S. Government Printing Office.
10. Samter, Max, editor: Immunological diseases, Boston, 1965, Little, Brown & Co.
11. Statistics, Journal of Venereal Disease Information **29**:356-357, Nov., 1948.
12. Wallace, Alwilda: Trends and uses of various tests in syphilis serology today, Technical Bulletin of the Registry of Medical Technologists **35**: Nov., 1965.
13. Annual Report of Notifiable Diseases, Statistics Canada, Ottawa, Canada, 1972.
14. U. S. Department of Health, Education, and Welfare: Morbidity and mortality **20(49)**:443-444, 1971.

PART B

ENTERIC DISEASES CAUSED BY BACTERIA

Infectious diseases of the gastrointestinal tract have existed for centuries. Some diseases were described by Hippocrates and his contemporaries. It appears probable that these diseases may have existed for many years before they were recognized as specific disease entities. Although there were many theories concerning the causes of enteric diseases, scientific knowledge concerning their etiology and epidemiology is largely a product of the twentieth century. Until the cause and method of transfer became known, effective control of them was impossible.

The pathogenic bacteria causing enteric diseases have many similarities, but there are also many dissimilarities among them and the way they affect the body. Research scientists are continuing to discover new strains of bacteria and to learn more about their behavior and their role in causing disease in man and animals.

Most of these diseases are caused by the ingestion of contaminated food and drink. The newer knowledge of sanitation and its role in prevention has helped to reduce the incidence of enteric disease and made effective control possible. Through scientific research, vaccines have been produced that aid in the prevention of some enteric diseases. Although the incidence of these diseases in the United States and Canada has been decreasing, sporadic cases and mild epidemics continue to occur. Enteric diseases remain endemic and epidemic in many parts of the world and exact a heavy toll in human lives. The major reservoir of infection is the gastrointestinal tract of man. Because of a highly mobile population and modern methods of transportation, constant vigilance is necessary to prevent outbreaks of enteric diseases.

19

ASIATIC CHOLERA

Etiology

The causative organism in Asiatic cholera is a gram-negative, motile, aerobic bacteria called *Vibrio cholerae.* The *Vibrio cholerae (Vibrio comma)* is described as a comma-shaped rod, but it may be found as a long spirillum form. Included among the vibrios is the El Tor strain, which has been identified as causing paracholera. There are numerous strains of the vibrios, and their role in causing disease has not been completely established.

Epidemiology

Some authorities believe that methods of transmission of the *Vibrio cholerae* have not been clearly established, but the present evidence indicates that man is the only reservoir of infection. The disease is transmitted by the anal-oral route, and the causative organism may be identified in the feces of patients, convalescent carriers, and asymptomatic individuals. During the acute stage of the disease, the organism is present in vomitus but is not present in the urine. Vehicles for transmission include contaminated water supplies, milk, fruit, and vegetables. The transmission is to persons with poor personal hygiene in areas where sanitation is deficient.

The *Vibrio cholerae* is easily destroyed by acid disinfectants such as phenol preparations. The undiluted gastric juice in the stomach will usually kill the organism; however, when the pathogen is mixed with food and liquids, it may pass on into the intestine. The organism is killed by drying and in warm weather may be expected to die in about twenty-four hours. It has been found to survive in clothing for several days and to live for a week or longer during cold weather.

Throughout the centuries, cholera has killed millions of people. The last epidemic in the United States occurred in 1873; however, New York City reported an incident of cholera being imported in 1911. From 1971 to the end of 1972, no cases of cholera were reported by the Vital Statistics of the U. S. In August 1973 one case of cholera was recorded in Texas; the patient recovered. In Canada between 1971 and 1973, no cases were reported by Statistics Canada; however, during 1974, one case was reported. In 1973, thirty countries or territories reported a total of about 75,000 cases, as compared to 67,000 in 1972. The actual number of cases is believed to be even higher, since reports of outbreaks in some countries could not be officially confirmed. Twenty-five imported cases occurred in four European countries. The disease continues to be so widespread in parts of the world that Dubos and Hirsch have stated that much of the world's population is confronted by grave risk of exposure.[1] After a temporary lull in 1967 and 1968, the disease became widespread in some Mediterranean and neighboring countries. In 1970 it invaded west Africa. In 1973 five countries were newly affected by cholera: three in Africa, one in Asia, and one in Europe (Italy). In 1974 it invaded Portugal, and within four months, 386 cases were reported with eight deaths. The disease is endemic in India, Pakistan, China, Malaysia, the East Indies, the Philippines, Korea, and New Guinea.

Incubation period

The incubation period of cholera ranges from twenty-four hours to five days.

Diagnosis

Diagnosis is made by bacteriologic examination of stools, using a slide or culture technic.

Clinical manifestations

Cholera occurs with an abrupt onset that is very acute. There is profuse vomiting and violent, painless diarrhea. Within the first few hours the fluid loss may be great enough to result in severe dehydration and acidosis. The number of stools gradually increase and contain white particles, which have prompted the term *rice-water stools.* There is severe cramping of the feet and extremities, the blood pressure falls, the temperature is subnormal, the skin is cold and clammy, the eyes are sunken, and there is oliguria and collapse. The patient may die within a few days, or recovery may occur rapidly. Many cases are asymptomatic and have only mild diarrhea, distinguishable from other diarrheas with only laboratory diagnosis.

Treatment

According to Modell, there is no specific drug that greatly affects the course of the disease.[2] A number of drugs are used, including the tetracyclines, chloramphenicol, and oxytetracycline. Administration of the chemotherapeutic drugs decreases the number of *Vibrio cholerae* organisms in the stools. The most important aspect of therapy is the intravenous administration of isotonic saline solution, which is a major factor in preventing death from the disease. Water, salts, and alkali must be replaced. It has been proved that the presently available cholera vaccine gives only partial protection for about three to six months and does not prevent people from becoming carriers. In 1973 the world health organization reported on field trials of a new bacterial cholera vaccine. The possibility of a new vaccine offering better protection for a longer period is still being investigated.

Nursing care

The nursing care of the patient with cholera includes isolation and strict medical asepsis. A gown and gloves should be worn, and thorough handwashing should be rigidly carried out. Only essential nursing procedures should be performed. Terminal disinfection and disinfection of stools and oral secretions are the same as for other enteric infections.

Prevention and control

Cases should be reported and an epidemiologic investigation of source and contacts carried out. The World Health Organization requires the reporting to them of the appearance of the disease in a previously noninfected area. All contacts should be examined and immunized. Contacts should be quarantined for five days from the last known exposure. Screening and eradicating flies, disinfecting the patient's clothing by autoclaving or by soaking in a disinfecting solution, and avoiding the consumption of raw fruits and vegetables should be practiced. Cholera occurs among economically deprived people where crowding and unsanitary conditions exist. Ideal control conditions may be a luxury that cannot be afforded.

In addition to case reports the International Sanitary Regulations require persons arriving from cholera-infected areas and countries by land, sea, and air to have a valid certification of vaccination against cholera.

REFERENCES

1. Dubos, Rene J., and Hirsch, James G., editors: Bacterial and mycotic infections of man, ed. 4, Philadelphia, 1965, J. B. Lippincott Co.
2. Modell, Walter, editor: Drugs of choice, 1974-1975, St. Louis, 1974, The C. V. Mosby Co.

20

BRUCELLOSIS (UNDULANT FEVER)

Etiology

Brucellosis is caused by a small, gram-negative, nonsporulating, motile coccobacillus called "Brucella." Three strains of the organism have been identified as follows: (1) caprine strain causing *Brucella melitensis* in goats, sheep, cattle, and swine; (2) bovine strain resulting in *Brucella abortus* in horses, dogs, sheep, and cattle; and (3) porcine strain causing *Brucella suis* in swine primarily and also in cattle and horses. All three strains are pathologic for man. *Brucella abortus* is less likely to occur in man. Bacteriologically and serologically all three strains are closely related; therefore, all have been classified under the generic name *Brucella.*

Epidemiology

Brucellosis has been known by a variety of names. In 1887 Bruce discovered the disease in goats on the island of Malta, where it was known as Malta fever. It has also been known as gastric remittant fever, Neapolitan disease, goat fever, and more commonly as undulant fever. The disease was finally given the name brucellosis in honor of the work done by Sir David Bruce. *Brucella abortus,* which occurs in cattle, is known as Bang's disease.

Brucellosis is a disease of animals that may be transmitted to humans but is rarely transmitted from man to man. The largest number of cases result from accidental inoculation of laboratory workers and through cutaneous abrasions in persons handling infected animals, their carcasses, or infected excreta. The organisms may gain entrance to the body through the gastrointestinal tract by the ingestion of infected milk and/or infected milk products. Some studies have indicated that infected milk has been consumed over a considerable period of time without causing serious disease. There has also been some evidence that the *Brucella* organisms may gain entrance to the body through the respiratory system. On gaining entrance the microorganisms travel from the site of entry by way of the blood and lymph channels. The bacilli tend to localize in the lymph nodes in all the various organs.

Brucellosis poses an occupational hazard to persons working in slaughterhouses, farmers, meat packers, stock handlers, veterinarians, and laboratory personnel. Since more than one half of the population is susceptible to the disease, the consumption of unpasteurized milk is considered hazardous.

The disease may be contracted at any season of the year; however, the incidence appears to be greatest during the summer months.

Most cases of brucellosis occur in persons between 12 and 60 years of age, with the majority before 45 years of age. Studies indicate that children under 10 years of age rarely contract the disease; however, if they do become infected, the course of the disease does not differ from that in the adult. The sex ratio indicates that about four cases occur in males to one case in females, although some reports claim that overall incidence is about equally divided.

The United States Department of Health, Education, and Welfare reported 183 cases in 1971. In Canada during this same period eight cases were reported by Statistics Canada. In 1972, 196 cases were reported in the U. S., and sixteen cases in Canada. In 1973, the number of cases in the U. S. totaled 202, while Canada had a total of seven cases. During 1974, 181 cases were reported by the U. S. Communicable Disease Center, while in Canada twenty-four cases were reported during this same period. Statistics Canada reported one death from the disease during 1971. Between the years 1960 and 1969, the Vital Statistics of the U. S. reported fifty-four deaths from the disease. Brucellosis occurs in all European countries except Denmark, and it is endemic in Mexico, South America, Russia, and North Africa.

Incubation period

The incubation period of brucellosis is variable and may range from five to thirty days.

Clinical manifestations

Brucellosis is a systemic febrile disease marked by remission and exacerbations. The onset may be acute or insidious, and chronicity may occur. The disease may be present without symptoms or may be fulminating in type, resulting in death. Brucellosis attacks every organ and tissue of the body, and as many as 150 different symptoms have been associated with the disease. Diagnosis is frequently difficult because of the wide variety of symptoms, and as a result it is believed that many cases are missed.

Ths disease is characterized by a long, irregular, intermittent fever, which may range from 101° to 105° F. during the first week of illness. After several weeks the temperature falls by lysis. There is aching of the head, back, and extremities, splenomegaly, and enlargement of the liver. There is profuse perspiration with a sour odor, spongy bleeding gums, and anorexia. There may be nausea, vomiting, abdominal pain, and general malaise.

Neurologic symptoms are characteristic of the disease and occur in the form of depression or hysterical episodes. Constipation or diarrhea may be present, and bleeding may occur from ulceration of the intestinal mucosa.

Diagnosis

The diagnosis of brucellosis is made on the basis of clinical findings and occupational history and is confirmed by bacteriologic and serologic isolation of the *Brucella* organism. Laboratory methods include agglutination tests, blood cultures, cultures of feces and urine, sputum examination, and biopsy of lymph nodes or bone marrow secured by sternal puncture. Intracutaneous tests have been found useful in determining the presence of antigenic substances in the individual, but they do not provide evidence of an active infection.

Treatment

Treatment consists of bed rest with minimal activity and the administration of drugs for relief of pain and tetracycline drugs. The tetracyclines are bacteriostatic in action and are broad-spectrum antibiotics. They may be administered orally or parenterally and must be continued for three to four weeks. Although corticosteroid drugs in combination with antibiotic drugs may reduce toxic reactions, it is generally agreed that their use should be limited because of the danger of peripheral vascular collapse.

Nursing care

The nursing care of patients with brucellosis differs little from that of patients with typhoid fever. Frequent bathing helps to relieve the odor from the perspiration, reduce the temperature, and provide comfort for the patient. Meticulous skin care and mouth care are important. Heat may be applied to painful joints. The patient may need encouragement to eat, and records of food and fluid intake should be maintained. The diet may be semifluid or as tolerated by the patient. In the chronic state the diet may be low fat, high protein, or high carbohydrate with vitamin supplements.

The patient should be isolated, and stools, urine, and vomitus disposed of as in typhoid fever. The *Brucella* is killed by direct sunlight, and preparations such as phenol, benzalkomium (Zephiran), or the hypochlorites will ensure adequate disinfection.

The patient should be in quiet, pleasant surroundings. Because of his neurologic symptoms he must be protected from injury and given encouragement, and after the acute symptoms have ceased diversionary interests and activities should be provided.

Prevention and control

All cases of brucellosis should be reported and epidemiologic investigation of the source of the disease made. The major factor in control is the control of the disease in animals. The recommended measures include testing of dairy herds, pasteurization of all milk, immunization of young animals, and interstate and international control of all domestic animals and feed materials. All animals with positive serology should be slaughtered. There is a need for education in the care, handling, and disposal of the products of aborted animals and for thorough disinfection of the contaminated area.

21

BACILLARY DYSENTERY (SHIGELLOSIS)

BACILLARY DYSENTERY (SHIGELLOSIS)

Etiology

This is a pathologic term for any form of diarrhea due to intestinal bacilli.

Shigellosis is caused by one of the strains of *Bacillus dysenteriae,* identified as of the genus *Shigella.* The four main groups are classified as *Shigella dysenteriae, Shigella flexneri, Shigella boydii, and Shigella sonnei,* any one of which may cause the disease. The term "bacillary" is used to distinguish dysentery due to these bacteria from dysentery due to protozoa (amebic dysentery), and from viral and other forms of dysentery. The organisms are gram-negative, nonsporulating, nonmotile rods that closely resemble the *Salmonella typhosa.* Endotoxins produced by the organism affect the intestinal mucosa. An exotoxin may give rise to neurologic symptoms, and the endotoxin is believed to result from disintegration of the organism rather than being produced by it.

Epidemiology

Very little was known concerning dysentery and its causative organisms until the begining of this century. The first discovery was made by Shiga, a Japanese scientist, during an epidemic in Japan in 1898. Following Shiga's work, other strains of the organism were isolated, identified, and named after the men who discovered them.

Bacillary dysentery has been known to exist in institutions such as mental hospitals, jails, and orphanages for many years. Environmental factors such as crowding and poor sanitation increase the incidence of the disease.

The disease is spread by feces, fingers, flies, contaminated milk, food and water, and by any article that has been in contact with the feces of a patient or carrier. The microorganisms enter through the mouth.

Dysentery may occur during any season of the year, but it is more prevalent during the summer months. It occurs in all age groups. It has not disappeared from modern communities as has typhoid fever. It is constantly with us as it is spread in great part by the feces on the soiled hands of unknowing and unsuspected ambulatory cases and carriers, or through contaminated wells. Most patients attribute the diarrhea to "something I ate." This infection may prove fatal to children. Adults with diarrhea should avoid contact with children.

The incidence of shigellosis cannot be accurately determined, since cases are generally reported only during epidemics. Many sporadic cases probably go unreported. In 1971 Statistics Canada reported 1350 cases, while the U. S. Department of Health, Education, and Welfare reported 16,143 cases. In 1972, 20,207 cases were reported in the U. S. During the same period Canada had 1290 cases. In 1973, the U. S. had a total of 23,818 cases, while Canada had 1912 cases reported. For 1974 no statistics were available for the U. S., however, for the same period 2369 cases were reported by the Public Health Section, Health and Welfare Division, Statistics Canada. The disease is endemic over all of North America, Europe, and in the tropics.

Incubation period

The incubation period is variable, usually between one and seven days, with an average of about four days.

Clinical manifestations

This disease may vary greatly in severity from a very mild disturbance to severe and fatal dysentery.

Shigellosis is characterized by an acute onset with abdominal pain, accompanied by painful diarrhea and griping. The stools contain mucus, pus and are often blood tinged due to ulcers forming in the large intestine. Rectal irritation and tenesmus are usual symptoms. The temperature may rise from 100° to 103° F., and moderate leukocytosis may be present. Vomiting may or may not occur. In severe cases headache and prostration may be present.

Diagnosis

The diagnosis of shigellosis is based on clinical findings and bacteriologic examination. The causative organism may be found in the feces during the acute stage of the disease, which is usually four or five days. Specimens secured from feces or by the use of a rectal swab must be cultured immediately, since the shigella organism dies very quickly. Agglutination tests may be carried out, but they are not very satisfactory for diagnostic purposes.

Treatment

Shigellosis is a self-limiting disease. In mild cases recovery may be expected in about ten days, whereas in more severe cases the disease may be prolonged for two or three weeks. Chronicity may occur, continuing for months or even years. Specific drug therapy includes the well-absorbed sulfonamides, with sulfadiazine being the drug of choice. In case of resistance to the sulfonamides, antibiotic therapy may be substituted. Camphorated tincture of opium (paregoric) and adequate electrolyte replacement is indicated. The diet should be low residue, and milk and cream should be eliminated.

Nursing care

The nursing care of patients with shigellosis is the same as that for all patients with enteric disease. The patient should be isolated and strict medical asepsis carried out. A gown should be worn when giving any nursing care. Accurate records of fluid intake should be maintained. If stool specimens are secured for bacteriologic examination, the nurse should understand the importance of immediate transfer of the specimen to the laboratory. Routine nursing care should be planned to conserve the patient's strength. Disinfection of bowel discharges should be carried out the same as for typhoid fever.

Prevention and control

All cases should be reported. In case of epidemics epidemiologic investigation of possible sources should be made, including food handlers. Cases should be isolated until at least two negative stool cultures are obtained at twenty-four-hour intervals. Both concurrent and terminal disinfection should be carried out. Preventive measures include pasteurization of milk, safety of water supplies, screening against flies, thorough washing of fruits and vegetables, and education in handwashing before meals and after toilet.

INFANTILE DYSENTERY (DIARRHEA)

Infants and young children may become infected with any of the enteric bacteria group of pathogenic organisms. The occurrence of such infections are commonly known as infantile diarrhea, summer diarrhea, and diarrhea of the newborn. Any diarrhea occurring in infants is potentially serious, but epidemic diarrhea in newborn infants, particularly in hospital nurseries, is always a matter of grave concern.

Studies conducted during outbreaks of diarrhea among newborn in nurseries indicate that certain strains of *Escherichia coli* are a frequent cause of the infection. *E. coli* is a gram-negative, nonspore-forming, usually motile, anaerobic, short rod that may on some occasions group itself to form chains. The normal habitat of the organism is the intestinal tract of man, where it is usually considered to be beneficial. However, under certain conditions it may become pathogenic and manifest itself in various kinds of infections.

The source of the infection is man, and its spread is from person to person. Nursery-acquired infection is generally the result of carelessness among professional and other personnel involved in infant care. There has been some indication that an infant may be infected by the mother during the birth process.

The disease is widespread in North America and in Europe, and the mortality among infants may be as high as 40% to 60%. In 1972, Canada reported fifty-five cases with thirteen deaths. For the same year, ten states reported 190 cases. No statistics on the death rate are available. In 1973, fifteen states reported 212 cases. Again, no statistics on the death rates are available.

The incubation period varies between one and six days. Diagnosis is confirmed by identification of the specific strain of the organism through bacteriologic examination of stool cultures.

The onset of infantile diarrhea is sudden, with severe diarrhea or loose watery stools. The infection is acute, is highly communicable, and spreads rapidly. The stools may be yellow, turning to green and containing very little mucus or blood. Dehydration is usually severe, with acidosis, vomiting, and fever. When prompt treatment is available, the infant may be expected to recover in about one week.

Treatment consists of the administration of antibiotics and replacement of electrolytes. Antibiotics frequently used are tetracyclines, chloramphenicol, and neomycin, the latter being the drug of choice. Treatment is generally continued over a ten-day period. In case of drug resistance or inadequate treatment, relapse may occur. Nothing is given orally unless ordered by the physician, and the infant must be kept warm and free from drafts.

Infected babies must be isolated and strict aseptic technic carried out. Thorough concurrent and terminal disinfection is extremely important. The *E. coli* organism is resistant to many disinfectants as well as to sunlight. It seems fairly certain that airborne transmission of the infection may occur. Extreme caution must be exercised in the use of common facilities such as scales and bathing equipment and in the care of contaminated diapers or other clothing, all of which should be carefully handled and disinfected.

22

FOOD INFECTION (SALMONELLA)

Food poisoning, a commonly used term, should be differentiated from *food infection.* Food poisoning results from the formation of a bacterial toxin, that is, staphylococcus enterotoxin and *Clostridium botulinum* toxin. Poisoning may also be caused by certain chemicals.

Etiology

Food infection is caused by a species of *Salmonella* bacillus. About 800 different species of the salmonella organism have been identified, and almost all will produce disease in man and animals. *Salmonella typhimurium* is the commonest species causing food infection in the United States and Canada. The specific cause is an endotoxin produced by the salmonella organism.

Epidemiology

Infections caused by the ingestion of contaminated food probably existed for centuries before the cause became known. The discovery and isolation of *Salmonella* is the work of twentieth century bacteriologists. Outbreaks of food infection occur worldwide, and there has been an increase in the incidence of such infections during the past few years. The increase has been attributed to the modern methods of production and distribution of foods that are infected in their natural state.[2] Studies have shown that the salmonella organism is present in a high proportion of human and animal food products.[4] Many types of food have been incriminated as causing food infection, including meat pies, corned beef, sausage, fowl, dried eggs, cheese, ice cream, and cream pies. Abrahamson reports that adequate regulations do not exist concerning the processing of frozen ready-to-eat products. These products offer the greatest hazard to public health efforts in controlling infections. Precooked foods are often not heated sufficiently to kill the pathogens in them.[1] Recent studies indicate that chilled ready-to-eat foods such as salads and desserts found in markets and delicatessen stores are frequently contaminated beyond bacteriologic safety.[3]

It has been estimated that only a fraction of the actual number of cases of food infection are reported; therefore, statistics are not reliable in assessing the total problem. Outbreaks usually occur after public gatherings such as weddings, family reunions, or picnics, as well as in restaurants following banquets.

The transmission of the *Salmonella* causing food infection is by the feces of man and animals. Human carriers are believed responsible for a large number of cases. Outbreaks occur most frequently during warm months, particularly when there is a lack of proper refrigeration. The infection attacks all age groups. Carelessness is a prime factor in many outbreaks and involves inadequate handwashing and washing of fruits and vegetables that are consumed raw.

The U. S. Department of Health, Education, and Welfare reported 21,928 cases in 1971. In Canada during this same period 1729 cases were reported by Statistics Canada. In 1972, 22,151 cases were reported in the U. S., and 2441 cases in Canada. In 1973, the number of cases in the U. S. was 23,818, while Canada had a total of 4261 cases. During 1974, 3846 cases were reported by the Public Health Section, Health and Welfare Division, Statistics Canada. During the first twenty-five weeks of 1974, the U. S. Communicable Disease Center reported 11,450 cases. Between 1960 and 1969 deaths resulting from Salmonellosis (including Paratyphoid fever) totalled 722 in the U. S. In Canada during 1971, no deaths occurred from Salmonellosis.

Incubation period

The incubation period is short, from seven to seventy-two hours. There appears to be a relationship between the size of the dose of pathogenic organisms and the onset of symptoms. When the dose is large, the incubation period is shortened.

Diagnosis

The diagnosis of *Salmonella* food infection can usually be made from the history and clinical symptoms. Stool cultures may be taken; however, the patient is usually convalescent before reports are available. Blood cultures in food infection are negative.

Clinical manifestations

The infection is frequently explosive in onset with vomiting and diarrhea. There are usually headache, chills, slight elevation of temperature, and abdominal pain and tenderness. Dehydration may occur when the vomiting and diarrhea are severe, in which case the temperature may be elevated to as much as 105° F. The patient may suffer from varying degrees of prostration. Stools and vomitus are watery, and vomitus may be tinged with blood or bile. There is no blood in the stools. Neurologic symptoms such as dizziness may be present. Recovery usually occurs within three to four days, but in severe infections death may occur within twenty-four hours.

Treatment

Salmonella food infection is generally self-limiting, and many mild cases are cared for at home. Patients with severe infections may be cared for in the hospital. Treatment at the onset may include gavage to remove any infected material from the stomach, electrolyte replacement, bed rest, heat to the abdomen, and mild sedation. Drug therapy has not given significant results. Diet is limited to clear liquids, with easily digested foods added as the patient improves. Persons found to be carriers may be treated with chloramphenicol.

Nursing care

Since the patient may feel acutely ill and exhausted, every effort should be made to provide rest in a comfortable quiet environment. Adequate ventilation and room deodorizers may add to the patient's comfort by controlling disagreeable odors resulting from diarrhea. Only essential nursing duties should be performed, and fluids should be given only as tolerated. Records of intake and fluid loss should be maintained. Vital signs should be checked every four hours. The care of feces and contaminated linens should be practiced the same as for other enteric infections. Isolation is unnecessary, but thorough handwashing is important.

Prevention and control

Cases should be reported and epidemiologic investigation carried out in epidemics to determine the source of the infection. Food handlers in hospitals and other institutions should be trained and supervised in proper handwashing practices, including cleanliness and trimming of the fingernails. Public education in the care, handling, and refrigeration of frozen foods should be given. Frozen foods should be thawed in the refrigerator and not in the open air, and cooked foods should not be left to cool in the open air. If eggs are washed, they should be used the same day.[4] By the end of 1973, laboratories in twenty-nine countries around the world were providing data for the world health organization's program for the surveillance of *Salmonella*. In most countries taking part in the program there are indications of an increase in the incidence of *Salmonella* causing food infections.

REFERENCES

1. Abrahamson, A. E.: Administrative microbiological standards for sanitary control of frozen foods, Public Health Reports **81**: 83-86, Jan., 1966.
2. Huckstep, R. L.: Typhoid fever and other Salmonella infections, Edinburgh, 1962, E. & S. Livingstone Ltd.
3. Rasmussen, Carol A., and Strong, Dorothy H.: Bacteria in chilled delicatessen foods, Public Health Reports **82**:353-359, April, 1967.
4. Werrin, Milton, and Kronick, David: Salmonella control in hospitals, Am. J. Nurs. **66**:528-530, March, 1966.

23
TYPHOID FEVER

Etiology

Typhoid fever is caused by *Salmonella typhosa* and is the most serious of the enteric infections caused by the *Salmonella* group of bacteria. The disease is common only to man; however, experimentally it has been possible to transmit the disease to chimpanzees. As with other organisms of the *Salmonella* group, *Salmonella typhosa* is a gram-negative, nonsporulating, motile bacillus. Most of the organisms will be killed when exposed to a temperature of 60° C. for fifteen to twenty minutes; however, they have been found to survive for relatively long periods of time under natural conditions, for example, one week in sewage-contaminated water (Fig. 19).

Epidemiology

Typhoid existed centuries before Christ, but it was not until the middle of the nineteenth century that the name "typhoid" was given to the disease. For many years it was believed that typhoid fever and typhus fever were the same disease.

Typhoid fever (enteric fever) is a disease of humans. The bacilli must be swallowed. The causative organism is excreted in the feces and urine of patients suffering from the disease or by human carrier of the disease. The role of the carrier has been dramatically portrayed in the history of "Typhoid Mary" who was responsible for several hundred cases of typhoid fever between 1901 and 1914, and who cleverly evaded public health officials during the period.

The typhoid bacillus gains entrance to the body by the ingestion of contaminated water, milk, and other contaminated food products. For many years water was the chief vehicle for causing epidemics of typhoid fever. Even after public water supplies became available, frequent epidemics resulted from cross-connections between water and sewage lines. Water as a vehicle for transmitting the disease was not brought under control until methods for water purification were established. Transmission through

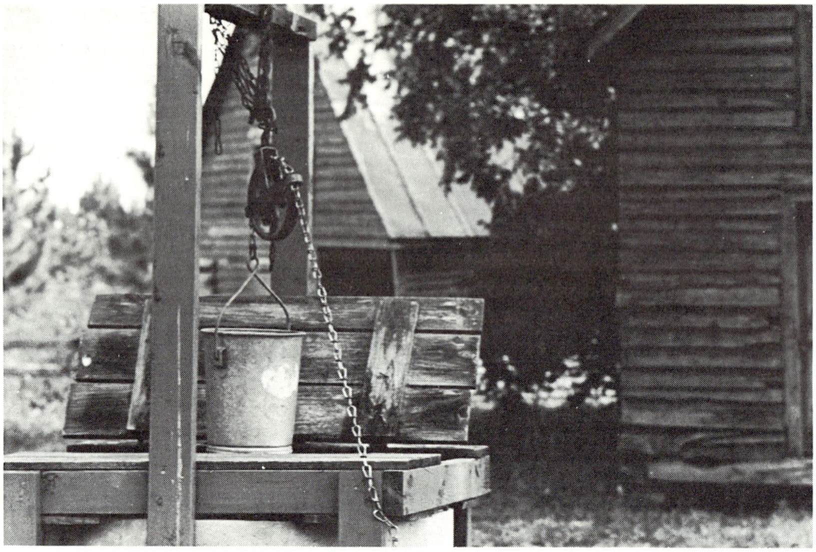

Fig. 19. Open wells are often contaminated by pathogenic microorganisms.

food, including milk, may result from carriers and missed cases of the disease. Epidemics have also occurred recently from shellfish that were grown in infected water. Flies have always been considered a hazard in carrying the disease. Unsanitary disposal of excreta, lack of screening, and exposed food allow flies to carry excreta on their feet to food. Public education, water purification, sewage disposal plants, and industrial and governmental cooperation together with modern immunization procedures have almost eliminated the environmental hazards and protected the individual from the disease. The chief danger is from the typhoid carrier, or a person already ill with typhoid.

Typhoid fever may occur during any season of the year; however, the greatest incidence occurs during the warm months. Persons of any age may contract the disease. Cases are about equally divided between the sexes, although carriers are about five times more common among women than men. Top states that about 80% of the known carriers are women. Usually the female carrier is past 40 years of age and frequently is found to have cholecystitis and cholelithiasis.

Although most physicians and nurses may never see a case of typhoid fever during their professional career, the disease continues to be a worldwide problem and we should all be aware that it could become a scourge once again. In the United States and Canada typhoid fever is mainly a rural problem. In rural areas where open wells, springs, and unsanitary excreta disposal conditions exist, typhoid fever may be encountered (Fig. 20). The disease continues to be a public health problem in underdeveloped countries of the Far and Middle East, in Central and South America, and in parts of Europe.

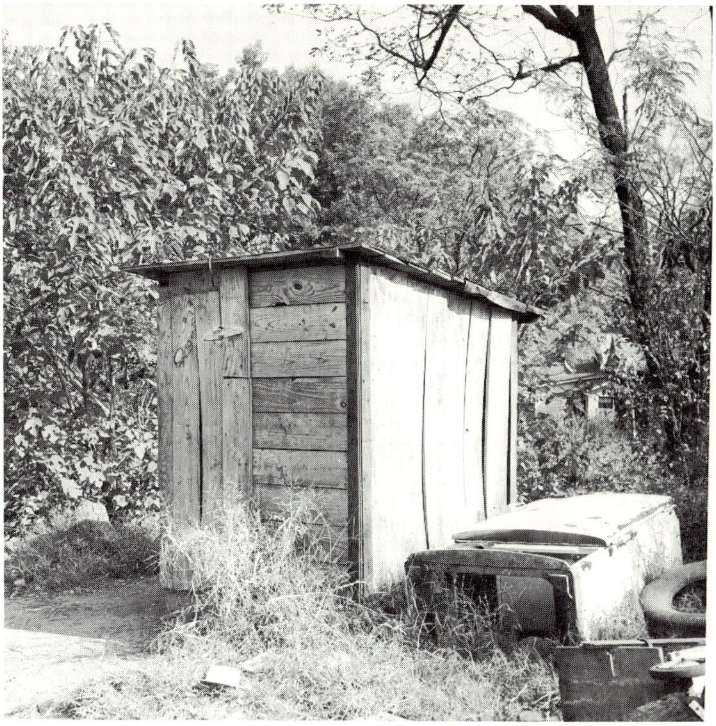

Fig. 20. Flies from unsanitary privies may carry disease organisms on their feet and deposit them on food.

The United States Department of Health, Education, and Welfare reported 407 cases in 1971. In Canada during this same period, ninety-nine cases were reported by Statistics Canada. In 1972, 398 cases were reported in the U. S., and 108 cases in Canada. In 1973, the number of cases in the U. S. was 680, while Canada had a total of 101 cases. During 1974, 414 cases were reported by the U. S. Communicable Disease Center. During this same period 116 cases were reported by Statistics Canada. Between 1960 and 1969, 122 persons died from this disease in the U. S. During 1971, one person died of typhoid fever in Canada.

Incubation period

The incubation period is variable—usually ten to fourteen days. It may be as short as seven days or as long as twenty-one days.

Diagnosis

Accurate diagnosis of typhoid fever is dependent on the isolation and identification of the *Salmonella typhosa* organism. There are currently four diagnostic procedures for typhoid fever: the Widal test, and blood, stool, and urine cultures. Blood cultures during the first week are estimated to be from 80% to 90% positive and are considered to be the most significant diagnostic procedure during the early period of the disease. By the second week after the onset of the disease the agglutination reaction in the patient's blood is usually positive. The Widal test is used to detect the presence of these agglutinins. Stool and urine examinations may be done early in the disease and the organism isolated. The number of positive stools tend to increase during the second and third weeks. Stool and urine cultures are done at intervals during the course of the disease. Occasionally it may be possible to isolate the organism from vomitus. A complete blood count is usually done on the admission of the patient to the hospital but is not considered diagnostic for typhoid fever.

Clinical manifestations

The causative organism invades the bloodstream by way of the lymphatic tissues and is carried to all parts of the body. Early symptoms may be vague with headache, anorexia, and malaise. As the disease progresses, there are joint pains, abdominal discomfort, vomiting, and usually constipation, although there may be diarrhea. Cough and bronchitis occur in about 50% of the cases. During the first week the temperature rises in a stepladder pattern until it reaches about 104° F., where it remains until near the end of the third week, after which it falls by lysis. The temperature is irregular, with about a 2° remission in the morning. The pulse rate is slow in relation to the temperature. The tongue and mouth become dry, and sordes appear about the teeth and lips. There may be urinary retention and abdominal distention, and splenomegaly usually develops. The patient appears dull and apathetic. After the first week, a rose-colored eruption (rose spots) appears on the abdomen and chest, and in most cases there is some degree of leukopenia. The lymphoid follicles (Peyer's patches) in the lower ileum, occasionally extending further into the small intestine, become inflamed and hyperplasia occurs. The condition is usually followed by necrosis and ulceration of the lesions. After the fourth week healing may take place, or hemorrhage and even perforation of the intestinal wall may occur.

The diagnosis of typhoid fever is frequently complicated by the wide range of symptoms and the pathologic changes that may occur in every organ of the body. In about 98% of the cases an attack of typhoid fever renders the patient immune for the rest of his life.

Treatment

A number of drugs have been tried in the treatment of typhoid fever; however, chloramphenicol is currently the drug of choice. The clinical symptoms of the disease disappear in three or four days after treatment with chloramphenicol; however, bacteriologically the patient remains infectious. Relapse tends to occur more frequently when drug therapy is discontinued too early. Other treatment includes maintaining electrolyte balance, mild sedation to control mental confusion, and meeting dietary requirements.

Complications

Complications in typhoid fever may involve any body system and may range from mild involvement to serious or fatal conditions. Among the more serious complications are pneumonia, cholecystitis, hemorrhage, and intestinal perforation.

Nursing care

The patient must be isolated until at least three negative stool cultures twenty-four hours apart have been secured. Strict medical asepsis must be carried out. A nurse caring for a patient with typhoid fever must consider all the patient's secretions and excretions as being cultures of typhoid bacilli. A gown must be worn when any nursing care is administered. All stools, urine, vomitus, and bath water must be disinfected unless disposed of in a municipal sewage system. The rectal temperature should be taken every two to four hours during the acute stage of the disease, and the pulse rate must be checked at frequent intervals. Tepid or alcohol sponges should be given for an elevated temperature, but care should be taken to conserve the patient's strength and to avoid chilling the patient. Antipyretic drugs should not be administered for fever. The skin must be protected by frequent turning of the patient and proper positioning, since it is especially susceptible to skin infections and decubiti. Mouth care should be given at regular intervals. The patient should be encouraged to take adequate fluids by mouth. If fluids are administered parenterally, caution must be exercised, since overloading the vascular system may lead to cardiovascular complications. The patient should be fed and should not be allowed to sit up.

Abdominal distention should be guarded against, since it thins the intestinal wall and may contribute to hemorrhage or perforation of intestinal ulcers. Small low enemas may be given and glycerin suppositories or mineral oil to avoid constipation. All stools should be examined for evidence of blood, and any bright blood must be reported at once. Specimens may be sent to the laboratory for examination for occult blood. The patient should be observed for bladder distention and retention of urine, and catheterization may be necessary. During the acute stage the patient is drowsy and lethargic, and incontinence may occur.

The patient should be in quiet, pleasant surroundings and visitors reduced to a minimum. Since mental confusion and delirium may occur, the patient should be protected from injury. Careful observation of the patient at all times is important. Chills, abdominal pain, increase in pulse rate, and chest pain may foretell serious complications, and the physician should be notified without delay. Perforation gives rise to sudden momentary abdominal pain and then ceases. Therefore, the nurse should be alert to the seriousness of any slight abdominal pain.

Prevention and control

All cases of typhoid fever must be reported, epidemiologic investigation made, and the source of the disease thoroughly investigated. All family contacts should be examined and immunized and should not be employed as food handlers. Patients convalescing should be kept under observation for a sufficient time to determine complete recovery.

Prevention of typhoid fever depends on control of factors that cause the disease, that is, control of water supplies, proper disposal of excreta, pasteurization of milk, identification and control of typhoid carriers, public education, and inoculation of persons planning foreign travel. The administration of typhoid vaccine has been one of the most important factors in the control of typhoid fever. In the twenty-nine countries supporting the World Health Organization's surveillance program of *Salmonella,* there are indications of a decrease in the incidence of *Salmonella* causing typhoid and *paratyphoid fevers,* but an increase in all other *Salmonella.*

24
PARATYPHOID FEVER

Etiology

Paratyphoid fever is caused by any one of three types of *Salmonella* organisms. *Salmonella paratyphi A* is caused by *Salmonella paratyphi; Salmonella paratyphi B* is caused by *Salmonella schottmülleri;* and *Salmonella paratyphi C* is caused by *Salmonella hirschfeldii.* The first of these organisms was identified in 1896, which was also the first time that the name "paratyphoid fever" was used.

Epidemiology

Paratyphoid fever resembles typhoid fever, but is milder in its symptoms and shorter in duration.

Paratyphoid fever is less likely to be caused by contaminated water supplies but more likely to be caused by prepared foods, including meat pies, synthetic milk and cream products, and shellfish. There is a greater danger of missed or undiagnosed cases because frequently it resembles food infection. The reservoir of infection is man, and the causative organism is discharged in the feces.

In 1971, the Public Health Section, Health and Welfare Division, Statistics Canada reported twenty-four cases. In 1972, fifty-three cases were reported by Statistics Canada; while in 1973 forty-six cases were reported. During 1974, sixty-nine cases were reported in Canada. Paratyphoid fever is not a Specified Notifiable Disease in the United States, so no statistics are available.

Incubation period

The incubation period varies between one and ten days.

Clinical manifestations

The onset of paratyphoid fever may be abrupt, with chills, headache, aching, vomiting, diarrhea, abdominal discomfort, bronchitis, and elevation of temperature. The lymphatic tissue throughout the entire intestinal tract is involved, and hemorrhage and perforation is a possibility. The temperature reaches its peak more quickly than in typhoid fever but is characterized by similar remissions. The pulse may be irregular and slow.

The diagnosis, treatment, and nursing care in paratyphoid fever are the same as those in typhoid fever. Preventive and control measures are identical with those for typhoid fever.

25

ANTHRAX

Anthrax has existed for centuries, being described by Hippocrates about 300 B.C. It is primarily a disease of domestic animals such as cattle, sheep, goats, horses, and swine, but it is easily communicated to man. Wild animals including deer, rabbits, and bears may become infected. The cause of the disease was unknown until 1877, when Koch and Pasteur identified the specific bacteria and the cause of anthrax. In 1881 Pasteur applied the principle of vaccination when he inoculated fifty sheep with anthrax vaccine. The original pasteurian vaccine has been replaced by a nonencapsulated spore vaccine that has many advantages over the original pasteurian vaccine.

Etiology

Anthrax, an acute infectious disease, is caused by the *Bacillus anthracis,* a gram-positive, nonmotile, encapsulated bacterium. The somewhat large organism may occur singly or in short chains. The specific bacterium is both aerobic and anaerobic, and in the presence of oxygen it forms spores. The spores are not formed while the organism is in the body of the animal, but germination does occur. When the organism leaves the body and is exposed to air, sporulation occurs.

The *Bacillus anthracis* persists in the soil for years, and in areas where the disease is endemic the spores may be disseminated over wide areas. Animals grazing over contaminated areas ingest the organism with the forage. By-products of infected animals such as bone meal may also transmit the disease.

The causative organism in vegetative form is readily destroyed within the host, but outside the body the spores are resistant to the usual disinfectants, drying, and heat. As with all spores, moist heat in the form of autoclaving is the most dependable method of destruction.

Epidemiology

Anthrax is an acute infectious disease transmitted to man. The disease in humans has been known as "woolsorters' disease," "ragpickers' disease," and "Mal de Trieurs de Laine." Other names given to the disease are malignant pustule and malignant edema. The disease is, essentially, an occupational disease confined to those persons who handle animals and animal products such as, hair, wool, and hides. Veterinarians, farmers, and slaughterhouse workers are at risk from handling infected animals.

Periodic epidemics of the disease occur in various areas of the world, including the United States and Canada.

Human anthrax is endemic in Iran, where poor socioeconomic factors and primitive methods of handling wool, leather, meat, and bones exist. Because of poverty, people are forced to eat diseased animals, and infection frequently occurs from handling infected animals. The United States Department of Health, Education, and Welfare reported five cases in 1971, two cases in 1972, and two cases in 1973. In Canada between 1971 and 1974 no cases were reported by Statistics Canada. In the U. S. the reported death rate between 1960 and 1969 from this disease was one person. During this same period no deaths from this disease occurred in Canada.

Although reporting is required in the United States, Canada, and most other countries, it is possible that many cases occur in remote rural areas of some countries where doctors or transportation facilities do not exist. It has been estimated by Dubos that from 20,000 to 100,000 cases occur annually in the world.[1] There is also evidence that subclinical infections exist.

Transmission

Three routes of infection have been identified: cutaneous anthrax, inhalation anthrax, and gastrointestinal anthrax.

The cutaneous form of the disease is transmitted by handling contaminated animal hair, hides, and wool. It may also be contracted from infected animal tissues or manufactured products such as shaving brushes and bone meal. Pulmonary anthrax results from inhaling spores, whereas the gastrointestinal form is the result of ingestion of contaminated, improperly cooked meat or bones. The most common route of infection is through wounds or abrasions of the skin—the cutaneous route.

Incubation period

The average incubation period for anthrax is two to four days, but it may be as long as seven days.

Clinical manifestations

Nearly all cases of anthrax in man are of the cutaneous type and generally follow an injury of the skin. The disease begins with the appearance of a red macule with edema. After one to four days, central vesiculation occurs, and after rupture a black necrotic indurated lesion exists. In about three weeks the crust separates, and the area gradually fills with granulation tissue leaving a scar. In some cases severe edema may be the only symptom, and if it affects the mouth and larynx, suffocation and death may occur.

The cutaneous lesions of anthrax are not painful, but tenderness of the regional lymph nodes is common. Constitutional symptoms such as elevation of temperature and leukocytosis may be present.

Pulmonary anthrax is rare, but it occasionally occurs. The spores and bacilli are inhaled into the lungs, causing severe pulmonary edema, hemorrhage, pneumonia, and death. Symptoms include malaise, cough, high elevation of temperature, increased respiratory rate, stridor, diaphoresis, and myalgia. Septicemia, pleural effusion, and meningitis may complicate the infection.

Gastrointestinal anthrax is rare. It results from improperly cooked infected meat and bones. A large pustule develops, usually in the terminal ileum, with necrosis, edema, and hemorrhage. The edema may be severe enough to cause an obstruction of the bowel.[3]

Diagnosis

The diagnosis of cutaneous anthrax is made from stained smears. Material should be taken from beneath an unopened vesicle. After necrosis occurs it may be difficult to isolate the organism. Cultures and inoculation of mice or guinea pigs may be done to confirm diagnosis. Diagnosis of pulmonary anthrax is more difficult, but smears of blood, sputum, or spinal fluid may be used to identify the organism.

Treatment

The drug of choice in the treatment of anthrax is procaine penicillin. Tetracycline or oxytetracycline has been reported to give good results.[2]

Nursing care

The nursing care of the anthrax patient requires extreme precautions. Because of the presence of spores, strict medical asepsis must be carried out. Dressings from lesions must be wrapped in paper and burned immediately. The nurse may use gloves. All nondisposable equipment, including bed linens, gowns, and towels, must be autoclaved prior to laundering. Feces, urine, sputum, and other excreta should be disinfected at once to prevent the formation of spores. Patients should remain isolated until lesions are clean and bacteriologically negative for *Bacillus anthracis*.

Prevention and control

The use of human anthrax vaccine has been reported to give good results among persons in high-risk occupations. Prevention of the disease among animals falls within the scope of veterinary medicine and is necessary to prevent the disease in man.

Cases of anthrax should be reported and the patients isolated. Concurrent and terminal disinfection should be carried out. Autoclaving or burning should be utilized to assure the destruction of spores. Epidemiologic investigation of all human cases to determine the source and prevent further spread is indicated. International control prohibits the importation of bone meal unless it is properly sterilized. The sterilization of animal products used by industry and the elimination of environmental industrial hazards are frequently augmented through consultant and advisory service from state departments of industrial hygiene.

REFERENCES

1. Dubos, Rene J., and Hirsch, James G., editors: Bacterial and mycotic infections of man, ed. 4, Philadelphia, 1965, J. B. Lippincott Co.
2. Modell, Walter, editor: Drugs of choice, 1974-1975, St. Louis, 1974, The C. V. Mosby Co.
3. Kohout, Elfriede, Sehat, Abolghassen, and Ashraf, Mansur: Anthrax; a continuous problem in southwest Iran, Am. J. Med. Sci. 247:565-573, May, 1964.

26

BOTULISM (FOOD POISONING)

Botulism is not an infectious or a communicable disease but a poisoning caused by the ingestion of a neuroparalytic toxin. Fortunately the disease is rare, but its occurrence is dangerous and tragic.

Etiology

The neuroparalytic toxin is produced by *Clostridium botulinum.* The organism belongs to the genus *Clostridium.* In addition to botulism the genus includes the organism that causes tetanus and those that cause gas gangrene.

Clostridium botulinum, the cause of food poisoning, is a gram-negative, anaerobic, spore-forming rod. The toxin is the most deadly of poisons—the mere tasting of foods containing it has been known to cause death. A mere ½ pound of toxin could wipe out the population of the world. The large oval spore located near the end of the rod gives it a swollen appearance. There are two species of the botulinum organism that produce toxins, *Clostridium parabotulinum* and *Clostridium botulinum.* Both species have been divided into types designated A, B, C, D, E, and F, according to the specific toxin that they produce. Types A and F cause most intoxications in man, and only occasionally type B. This demonstrates an individual susceptibility in man to the different types of toxin. Mortality rates are closely related to the specific type of toxin. Types C, D, and E rarely affect man.

In nature the *Clostridium botulinum* organism is found in the soil, most frequently in virgin soils. It is also found in vegetable matter. The organism is not present in human feces but has been found in the feces of domestic animals where the disease is enzootic.[1]

Epidemiology

Botulism was first recognized in Germany about 200 years ago, where it was known as "sausage poisoning." It was caused by the ingestion of large blood sausages that had been improperly smoked and stored too long before consumption. In 1897 Von Ermengen, a Belgium bacteriologist, identified the causative organism. The disease occurs sporadically on a worldwide basis. In the past, commercially processed foods, smoked or salted fish, ham, and spiced or potted meats have been responsible for outbreaks of the disease. Because of improved processing methods, most outbreaks now result from home canning. Vegetables, including string beans, corn, and peas, have frequently been incriminated.

In 1970, twelve cases of diagnosed botulism were reported in the United States. In 1971, the Public Health Section, Health and Welfare Division, Statistics Canada reported ten cases. During this same period twenty-five cases were reported by the U. S. Department of Health, Education, and Welfare. In 1972, nine cases were reported in Canada, and twenty-two cases in the U. S. In 1973 Statistics Canada reported seven cases, while the U. S. had a total of thirty-four cases. During 1974, nine cases were reported by Statistics Canada. During the first twenty-five weeks of 1974, twenty-five cases were reported by the U. S. Communicable Disease Center. In the U. S. the reported deaths between 1960 and 1969 for this disease totaled seventy-one. No statistics for deaths in Canada during this same period are available.

There is no natural immunity to the poisoning, and immunity does not follow one attack. All ages, races, or economic groups may be attacked.

Incubation period

The incubation period varies from less than twenty-four hours to several days after ingestion of food containing the toxin. The toxin is so lethal that a minute amount of food containing the toxin may cause early death.

Clinical manifestations

The poisoning begins with nausea and vomiting, followed by abdominal distention and discomfort. Diarrhea rarely occurs, but complete constipation is common. Within twelve to twenty-four hours nerve paralysis begins to develop with fuzzy, dim, and double vision. Botulism toxin blocks the myoneural junctions of the nerves so that paralysis occurs. The paralysis progresses downward from the eyes. There is ptosis of the eyelids and difficulty in swallowing and speaking. The gait is unsteady and there is weakness of the extremities. Symptoms progress to respiratory and cardiac paralysis and death. In case of recovery, residual paralysis may continue for several months. The prognosis is closely related to the diagnostic ability of the physician and the speed with which treatment is secured.

Diagnosis

The diagnosis is made by identifying the toxin in the patient's serum, isolating the micro-organism, and identifying the toxin in the food ingested by the patient.

Treatment

The *Clostridium botulinum* does not invade the tissues, but the toxin is absorbed and reaches the bloodstream through the upper gastrointestinal tract. The toxin may be activated in the presence of acid, but it becomes unstable in the presence of alkaline conditions. The amount of toxin that may be absorbed through the stomach wall depends on the resistance of the toxin to stomach acid. If medical treatment is secured early, lavage with a solution of sodium bicarbonate to empty the stomach is indicated.

After a negative skin sensitivity test, 50,000 units of bivalent botulinus antitoxin (A and B types) or polyvalent botulinus antitoxin (A, B, and E types) are administered intravenously in 1000 ml. of 5% glucose in saline solution. Epinephrine should be readily available in case of anaphylactoid reaction.

In the presence of pharyngeal paralysis nothing is given by mouth, and the patient is maintained on intravenous fluids. If paralysis persists, feeding by gavage may be given. Mild sedation is given to relieve anxiety and a broad-spectrum antibiotic to combat pneumonitis is administered. A respirator such as the Bird should be available in case of respiratory distress. Small saline enemas may be given to relieve the severe constipation.

Nursing care

The patient is placed on absolute bed rest. Isolation and medical asepsis are unnecessary. All nursing care procedures such as turning or changing bed linens are eliminated. The laryngeal paralysis allows saliva to collect in the mouth and throat, and unless removed, it may be aspirated and cause pneumonia. The patient must not be left alone, and absolute quiet should be maintained. The patient does not lose consciousness, and persons who are near him should guard their conversation.

Prophylaxis

Persons who have eaten the incriminating food and are asymptomatic may be given botulinus antitoxin intramuscularly. Pentavalent (A, B, C, D, and E types) botulinum toxoid, aluminum phosphate absorbed for human immunization, is available from the National Communicable Disease Center, Atlanta, Georgia.

Prevention and control

All cases of botulism or suspected cases should be reported, and an investigation should be made to determine the source of the poisoning. All persons who may have been poisoned should be located for prophylactic treatment. Education of housewives concerning proper canning and refrigeration methods and signs that may indicate food spoilage should be provided.

REFERENCE

1. Dubos, Rene J., and Hirsch, James G., editors: Bacterial and mycotic infections of man, ed. 4, Philadelphia, 1965, J. B. Lippincott Co.

SECTION THREE

Viral diseases

CHARACTERISTICS OF VIRUSES

Viruses are ultramicroscopic intracellular parasites that invade plants, insects, and animals including man. They also invade bacterial cells, where they are known as bacteriophages.

It is believed that viruses may have always existed but were not recognized as infectious parasites until 1898. The first virus to be discovered as the cause of disease in humans occurred in 1902, when it was identified as the cause of yellow fever.

Virology, the study of viruses and viral diseases, belongs to the twentieth century. The electron microscope has made it possible to visualize and identify very small viruses, and new laboratory technics such as tissue culture have given impetus to research in viruses and diseases caused by them. Although much is known about viruses, there is a great deal that remains unknown.

Many viruses are selective and will penetrate and multiply only in a suitable host. However, in the laboratory some have become adapted to living under conditions other than their preferred living host. As long as the virus remains outside the cell (extracellular), it is unable to perform any metabolic activities; however, in the presence of a suitable host it has the power to attach itself to the living cell and to penetrate the cell. When the virus gains entrance to the cell, it begins the process of intracellular multiplication. When the virus invades the cell, the normal activities of the cell are interrupted and the virus utilizes the normal cell metabolism for the materials necessary to manufacture new virus material.

All viruses consist of an inner core containing a single nucleic acid that is identified as deoxyribonucleic acid (DNA) or ribonucleic acid (RNA), which is surrounded by a protein coating. The viruses that cause disease in man contain either DNA or RNA, whereas plant viruses contain only RNA. It is the nucleic acid that is infectious and not the protein coating.

Viruses vary in shape but follow a fairly consistent gradation in size. The largest viruses are the cause of several diseases, including psittacosis and lymphogranuloma, whereas poliomyelitis is caused by one of the smallest viruses. Viruses also vary in their ability to survive outside the body. Some are easily destroyed by ordinary disinfectants and heat, whereas others, such as the smallpox virus, survive drying and remain viable for several days. The hepatitis virus may remain viable for months and requires autoclaving for its destruction. Hepatitis is occasionally transmitted to a recipient of blood in which the living virus has remained viable for many weeks.

Viral diseases are transmitted by direct and indirect contact. Some, such as yellow fever, result from inoculation by an insect vector, others result from droplet infection as in measles, and some result from contamination by body excretions, saliva, and feces.

Diseases caused by viruses are usually self-limiting, and the sulfonamide and antibiotic agents do not alter the course of the diseases caused by small viruses. Some large viruses may be treated satisfactorily with broadspectrum antibiotics. Gamma globulin may provide passive immunity in some diseases, but it does not kill the virus. In some viral diseases such as measles one attack renders the individual immune to further attacks of the same disease. Through tissue culture methods and the process of virus adaptation, mutants of selected viruses having low virulence and stability have been produced that are now used to produce vaccines for active immunity in a number of viral diseases.

CLASSIFICATION OF VIRUSES

The best method for classifying viruses has not been completely resolved. Therefore, several methods are currently in use. A large number of viruses have been identified, and others are gradually being added to the list; consequently, in addition to major groups there are subgroups and in some situations, intergroup classification. As new viruses are isolated and identified, it is likely that further changes in classification will occur. Table 8 gives a rather general classification of viruses, with some of the diseases caused by them, together with the kind of nucleic acid responsible for the infectious process.

Table 8. Modified classification of viruses that cause diseases in man

Virus group	*Nucleic acid*	*Diseases*
1. Enterovirus Group		
a. Poliovirus	RNA	Poliomyelitis (3 serotypes)
b. Coxsackie virus A and B	RNA	Causes a number of febrile disorders of alimentary tract
c. ECHO virus	RNA	Infantile diarrhea, aseptic meningitis, gastroenteritis, and a number of febrile disorders, some with a rash
2. Rhinovirus	RNA	Common cold
3. Reovirus Group	RNA	Febrile disorders of respiratory and gastrointestinal tracts
4. Arborvirus Group B	RNA	Yellow fever and St. Louis encephalitis
Groups A and C and other small groups	RNA	Causes a number of diseases in humans
5. Myxovirus Group I	RNA	Influenza types A, B, and C
Group II	RNA	Mumps, Newcastle disease, parainfluenza 1, 2, 3, and 4, measles, and respiratory syncytial
6. Papovavirus Group	DNA	Papilloma (wart)
7. Adenovirus Group	DNA	Specific diseases undetermined
8. Herpesvirus	DNA	Herpes simplex and herpes zoster (human)
9. Poxvirus Group	DNA	Variola, vaccinia, and a number of unclassified important diseases, including rubella, rabies, and infectious hepatitis

27

CHICKENPOX (VARICELLA)

Etiology

Chickenpox is a usually mild, afebrile, highly communicable, annoying disease caused by a filtrable virus. Evidence supported by several researchers indicates that the virus causing chickenpox and herpes zoster are closely related and probably are the same herpes virus. The disease is characterized by a skin rash appearing in crops, which pass through a series of successive stages including the macule, papule, vesicle, and finally the crust. The prodromal period is short and may be completely unnoticed, the rash being the first indication of the disease.

Epidemiology

Chickenpox exists in all countries of the world. For many years chickenpox and smallpox were believed to be the same disease, and not until the middle of the nineteenth century were they identified as separate disease entities. The disease usually occurs as epidemics at intervals of several years, but it does not appear to have a cyclic pattern. This disease is not notifiable in Canada and was not notifiable in the U. S. until 1972. In 1972 164,114 cases were reported, while in 1973, the total rose to 182,927 cases.

Age and seasonal factors

Chickenpox is a mild disease of young children, although it may occur as severe cases in adults. Most children have acquired the disease before 8 years of age, with the greatest incidence occurring during the preschool years. The disease may occur at any age but is considered rare in adults. Most infants appear to have a passive immunity; however, the disease is not uncommon in infants, even when the mother has a history of chickenpox. Since chickenpox occurs during early childhood and frequently in a mild form, many adults are unable to verify a history of the disease.

The seasonal incidence varies among different environmental regions. In the colder climates the disease occurs during the winter and spring months, whereas in temperate climates epidemics may begin during the fall months, continuing through the winter and spring.

Transmission

The primary method of transmission is by direct or indirect contact. It is an airborne droplet infection. Transmission may occur one day prior to the appearance of the rash and after the first vesicles appear. After crusting of the final crop of lesions the disease is not considered infectious. In some instances transmission may result from indirect contact with articles freshly soiled by discharges from skin lesions or nose and throat secretions, and dissemination may result by way of air currents.

Communicability period

One day before onset and six days after macules appear.

Incubation period

The incubation period is from fourteen to sixteen days, and rarely the period may be longer than twenty-one days.

Clinical manifestations

The prodromal period is short, usually not longer than twenty-four hours, but in adults forty-eight hours is not uncommon. During this period there is general malaise, headache, vague myalgia, slight elevation of temperature to 102° F, and anorexia. The height of the temperature may vary, depending on the extent of the rash. In children the first indication of the disease may be the rash. The skin rash occurs in successive crops over a period of about five days; however, it is possible for new lesions to appear for as long as seven to twelve days. Each lesion passes through the stage of macule, papule, vesicle, and crust in rapid succession, so that all types of lesions may be present simultaneously. The rash tends to concentrate on the trunk first, then the neck, face, and proximal extremities, but to a limited extent on the palms of the hands and soles of the feet. The number of crops of lesions may vary from one to four or five. Vesicles also occur on the mucous membrane of the mouth and throat, where they rupture and disappear quickly. During the vesicular stage, pruritus is present, and scratching may result in infection and possible scarring. The disease is considered communicable until all lesions are crusted. Scabs fall off in about seven to fourteen days. Accompanying these manifestations is generalized lymphadenopathy.

Diagnosis and differential diagnosis

The diagnosis of chickenpox is considered in general to be a comparatively easy matter and is based on the clinical characteristics of the skin rash and history of exposure. Laboratory diagnosis may be made by tissue culture of vesicle fluid taken from a lesion during the first three days of the rash.

A problem of differential diagnosis concerns the individual who is partially immune to smallpox. Such individuals may have a mild case of smallpox that is misdiagnosed as chickenpox, resulting in outbreaks of smallpox.[1] Other diseases that enter into the problem of differential diagnosis include impetigo, various forms of urticaria, scabies, and herpes zoster.

Treatment (symptomatic)

There is no specific treatment for chickenpox. The disease is self-limiting, and treatment is based on symptoms. An antipruritic lotion may be used if the itching is severe. Mild sedation may be necessary to relieve itching. Antipyretic agents may be administered to lower fever. The possibility of adverse reactions from the use of steroids has been reported, either when used as therapy or when an individual is undergoing steroid therapy and contracts chickenpox. If secondary infections occur, antibiotics or chemotherapy may be given.

Secondary cases of chickenpox may be more severe than primary cases, and gamma globulin has been administered to exposed contacts to modify the disease. The duration of the incubation period is not affected by the use of gamma globulin.[2]

Complications

Staphylococcal or streptococcal infection may occur as secondary infection, and although such infections may be superficial, generalized conditions may result. Erysipelas and abscesses may also occur. Serious complications are rare because of the use of sulfonamide and antibiotic agents when indicated.

Nursing care

In the absence of serious complications, a patient with chickenpox is rarely admitted to the hospital. During the acute stage, bed rest is indicated with adequate hydration. Cool sponge baths and limiting the use of soap may be soothing. Dress the patient in loose clothing. Application of antipruritic agents to relieve itching may provide comfort. Diet is generally offered as tolerated. If lesions have occurred in the mouth, the patient will require frequent mouth care. If the patient is admitted to the hospital, he should be isolated until all lesions have crusted. A small child may need to be restrained to prevent scratching lesions and causing infection. Keep the child's fingernails short and clean. In the case of infants, in order to limit the possibility of infection, special care should be given to the anogenital area, where lesions may be present. Older patients will need to have their fears allayed regarding scarring. Postcrust scarring is rare.

Immunity

There is no active immunity available, and no passive immunity for the healthy child. For the ill child human immune serum globulin (ISG) or zoster-immune globulin (ZIG) may be given. There is no test for immunity.

Prevention and control

There are no preventive measures for chickenpox other than avoiding exposure if possible. Although procedures may vary, reporting is generally not required except in the case of adults. Children with the disease are excluded from school for seven days from the appearance of the rash. The expectant mother should avoid contact with this disease. Congenital varicella is usually fatal; however, infection of the small infant, contracted after birth, is likely to be very mild.

REFERENCES

1. Horsfall, Frank L., and Tamm, Igor, editors: Viral and rickettsial infections of man, ed. 4, Philadelphia, 1965, J. B. Lippincott Co.
2. Ross, Aaron H.: Modification of chickenpox in family contacts by administration of gamma globulin, N. Eng. J. Med. **267**: 369-376, Aug. 23, 1962.

28

INFECTIOUS MONONUCLEOSIS (GLANDULAR FEVER)

Etiology

Infectious mononucleosis, known as "Pfeiffer's disease," "glandular fever," or the "kissing disease" is an acute or subacute infectious self-limiting disease. However, it has recently been recognized as more than an insignificant condition of unknown etiology—it is an acute disease caused by the Epstein-Barr virus that presents a unique clinical picture. The wide variation of symptoms has led some to believe that there may be more than one form of the disease.

Epidemiology

Infectious mononucleosis most often occurs as sporadic cases or may be endemic. The disease has been recognized in Europe for many decades and is now reported throughout the world. The exact incidence is unknown, since no individual reports are required in most states and countries. It is believed that many subclinical cases occur in which no diagnosis is made or in which diagnosis is inconclusive. The disease may exist in many countries of the world, but it is overshadowed by more common communicable diseases. It is not a notifiable disease in either the United States or Canada. However in 1972, thirty-five states optionally reported 14,178 cases to the U. S. Communicable Disease Center. In 1973, thirty-two states reported 12,833 cases.

Age, sex, and seasonal factors

The disease may occur at any age, but it is uncommon in children under 1 year of age. Hoagland found in a study of 200 cases that all but two were under 30 years of age.[2] The disease has a prolonged course, and has a predilection for the younger generation—15 to 30 years of age. The peak occurrence is at 20 years of age.

Certain groups of individuals appear to be at greater risk than the general population. It has been recognized for some time that hospital personnel, particularly physicians and nurses, are at risk. Outbreaks of the disease occur with increased frequency where young people live together such as dormitories and communes.

Specific information as to racial and sex factors is somewhat lacking, but the disease seems to affect both sexes equally.

The disease may occur at any time of the year, but it is reported to be more prevalent in early summer.

Transmission

The precise method of transmission is unknown. The best evidence points to direct oral contact, such as in kissing, as a possible method, resulting in a salivary interchange—hence the name "kissing disease." The practice of passing a soft-drink bottle from person to person where there is an exchange of saliva is a possible method of transmission. It has also been suggested that a carrier state exists in healthy persons, and that the virus can be transmitted in blood transfusions. However, this has rarely been reported.

Incubation period

Opinions are not uniform concerning the incubation period. Some evidence indicates that the incubation period in children may be less than fourteen days, whereas in the adult it may be from thirty-three to forty-nine days.[2] There appears to be an average incubation period of four to fourteen days. It doesn't seem to be a highly contagious disease and cross-infections in hospitals have been strikingly absent.

Clinical manifestations

Three stages of symptoms have been identified: prodromal period (onset)—seven to nine days, period of "full blown" disease, and convalescent period. The clinical symptoms nearly always present in infectious mononucleosis are fever, sore throat, and enlarged lymph nodes. The onset, or "prodromal period," is insidious, lasting a few days. The patient experiences general malaise for about two days prior to a gradually developing fever, reaching 100° to 102° F, headache, chills, sore throat, increase in malaise, fatigue of general onset, and nausea. Photophobia may occur. All symptoms are present by the fourth day.

The enlarging of the cervical, axillary, and inguinal lymph nodes, signal the beginning stage of the "full blown" disease, which lasts from the fifth to the twentieth day. Lymph nodes in the neck occasionally enlarge sufficiently to cause a condition similar to the "bull neck" seen in diphtheria. By the second week mild jaundice occurs in about 10% of patients. The liver may also be enlarged, and liver involvement may show up in abnormal liver function studies. Hepatitis, with or without jaundice, may be present. About 75% of the patients have some degree of splenomegaly. Supraocular edema frequently occurs and gives the patient an Oriental appearance. Sagging and puffiness of the eyelids may be noted in about 50% of patients, but this disappears in three to four days. The sore throat has a characteristic appearance. On examination, the throat is mildly congested, and there is a thick, pearly white membrane on the tonsils that is firmly adherent to the underlying structures. The membrane does not spread or undergo necrotic changes. Minute petechiae are spread about the border of the hard and soft palates, but in general are grouped in the midline. The petechiae appear near the end of the first week, and disappear in two or three days. Tonsillar ulceration may occur. From 10% to 15% of patients may develop a mild skin rash that is characteristic of rubella.

The third stage of symptoms, the convalescent period, is usually protracted, and is associated with some degree of prostration. The lymphadenopathy, fever, and other physical signs gradually subside, and the blood picture returns to normal. Convalescence may require as long as three months. Symptoms may reappear during this period.

Some 10% to 15% of the patients may have ECG evidence of myocardial involvement. Neurological complications are rare and vary from encephalitis to ascending polyneuritis. Rarely, there may be hemolytic anemia, spontaneous splenic rupture, and respiratory obstruction. True rubelliform rash of infectious mononucleosis is rare, but urticarial drug rashes are frequent, due to antibiotics being used in the treatment of the sore throat.

Diagnosis

Laboratory examinations are not always conclusive, but they do provide assistance in diagnosis.

Blood count. By the end of the first week there is an increase in the leukocytes count of between 15,000 and 30,000 per cubic millimeter of blood. A large number of lymphocytes are present. Lymphocytes normally constitute 25% to 30% of the leukocytes, but their number may rise to 60% or more of the total count. Atypical lymphocytes are present.

Serological examination. A serological examination shows high titers of agglutinins against sheep red blood cells. Titers measured in normal persons are usually 1:28. Titers measured in patients with infectious mononucleosis rise to 1:224 or higher. The laboratory examination for this titer is called the Paul Bunnell test. If infectious mononucleosis is present the test will have a positive reaction.

Treatment

There is no specific treatment for infectious mononucleosis. Treatment is symptomatic and supportive. In severe cases steroid therapy has been used, and although it has no effect on the disease process, it tends to shorten the period of hospitalization. In the use of steroid therapy the physician must weigh its value against the hazards involved. Steroids may be indicated in a patient with threatened respiratory obstruction or in a patient with hemolytic anemia.

Antibiotics do not affect the course of this disease, but they may be used to fight secondary infections such as "strep throat."

If it is necessary to reduce the fever, aspirin seems to be the drug of choice. Bed rest is recommended during the acute febrile stage.

Complications

Complications from infectious mononucleosis are rare. Because most of the subjective manifestations and physical signs are mild or moderate, the outlook in this disease is good. Infectious mononucleosis seems to be a self-limited disease. Recovery is the rule. Relapses are fairly frequent, but recurrences are rare.

One of the most frequent clinical manifestations is splenomegaly. This enlargement of the spleen increases its vulnerability to injury. Splenic rupture is one of the serious complications, and requires rapid surgical intervention.

Another complication that may necessitate surgery, if severe enough, is extreme pharyngeal hyperplasia. In some patients the pharyngeal inflammation and edema may be severe enough to cause a partial obstruction making breathing difficult and swallowing impossible. For such respiratory distress, a tracheostomy may be performed.

Liver involvement may give rise to acute hepatitis that must then be treated symptomatically.

Nursing care

Many patients with mild attacks of the disease will be treated as outpatients. The hospitalized patient is placed on bed rest, which is continued for two or three days after the temperature returns to normal. Adequate hydration should be maintained, and diet should be soft or as tolerated. Warm saline throat irrigations provide relief from sore throat, and an analgesic may be ordered for relief from discomfort of the enlarged nodes and sore throat. Secretions from the nose and throat should be collected in tissues and cared for the same as in all communicable diseases. Isolation of patients and special handling of dishes and excreta appear to have no value, although some authorities recommend extra care in the handling of nasopharyngeal secretions. Other care is the same as for any patient with a febrile disease.

Prevention and control

There is no known prevention for infectious mononucleosis. Isolation of patients is unnecessary, but precautions should be exercised in the care of nose and throat secretions, and handwashing should follow patient care. Case reporting is generally required only in epidemics.[1]

REFERENCES

1. Gordon, John E., editor: Control of communicable diseases in man, ed. 10, New York, 1965, American Public Health Assn., Inc.
2. Hoagland, Robert J.: Clinical manifestations of infectious mononucleosis; report of 200 cases, Am. J. Med. Sci. **240**:21-29, Jan., 1960.

29

INFLUENZA (EPIDEMIC)

Etiology

Influenza is a persistent viral disease of mankind, causing great economic losses, acute illness, and death. It occurs periodically in epidemics that may vary from small outbreaks to pandemics.

Three types of human influenza viruses, A, B, and C were recognized in 1933, 1940, and 1947 respectively. Only type A is associated with pandemics. The gravity of influenza is usually related to type A epidemics, and less frequently to type B virus. Type C has not been found to be associated with epidemics. In the past forty years influenza pandemics have tended to occur at intervals of approximately ten years, and epidemics of varying intensity have been reported every two to three years.

The influenza pandemic spreads from a single focus of disease. Over the centuries, many, but not all, pandemics have emerged from within the Orient.

Epidemiology

Influenza is always present, with sporadic outbreaks and epidemics occurring in various parts of the world. The number of families of influenza virus are unknown, and the infinite number of antigenic strains is unknown. It is believed that widespread immunity to a particular strain develops over a ten-year period, after which a new antigenic strain arises with the capacity to multiply and infect a nonimmune population.[3] An unknown factor is whether or not these various antigenic strains may not always have been in existence. The appearance of epidemics caused by different strains has not altered the basic clinical or epidemiologic characteristics of influenza A. Serious pandemics such as those of 1918 to 1919 and 1957 to 1958 usually occur in cycles of about thirty to forty years, whereas epidemics characterize the interpandemic years.[1] Epidemics usually reach a peak incidence in about three weeks and run a complete course in three or four weeks. In a matter of a few months, influenza epidemics may spread from one end of the world to another. The spread is greatly encouraged by the increasing speed and proportions of modern intercountry travel. Once implanted in a receptive population, factors such as wet and cold weather, indoor life, common transport aggregations, which intensify the frequency of contacts, may trigger the epidemic wave.

Influenza is not a notifiable disease in either the U. S. or Canada, so no accurate statistics are available. However, in the U. S. in 1970, 3707 deaths were reported to have occurred as a result of influenza. Between 1960 and 1969 41,843 deaths were recorded by the Vital Statistics of the U. S. with an annual death rate of 4184 persons.

Age and seasonal factors

Influenza occurs among all age groups, and attack rates vary widely during different epidemics. Surveys made during the decade of 1940 indicated that the highest attack rate occurred among children 0 to 9 years of age, whereas in 1957 the highest incidence was in persons 15 to 19 years of age. During the Asian influenza pandemic in New York City, among 750,000 persons affected, the highest attack rate was among children.[4] Studies made in countries other than the United States indicate that rates are higher among school-age children. The fact that rates are higher among children than among adults is attributed to their more limited contact with the infectious agent and, therefore, their decreased resistance.

From the standpoint of mortality, certain groups of persons appear to be at greater risk. These include very young persons, aged persons, pregnant women, and persons with chronic debilitating diseases, especially cardiovascular-renal diseases.

Epidemics of influenza usually begin in the fall and extend into the late spring, but they may occur at any time of the year. There appears to be a tendency for major epidemics to occur at cycles of two to three years, with pandemics occurring at longer intervals, approximately every ten years.

Transmission

The reservoir of the virus is man. The transmission of influenza virus is not completely understood. The best evidence is that transmission results from airborne droplet infection from discharges from the nose and throat of the infected person. Contact may be through direct or indirect transmission. The disease is rapidly disseminated where there is crowding, such as in military camps, institutions, and schools.

Incubation period

The usual incubation period is from twenty-four to seventy-two hours.

Communicability period

Although the communicability period is not known, it is possibly during the early and febrile stages.

Clinical manifestations

Regardless of the strain of influenza virus, the symptoms are essentially the same. However, the disease may occur as a mild form or it may be severe.

The onset is invariably sudden with chills, fever, headache, muscle pains, and cough. During the acute phase of uncomplicated influenza, symptoms are largely constitutional with limited physical findings. There is a rapid rise in temperature, varying from 101° to 104° F., and upper respiratory symptoms are usually less severe than in other types of respiratory infections. There may be laryngitis and hoarseness with a hacking type of unproductive cough, but rarely is there a sore throat although some irritation may be noted. In the absence of complications symptoms usually subside in three to five days, but the patient may complain of fatigue and weakness for varying periods after the disease has subsided.[3] If the infection is severe and spreads to the lower respiratory tract, air hunger may develop.

Diagnosis

Diagnosis can usually be made on the basis of clinical symptoms, particularly during epidemics. Sporadic cases may present diagnostic problems, since illnesses characterized by coryza, pharyngitis, bronchitis, and diseases caused by adenoviruses may present symptoms similar to those of influenza.

Diagnosis may be made or confirmed by laboratory isolation of the virus or through serologic examination to determine the presence of antibody. Individuals who have recovered from influenza will have antibodies to the particular virus. A blood sample taken during the early days of the infection will show the presence of these antibodies; however, the particular strain of virus cannot be determined by the serologic test. A second blood sample taken about two weeks later is compared and evaluated in relation to the first test. Horsfall believes that expensive laboratory diagnosis should be reserved for epidemic conditions, subject, of course, to any special condition that might warrant such an examination.[3]

Treatment

There is no specific treatment for uncomplicated influenza. Therapy is based on symptoms. Complete bed rest should be provided for the patient. Patients should be protected from bacterial infections that might complicate the influenza infection. For this reason it is believed that patients should remain at home rather than be hospitalized. Increased fluid intake should be provided, a sedative cough mixture such as elixir of terpin hydrate may be used, and an analgesic such as codeine or aspirin to relieve aching may be indicated. Patients should remain in bed for two to three days after return of the temperature to normal. Antibiotics and sulfonamides may prevent secondary infection.

Complications

Complications resulting from influenza are generally few. Experience has shown that in severe epidemics and pandemics serious and fatal complications do occur. Individuals designated as high risk are most likely to be victims of fatal complications. Among the most frequent complications are influenzal or staphylococcal pneumonia, bronchitis, and bronchiolitis. Patients with chronic disease such as cardiovascular-renal disorders, diabetes mellitus, bronchopulmonary disease, and immunodeficiency, as well as infants, and pregnant women, especially those with a history of rheumatic fever, are considered at risk. All these people should be given priority for protection by vaccination. The "excess mortality" is due almost exclusively to pulmonary bacterial complications, and may represent in the "flu year" as many as six times the number of deaths in the intervening period.

Nursing care

Isolation of patients with influenza is unnecessary, but the exposure of well persons should be avoided. In turn, the patient should be protected from persons with bacterial infections. The patient on bed rest should not be allowed out of bed, and all nursing care should be given. The patient should be in a quiet comfortable room that is free from drafts and has a high humidity. A vaporizer may be used to increase humidity. The bed and sleep clothing should be kept dry to avoid chilling the patient. This is especially important if the patient is receiving an antipyretic such as aspirin, which may cause excessive diaphoresis. Nose and throat secretions should be collected in tissues and burned. Alcohol or tepid sponges may be given to reduce the fever. Frequent oral care and an antiseptic mouthwash will prevent fetid breath odors. Oily sprays and drops should not be used in the nose. The temperature should be taken every two to four hours, depending on the extent of elevation, and pulse and respiratory rates should be taken frequently. Blood pressure should be taken at least once a day and more often if indicated. The patient should be offered and encouraged to increase fluids and given a liquid diet during the acute stage of the disease, with a gradual return to a regular diet. Intake and output should be recorded, and the patient should be carefully observed for changes in pulse or respiratory rates, cyanosis, or productive cough with blood-streaked sputum, which should be reported to the physician immediately. Although most patients have an uneventful recovery, nursing care will be a major factor in preventing complications.

Prevention and control

The main body defense mechanism against influenza viruses is the production of antibodies to various proteins present in the virus, particularly a surface protein, the hemagglutinin, which allows the virus to attach itself to the host cell membrane, thus triggering the infection. The presence of such an antibody repels any new invasion against antigenically modified viruses.

Although intensely studied, the treatment or prevention of influenza through drugs such as interferon or interferon inducers, has not yet reached a level of practicability in the control of the disease. The way to control influenza appears to lie in simulating the natural immune defense mechanisms through the use of safe and potent vaccines prepared with appropriate strains of viruses.

Two types of influenza vaccines are now available: killed concentrated and partially purified for parenteral administration, and live attenuated vaccines for instillation into the upper respiratory pathways. Used wisely, they can give up to 80% protection in the interval between the emergence of new varients of virus. The immunity is short-lived, lasting usually from two to twelve months. Vaccinated persons may get influenza unless vaccination is repeated frequently. The infecting virus strain tends to vary continually, so that a vaccine effective today may be ineffective tomorrow.

The vaccine should be administered early before the influenza season and should be given to all high-risk individuals and to persons engaged in essential services, including hospital personnel. Immunization of the total population is not encouraged at this time.[2] Individual case reports are not required. In case of epidemics, reports are usually mandatory.

World Health Organization (WHO)

The WHO influenza program was established in 1947. This program's prime function consists of rapidly isolating and determining the characteristics of new influenza strains in order to make available for research and production laboratories the strains showing substantial variations from the current strains.

Two WHO internal reference centers for influenza in London, England, and Atlanta, Georgia, and twelve national centers in sixty-one countries are carrying out influenza surveillance activity. The Center for Influenza in Atlanta, in collaboration with the World Influenza Center in London, prepares and distributes diagnostic reagents annually to all national influenza centers to be used as reference. The material includes samples of recent influenza viruses and specific antisera.

One of the major problems to be solved by the WHO influenza program is the interval of two or three months between isolation of the new strain of virus and vaccine production.

Control of influenza in the individual person can be achieved with reasonable success; but control of world spread of the disease is still unattainable.

REFERENCES

1. Davenport, Fred M., and Hennessy, Albert V.: The clinical epidemiology of Asian influenza, Ann. Int. Med. **49**:493-501, March, 1958.
2. Gordon, John E., editor: Control of communicable diseases in man, ed. 10, New York, 1965, American Public Health Assn., Inc.
3. Horsfall, Frank L., and Tamm, Igor, editors: Viral and rickettsial infections of man, ed. 4, Philadelphia, 1965, J. B. Lippincott Co.
4. Rogers, Fred B.: Studies in epidemiology; selected papers of Morris Greenberg, New York, 1965, G. P. Putnam's Sons.

30
THE COMMON COLD

The whole, rather vague, clinical picture known as the "common cold" has been for many decades confused with the somewhat similar manifestations displayed in influenza. These two diseases are often distinguishable from each other only with difficulty. Other names by which a cold is known are: head cold (rhinitis), sore throat (pharyngitis), and chest cold (tracheobronchitis). These names simply indicate the chief location of the infection.

The "common cold," in the traditional sense, is not a disease in itself. It is rather a collection of signs and relatively mild symptoms such as adenopathy, inflammation of the mucous membranes of the nose, pharynx, and bronchial tree, fever, headache, general malaise, copious watery exudate from the nose, muscular pains, sinusitis, lacrimation, conjunctivitis, sneezing, and coughing.

It is now clear from virological studies that we must deal with several viruses. These viruses are so small that they cannot, at the present time, be seen under the microscope, and pass through filters that normally stop bacteria. Scores of viral infections, one hundred or more, cause the spectrum of symptoms we call "the common cold."

However, viruses are not alone in causing cold symptoms. They may be caused by a wide variety of microorganisms ranging from viruses to fungi. Secondary causes such as fatigue, poor nutrition, and chilling of the body may play a part when the virus from another person with a cold has already reached the nasal passageways of its new victim.

Etiology

Here we will concentrate on the "viral" cold. As a result of advanced laboratory procedures, rapid progress is currently being made in the isolation and identification of agents causing cold-like manifestations. Among these agents are members of the myxovirus group, including classic influenza and mumps, and the parainfluenza group, of which at least four distinct groups have been isolated.

The virus apparently responsible for some of the most severe respiratory illnesses in infants and small children is the respiratory syncytical virus (RS).

The names of differentiated groups of viruses associated with cold-like diseases of the respiratory tract are rhinoviruses, coryzaviruses, reoviruses, ECHO viruses (ECHO virus 28 has now been isolated from a number of cases of the so-called common cold), and adenoviruses.

Age, race, and seasonal factors

Colds are always with us, with seasonal peaks and multiple epidemics in the fall and winter. Children are more susceptible than adults, with the exception of men and women in the older age groups, or in physically run-down states.

Although there are wide differences in incidence among individuals, and in relation to age, there seems to be no differences in relation to sex or race. The common cold with its complications probably causes a greater number of days of disability than any other medical condition.

Transmission

The organisms are carried in nasal and oral secretions. These secretions inevitably contaminate the atmosphere during talking, laughing, sneezing, coughing, and similar actions that produce droplets and droplet nuclei. Added to this is the spread of oral, nasal, and conjunctival secretions by hands, eating utensils, drinking glasses, careless handling of tissues (handkerchiefs), the use of common towels and drinking cups, kissing, and so forth.

Epidemiology

The common cold is a very prevalent condition with an average of three to four annual colds per person. The majority of colds occur during cold weather, but also at times of temperature changes, such as winter to spring.

Incubation period

Immunity is of very short duration as is the incubation period. Extraneous factors such as fatigue, chilling, emotional upset, exposure to irritating gases or allergies, all of which affect the nasal mucosa, are believed to lower the natural resistance, facilitating invasion by the virus. The period between infection and the beginning of symptoms is from one to three days. Colds are believed to be communicable only at onset, and for the first two or three days of the symptoms.

Pathology

Pathological changes consist of edema of the mucous membranes lining the nose and throat, followed by acute inflammation. The membranes pour out mucus, at first thin and clear, later thick and purulent. The inflammation extends to varying degrees into the sinuses, down the respiratory passages, or up into the ears.

Clinical manifestations

Although there is considerable individual variation in the symptoms, the majority include coughing, sneezing, chills, headache, fever, general malaise, watery eyes, dry scratchy throat followed by copious nasal discharge, and a sense of oppression in the upper chest. None of these symptoms are diagnostic in themselves; together they are a cold. In addition, children are apt to have prostration. The cold usually has a duration between four and fourteen days with the symptoms gradually subsiding. Regardless of treatment, an uncomplicated cold continues to produce a purulent nasal discharge. Often there is a cough with expectoration from ten days to three weeks.

Diagnosis

Diagnosis is usually made from the clinical picture. Frequently the diagnosis is presumptive. The virus causing the cold probably cannot be detected at the present time. No proof of cold antibodies in the blood of those afflicted have been found.

Treatment

Colds, while hard to prevent, are equally hard to get rid of. Treatment is primarily symptomatic. Cold vaccines that would include all the microorganisms causing the common cold may never be developed. Several cold vaccines have been developed, but it must be noted that a vaccine against one virus does not necessarily give protection against colds due to other viruses in the group.

Aside from vaccines, which, although effective, are somewhat limited in their usefulness, there are no known specific measures for curing or preventing this respiratory disease. Antihistamines are frequently used, but they do not cure the disease, they simply alleviate some of the symptoms. Present day antibiotics, such as penicillin, are helpless against viruses. They can however, combat secondary infections caused by bacteria, such as pneumococci or staphylococci. For this reason only are antibiotics frequently used in severe respiratory infections. Fever-reducing medications such as aspirin should only be used with the doctor's advice, as fever is often associated with recovery. To ease the symptoms and to shorten the period of discomfort, the patient should force fluids, eat a well balanced diet in moderate proportions, and get extra rest.

Complications

Although often neglected, infection with respiratory viruses can lead to serious difficulties. The inflammation of the nose and throat presents a favorable place to lodge for pneumococci, streptococci, influenza bacilli, and other organisms. Conditions such as pneumonia, tracheobronchitis, otitis media, sinusitis, and laryngitis may occur. Fever sores may occur but are not a serious complication.

Nursing care

A day or two of bed rest is perhaps the most important aspect of the care, since it restricts activity and controls contact with other persons, thus limiting the spread of the cold. Visitors should be restricted.

Fluids should be encouraged in large amounts. Lubricating oil, cream, or jelly around the nostrils and mouth will help relieve chapping and cracking. The patient should be instructed in the proper technique for discarding tissues soiled with nose and throat secretions. Hand washing must be stressed. If the patient has diaphoresis to any great degree, the bed linen and sleep clothes should be changed frequently to avoid chilling and to promote rest and comfort.

A quiet, comfortable room should be provided, free of drafts, and with a high humidity. The diet should be light during the acute phase of the disease and increased as tolerated.

Observation of any change in symptoms should be reported immediately as it may indicate a developing complication.

Aspirin may be ordered to relieve the initial malaise. Nasal decongestants taken by mouth, inhalation, or as nose drops give temporary relief; however, such measures should be used sparingly in the acute phase and not thereafter as they help to spread the infection into the lower respiratory tract. Antimicrobial drugs are not effective against cold viruses; they are used only to control secondary bacterial infections. Although most patients have an uneventful recovery, nursing care will be a major factor in preventing complications.

Prognosis

The prospect for recovery is usually good, however, colds may reoccur frequently in susceptible individuals if exposed to the infection. Chronic sinusitis and nasal polyps may develop if the person suffers from repeated colds. There are no residual affects in healthy individuals.

Prevention

Complete prevention is unrealistic among the multiple daily contacts each person has. At present, the best prevention is to avoid people with colds—if you can. To expect all people with incipient colds to stay in isolation is unrealistic.

31

MEASLES (RUBEOLA OR RED MEASLES)

Etiology

Measles is caused by a filterable virus presently classified with the myxovirus group. Precise classification remains to be determined. The reservoir of infection is man, and the highly febrile communicable disease is characterized by a maculopapular rash and Koplik spots appearing on the mucous membrane of the mouth.

Epidemiology

In 1971, Statistics Canada reported 7454 cases while the U. S. Department of Statistics reported 75,290 cases. In 1972, 32,275 cases were reported in the U. S. During this same period Canada reported 3136 cases. In 1973, the U. S. had a total of 26,690 cases reported, while Canada reported 10,911 cases. During 1974, 11,932 cases were recorded by Statistics Canada, while in the U. S. 21,726 cases were reported for the same period. Between the years 1960 and 1966 the average yearly death rate in the U. S. was 363 persons; however, between the years 1967 and 1969 the average yearly death rate dropped to forty-nine persons per year. Vital Statistics Canada reported eleven deaths in 1971.

Age and seasonal factors

Measles is primarily a child's disease. However, susceptible adults may contract the disease, although most adults will give a history of having the disease during childhood. Age factors among children vary from country to country, but nearly all children will have acquired the disease by the time they are 5 years of age.

Outbreaks of the disease usually begins late in the winter months, continuing into late spring. Although sporadic cases may occur during the summer months, epidemics are not characteristic of the warm months.

Incubation period

The incubation period is nine to fourteen days, with slight variations. The incubation period is about ten days from exposure to onset of fever, and about fourteen days from exposure to appearance of the rash.

Communicability period

The communicability period is four days before to five days after the rash appears.

Method of transmission

The virus is spread through direct contact and through the air by droplets and contaminated dust. The virus doesn't appear to survive long outside the body.

Clinical manifestations

Measles begins insidiously with signs of a common cold. There is coryza with nasal discharge, conjunctivitis with lacrimation, sneezing, and photophobia and the child may appear lethargic and irritable. These manifestations all appear before the rash erupts. The condition increases in severity with a hacking cough and temperature that reaches from 104° to 105° F. There may be increased respiratory rate and dyspnea. By the third or fourth day of illness, examination of the mouth reveals small pink macules in the back of the mouth. Each macule has a bluish white speck in the center of the areola (Koplik spots). The appearance of the Koplik spots precedes the appearance of the skin rash by about two days. The dusty-red skin rash, which becomes maculopapular, appears first at the back of the ears, on the upper neck near the hair line, and on the forehead. It gradually spreads downward with the greatest concentration on the face and trunk, although the rash may be moderately heavy on the extremities. There is a great tendency for the eruption to coalesce. The rash gradually assumes a brown appearance, and after three or four days it begins to fade on the face and progress downward. A very fine desquamation follows the disappearance of the eruption. By the second or third day of the rash all symptoms have reached their peak, and the child feels very ill. Thereafter the temperature falls rapidly, and all other symptoms begin to disappear so that the child feels comfortable within three to five days.

Diagnosis

The diagnosis of measles usually offers no major problem. A history of exposure and the characteristic Koplik spots, which appear in nearly all cases of measles, simplify the question of diagnosis. Laboratory examination to demonstrate a reduction in the number of leukocytes (leukopenia) may be of diagnostic value. Antibodies appear within two or three days after the development of the rash and reach a peak from two to four weeks later. The measles hemagglutination-inhibition antibody test is rarely used except in case of a questionable diagnosis.

A number of other diseases may present problems of differential diagnosis. These include scarlet fever, rubella, typhus fever, Rocky Mountain spotted fever, and an allergic reaction to drugs. Although all of these diseases are characterized by a rash, each is a separate disease entity, and careful evaluation of the symptoms usually elicits a correct diagnosis.

Treatment (symptomatic)

There is no specific treatment for uncomplicated measles. Treatment is symptomatic and supportive. Bed rest in a comfortable room, dimly lighted if photophobia is present, is indicated for all children with measles. The patient should be kept in bed for the duration of the fever. Fluids should be offered freely and a liquid diet given during the febrile period. Analgesics such as aspirin and a nonnarcotic cough mixture may be ordered; however, they may offer only limited benefit, since the disease is self-limiting.

Authorities agree that sulfonamides, antibiotics, and steroids do not alter the course of uncomplicated measles and that they have no effect in preventing complications. However, if complications have occurred these medications will help combat any infection. In nonimmune young children or children with chronic disease, immune human globulin administered within one week after exposure may prevent or modify the disease. It will be ineffective if given after symptoms develop. Immune serum or gamma globulin may be given to modify the illness and reduce complications.

Complications

Most children recover from measles with no complications. Those that do occur are the result of bacterial infection and are more likely to occur in infants and very young children. Children with a history of otitis media or mastoid infection are more likely to have a recurrence of the infection. Other possible complications include bronchopneumonia, tracheobronchitis, bronchiolitis, and nephritis. Reports indicate that encephalitis or encephalomyelitis, although rare, may occur in a small number of patients. Mortality rates from bacterial complications have been reduced sharply since the introduction of sulfonamide and antibiotic therapy. Complications vary with the severity of the disease. Measles is usually regarded lightly, but it is a potentially serious disease because of the infections that often accompany or follow it.

Nursing care

Most children with measles are cared for at home, and it is recommended that hospitalization should be avoided if possible to prevent exposure to bacterial infection. Whether the child is in the hospital or at home, every effort should be made to prevent exposure to bacterial infection. The patient should be isolated until five to seven days after the appearance of the rash. Medical asepsis and concurrent disinfection should be carried out. Unless care is taken, cross-infection is always a possibility. The room should be comfortably warm, well ventilated, free from drafts, and have increased humidity to relieve the cough. If photophobia is present, bright lights should be avoided, but complete darkness is contraindicated. The light in the room should be dimmed.

Secretions from the respiratory passages should be collected in tissues and burned. Warm compresses or irrigations with 2% boric acid solution or physiologic saline solution may be used to remove secretions about the eyes and relieve irritation resulting from conjunctivitis. Advise the patient to keep the hands away from the eyes. Keep children's nails short. The lips and nares may be kept moist with petroleum jelly. In young children mouthwashes are avoided as a precaution against aspiration into the bronchi or eustachian tubes. A vaporizer will supply moisture and help to thin respiratory secretions. In the case of young children great care should be exercised in placement of the vaporizer so that the child cannot reach it and be burned.

During the exanthem stage of the disease, soap should not be used in bathing the patient. Pruritus may be relieved by sponging with tepid water to which bicarbonate of soda or starch has been added. Tepid water, rather than alcohol, should be used for sponges to reduce fever and itching. Soothing lotions may also be used.

During the febrile period the diet should be liquid, and fluids should be encouraged to prevent dehydration. There should be a gradual return to a normal diet as the child convalesces.

Constipation may be avoided by the use of mild laxatives or small low enemas.

The patient should be observed for any evidence of earache such as rolling the head, pulling the ear, or discharge from the ear. Increase in temperature, cyanosis, dyspnea, croup, or convulsions may foretell possible serious complications and should be reported to the physician without delay.

Measles may cause a temporary upset in the child's normal growth and behavior patterns. A small degree of regression is not unusual in the young child and may be indicated by regression in toilet habits, eating patterns, or overdependence. Such regression is generally only temporary, and efforts should be made to prevent the behavior from becoming fixed. Therefore, severe discipline and calling attention to the behavior should be avoided.

Prevention and control

The only effective means of preventing measles in susceptible children is through immunization with measles vaccine. Gamma globulin may provide a passive immunity or modify the symptoms of the disease. In immune mothers, newborn infants generally have a passive immunity lasting for a few months after birth. Since active immunization is not recommended until 12 months of age, young infants may contract measles. Work has been done in splitting the measles virus and preparing a vaccine using only a fraction of the virus. Trials have indicated that the vaccine may be administered to newborn infants to extend the period of immunity and to protect all infants until live attenuated measles vaccine can be administered.[2]

Two strains of live attenuated measles vaccine are available: the Edmonston B strain and further attenuated Schwarz strain. The Edmonston B strain is prepared in two forms, in chick embryo or in canine kidney cell culture. The latter may be administered to children who are allergic to the protein of eggs. Gamma globulin is administered simultaneously with the Edmonston B vaccine to reduce the severity of reactions that may occur. Reaction to the Schwarz vaccine is comparable to that of the Edmonston B vaccine with gamma globulin. Therefore, gamma globulin is not administered with the Schwarz strain of vaccine.

Efforts to control measles in the community are difficult, since exposure frequently occurs early during the prodromal period before diagnosis has been established. Exposed children should be excluded from school for fourteen days after exposure. Most states and provinces require that cases be reported to the local health department.[1]

REFERENCES

1. Gordon, John E., editor: Control of communicable diseases in man, ed. 10, New York, 1965, American Public Health Assn., Inc.
2. New measles vaccine OK for very young, Am. J. Nurs. **66**:1490-1491, July, 1966.

32

RUBELLA (GERMAN MEASLES)

ACQUIRED RUBELLA

Etiology

Rubella or German measles, is often called three-day measles because even though the disease lasts from one to five days, the rash usually evolves over a three-day period. The disease is caused by a filterable pseudoparamyxovirus not completely classified at this time, but it is believed to be an RNA virus. Present evidence indicates that the virus causing rubella and that causing measles (rubeola) are unrelated, although the rash occurring in both diseases may result from the same or a similar rash agent. It has been proved that rubella may occur in the absence of any rash.

Epidemiology

Rubella is a mild, highly communicable, fairly common disease occurring as sporadic cases and in epidemics. In itself this disease is rarely serious. Distribution of the disease is worldwide, and in some countries fatalities result from it. Epidemics of the disease do not occur in regular cycles but may occur at intervals of three to seven years. The disease is self-limited and rarely produces complications. In 1971, the U. S. Department of Health, Education, and Welfare reported 45,086 cases, while Statistics Canada reported 12,567 cases for the same period. In 1972, 25,507 cases were reported in the U. S., and 2808 cases in Canada. In 1973, Vital Statistics of the United States reported 27,804 cases, while Statistics Canada recorded 3296 cases. During 1974, 11,654 cases were reported to the U. S. Communicable Disease Center, while Statistics Canada recorded 7705 cases. In Canada during 1971, two deaths occurred from this disease. During the ten-year span between 1960 and 1969, 200 deaths occurred in the U. S., while in 1970, eighty-nine persons died from the disease.

The first serious attention given the disease was in 1941, when it was discovered that rubella which occurs during pregnancy produces teratogenic effects in the offspring.

Age and seasonal factors

In the past, rubella has been considered a disease of school-age children, adolescents, and young adults. It rarely occurred in infants, and the incidence among young children was very low. There is evidence that the disease is occurring with greater frequency among younger children.[4]

The disease occurs most commonly in the fall, continuing through the spring months. The disease affects all sexes and races equally.

Communicability period

The disease is communicable during the prodromal period and for seven days after the appearance of the rash. The prodromal period is the interval between the onset of symptoms and the appearance of the characteristic rash. Recent studies have recovered the virus from the pharynx seven days prior to and seven days after development of the rash.

Transmission

The transmission of this disease is probably much the same as for measles. The virus is passed by direct contact or by contaminated dust particles and droplets in the air. These infectious droplets from the nose and throat secretions of the infected person are inhaled. In pregnancy, the rubella virus may cross the placental barrier and affect the fetus.

Incubation period

The incubation period is from fourteen to twenty-one days, but it may be less than fourteen days and longer than twenty-one days. It is usually eighteen days after exposure.

Clinical manifestations

Symptoms and their severity are variable. In some cases development of the erythematous rash may be the first indication of the infection, whereas in other cases enlargement and tenderness of the lymph nodes may be present for as long as seven days prior to the appearance of the rash. In other cases all of the symptoms commonly associated with the disease may be present without evidence of a rash. The postauricular, posterior cervical, and occipital lymph nodes are frequently involved. There may be malaise, coryza, headache, sore throat, mild conjunctivitis, and elevation of temperature. The fever may remain low grade or moderate, ranging from 101° to 104° F. The pale pink macular eruption begins about the hairline, gradually extending downward to the trunk and extremities. The macules are closely grouped together and appear as a scarlet blush that fades on pressure. The rash usually begins to disappear within forty-eight hours and may be completely gone by the third day, thus the name, three-day measles. However, the extent and duration of the eruption may vary from one to five days. With the appearance of the rash, other symptoms begin to disappear, except for the lymphadenopathy, which may continue for several weeks. A very fine desquamation of the skin usually follows the disappearance of the rash. Painful and even swollen joints occur, especially in young women. There are no Koplik's spots nor does the patient suffer with photophobia as in red measles.

Diagnosis

Clinical diagnosis of rubella is not always possible, since a number of other diseases may confuse the clinician. Among these diseases is scarlet fever, mild measles, roseola infantum, and infections caused by the Coxsackie and ECHO viruses, in which rashes may occur.

Opinions differ concerning the precise value of laboratory examinations for the diagnosis of rubella. The neutralizing antibody test is considered the most reliable. As in other diseases referred to, two samples of blood are secured. One sample should be taken as soon after exposure as possible and a second sample taken two or three weeks later. Rubella antibodies may be present by the third day of the rash, and the second test should show a rise in the antibody titer in the presence of rubella infection. It is recommended that neutralizing antibody tests should be performed on all pregnant women.

Treatment

There is no specific treatment for rubella, and therapy is symptomatic. Antipyretic agents such as aspirin may be ordered for fever and antipruritics or antihistaminics for pruritus if present. Bed rest for the duration of the disease may not be necessary for all patients. However, it is mandatory until the fever subsides. Activity should be reduced.

Complications

Arthritis affecting the hips, shoulders, knees, and ankles may accompany rubella. The complication appears to be self-limited, with a duration of three to twenty-eight days. If the patient with rubella complains of joint pain, bed rest is indicated.[3] Severe complications are rare. Encephalitis has been known to occur.

Rubella occurring during the first fourteen weeks of pregnancy results in serious defects in 15% to 20% of the offspring. The risk is 50% if the disease occurs during the first four weeks of pregnancy. It has also been shown that rubella during the first trimester of pregnancy increases the incidence of abortion and stillbirths.[2] Because an attack of rubella in childhood is rarely harmful, and probably confers lifelong immunity, it has been recommended by some that girls be purposely exposed to the disease between 6 and 8 years of age to avoid contracting it during pregnancy later in life. However, vaccination of all children is now the preferred procedure. It has been found that the rubella virus can live in the fetus throughout pregnancy and that the live newborn infant will have congenital rubella.

Nursing care

Most patients with rubella will be seen in the physician's office or in an outpatient clinic, but most cases will never be seen by any physician. Hospitalization is rarely required. If hospitalized, the patient should be isolated and concurrent disinfection carried out. Adequate hydration and a light diet should be provided. Nursing procedures for relief of pruritus and fever are the same as those for measles. Newborn infants with congenital rubella should be isolated and medical asepsis carried out. Because of the mildness of the disease, isolation of patients in the community is usually difficult.

Prevention and control

Vaccination of all children is now the preferred procedure for prevention and control. Immune human gamma globulin may be administered to very young children to modify the disease, but it should be given within four or five days after exposure. A single dose of active attenuated rubella virus vaccine for active immunization against the disease was found to protect between 90% and 95% of susceptible children when they were exposed to German measles. Vaccination of all children between 1 year of age and puberty will assure protection.

Most states, Canada, and some foreign countries require that all cases of rubella be reported to the health department. Isolation is recommended for seven days after development of the rash. Exposed children are not excluded from school, but daily inspection of such children should be made. Children with any elevation of temperature of 0.5° F. or more should be excluded and kept under further observation.[1]

CONGENITAL RUBELLA

Congenital rubella usually results when the mother has acquired rubella in the first three months of pregnancy. However, this is not always the case as congenital rubella can occur when the pregnancy has proceeded as far as twenty weeks. The incidence of affected babies varies with the month of pregnancy in which the mother contracts the disease. In the first month of pregnancy, 50% to 60% of babies will be affected, whereas in the fourth month, 4% to 5% will be affected.

The severity of defects also varies with the time that the mother contracts the disease. The earlier in the pregnancy the mother has rubella the more severely will the fetus be affected. After the twelfth week the defects tend to be less severe, only affecting the eyes and ears. This variation in severity is not absolute, as a single case of a severely affected child has been described when the mother had reached the sixteenth week.

Epidemiology

The National Center for Health Statistics, Vital Statistics of the U. S. reported sixty-eight cases in 1971, forty-two cases in 1972, 40 cases in 1973, and 47 cases during 1974. No statistics are available for Canada.

Characteristics

The triad of cataracts, deafness, and congenital heart disease was first described by Gregg, an Australian ophthalmologist, in 1941. Since then additional features have been noted, especially since reliable virological methods of diagnosis became available in the early 1960s.

In the newborn baby congenital rubella may manifest itself by a birth weight of under 2.5 kg. (5.5 lbs.), a purpuric rash associated with thrombocytopenia, x-ray changes in the long bones, enlarged liver and spleen, and congenital heart disease, usually a patent ductus arteriosus. Eye defects may be present at birth, but may not develop until the child is 2 years of age. Similarly, deafness may not be detected until the child is in its second year. Mental retardation may result from chronic meningo-encephalitis, and in many children the situation is worsened by the lack of secondary stimulation from visual and hearing loss.

Diagnosis

The condition may be suspected by the clinical manifestations and confirmed by the isolation of the rubella virus from a throat swab, cerebrospinal fluid, urine, or lens material obtained at the cataract operation. Isolation of the virus may occur months and even years after birth. This means the patient with congenital rubella remains infectious for a long period of time, unlike acquired rubella when the virus can be recovered for about only ten days after the rash appears.

Prevention

Gamma globulin is used to prevent the effects of congenital rubella, but does not prevent the defects from occurring.

Active immunization with live attenuated rubella virus vaccine was found to protect 90% to 95% of susceptible children when exposed to German measles. If it was given to all children between 1 year of age and puberty we would assure protection against rubella in pregnant women. For women of childbearing age, it is essential to test their serum and immunize those with no rubella antibodies. Such women should not become pregnant in the three months following immunization. Under no circumstances should a pregnant female be vaccinated. In some countries such as England, a program of immunizing mothers in the puerperium following the first pregnancy has been started. If they have no antibodies they are actively immunized with live attenuated vaccine early in the puerperium, and, again, advised not to become pregnant in the following three months.

There are special occupational groups of women who come in contact with rubella, such as nurses, social workers, school teachers, and doctors. These women should have their blood examined for antibodies, and those without antibodies should be immunized at least three months before they become pregnant.

Terminating a pregnancy is not the only way to prevent the birth of a child with congenital rubella; the risk of the child being affected may at the worst be only 60%. With the recent advances in vaccine production, a means of prevention is available, but this requires considerable care in its administration if congenital rubella is to be prevented.

Immunization

Passive immunization: recommended for nonimmune women during the first three months of pregnancy to protect the unborn child. Gamma globulin (antibodies) from the blood of immune persons is used.

Active immunization: live attenuated rubella virus vaccine is used.

Test for immunity: the hemagglutination inhibition test for detection of rubella antibodies is used.

ROSEOLA INFANTUM

This is an acute viral disease often confused with rubella (German measles). The disease consists of a three-day rash that typically occurs in infants about 12 months of age. The baby has a high fever, frequently accompanied by convulsions. The onset is sudden, and the fever remains high for three to four days. The rash appears after the fever and lasts one to three days. Diagnosis is difficult as allergies may confuse the clinician. Many of these infections remain subclinical.

REFERENCES

1. Gordon, John E., editor: Control of communicable diseases in man, ed. 10, New York, 1965, American Public Health Assn., Inc.
2. Krugman, Saul: Rubella—new light on an old disease, Am. J. Nurs. **65**:126-127, Oct., 1965.
3. Yanez, Jose E., Thompson, George R., Mikkelsen, William M., and Bartholomew, Lee E.: Rubella arthritis, Ann. of Int. Med. **64**:772-777, April, 1966.
4. Horsfall, Frank L., and Tamm, Igor, editors: Viral and rickettsial infections of man, ed. 4, Philadelphia, 1965, J. B. Lippincott Co.

33

MUMPS (EPIDEMIC PAROTITIS)

Etiology

Mumps (infectious or contagious parotitis) is caused by a filterable virus of the myxovirus group. The self-limiting, moderately communicable disease affects the parotid gland. If only one gland is affected, it is called "single mumps," and when other glandular tissues become involved, it is called "metastatic mumps." The natural reservoir of infection is man.

Epidemiology

Mumps has been known since the time of Hippocrates. The disease was thought to be caused by bacteria until 1934, when the filterable virus was isolated and determined to be the etiologic agent. The disease is worldwide in occurrence and generally is endemic in most large communities. Epidemic parotitis may occur where there are large concentrations of people. The Vital Statistics of the U. S. reported 124,939 cases in 1971, 74,215 cases in 1972, 69,612 cases in 1973, and 54,895 cases in 1974. During the ten-year span between 1960 and 1969, 394 deaths occurred in the U. S. In Canada, it is not a specified notifiable disease so no statistics are available.

It is estimated that from 30% to 40% of all cases of mumps are inapparent.[2]

Age and seasonal factors

Mumps is classified as a child's disease, but age factors are variable. In an immune mother it is believed that immunity may be transferred to offspring, resulting in passive immunity of the newborn infant. The correctness of this may indicate why the disease rarely occurs during infancy. Although most cases occur in children, nonimmune adults may contract the disease if exposed. Considerable attention is being focused on the pregnant woman who contracts mumps early during pregnancy. Sex differences may vary with the population affected.

The disease is endemic the year round, with most epidemics occurring in the late winter and spring months.

Communicability period

The communicability period is one to six days before the first symptoms appear until swelling disappears.

Transmission

Mumps is transmitted by direct contact and droplet infection. The reservoir is man. There is some evidence that the disease may be spread by droplet nuclei or indirect contact with articles freshly soiled by mouth and throat secretions. The virus may be present in saliva seven days before the onset of symptoms and until nine days after glandular swelling subsides. Mumps virus has been repeatedly demonstrated in the urine of patients with mumps within two weeks from onset and often longer. This necessarily alters the older concept of mumps as a disease requiring only those preventive precautions applicable to pathogens borne by respiratory secretions. Urine of patients with mumps, as well as their respiratory secretions, must be dealt with as infectious.

Incubation period

The incubation period for mumps is regarded as being from fourteen to twenty-eight days.

Clinical manifestations

The first symptoms of mumps may begin rather suddenly with headache, earache, loss of appetite, fever, and swelling of the parotid gland, which is located in front and below the ear. Swelling and pain occur either unilaterally or bilaterally. Sometimes all or some of the other salivary glands, such as the sublingual and submaxillary, may become involved.

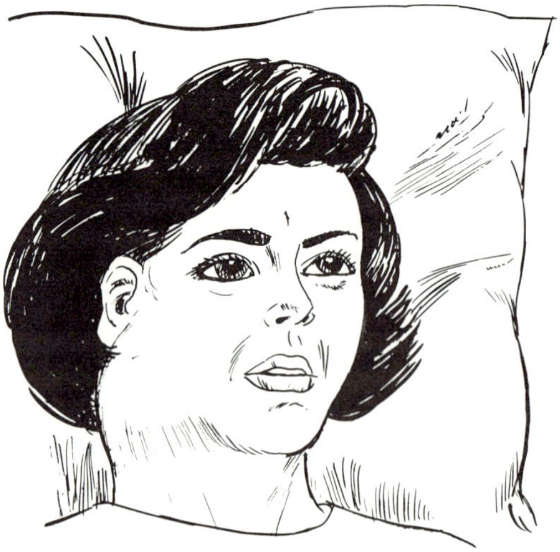

Fig. 21. Parotitis. Swelling of the parotid gland.

Pain is related to the extent of swelling of the gland, which usually reaches its peak in about twenty-four to forty-eight hours and continues for seven to ten days. The temperature usually remains only moderately elevated, but it may reach 104° F. during the acute stage of the disease. Occasionally enlargement of the gland may be the only symptom noted (Fig. 21). Children may have difficulty in swallowing. In many cases of mumps glandular involvement is so slight that it may pass unnoticed. A mild, unrecognized case of mumps actively immunizes the patient, but it also spreads the disease.

Diagnosis

Mumps can often be diagnosed by the enlargement of the parotid gland; however, other conditions affecting the gland may limit the accuracy of clinical diagnosis, and laboratory examinations may be necessary for confirmation. There are two tests that are helpful in diagnosis: (1) complement-fixation test, and (2) hemagglutination-inhibition antibody test. For reliable results two samples of blood are collected, one early in the disease and the other about two weeks later. To confirm the diagnosis of mumps the second test should show a significant rise in antibody titer. Diagnosis can also be made by tissue culture methods using oral secretions, urine, and cerebrospinal fluid.

Treatment and nursing care

As with other viral diseases, mumps is self-limiting, and there is no specific therapy for it. Treatment is symptomatic and supportive. The patient should be isolated, and on complete bed rest until all swelling of the parotid gland has subsided. Since most patients do not feel acutely ill, it is difficult for them to submit to isolation and complete bed rest. The nurse plays an important role in interpreting to the patient the need for bed rest and in helping to provide diversional interests. The application of heat or cold to salivary glands may provide relief from discomfort of swollen glands, and in some cases an analgesic may be required. Incidence of sterility from testicular swelling is in dispute; it is rare. When the testes are affected, a scrotal support should be provided and an ice bag applied. If the mammary glands in the female are involved, a supporting breast-binder should be applied. Concurrent disinfection of articles soiled by saliva and urine should be carried out. Swallowing is usually difficult, and liquids or a diet of soft foods should be given. Foods containing acid should be avoided, as they usually increase the pain in the glands.

Although death from mumps is of the greatest rarity, and serious complications are quite uncommon, the illness does cause considerable temporary discomfort and disability.

Complications

Most complications occur in individuals past puberty and may make their appearance before, during, or after parotitis. The commonest complications are orchitis and oophoritis. Other glandular tissues such as the spleen, pancreas, prostate, mammary glands, and thyroid may be affected. Some central nervous system involvement occurs in 30% to 50% of all cases; 99% recover. Symptoms appear late in the disease and may be those of meningitis, encephalitis, and encephalomyelitis, and the optic or trigeminal nerves may be involved.

The use of sulfonamide, antibiotic, and steroid agents are not effective in therapy, and the use of human immune globulin does not appear to provide substantial relief. Wise, in 1902, stated, "The bowels should be moved, a light diet given, and hygienic surroundings maintained."* By and large, the same probably holds true today.

Prevention and control

Most authorities believe that no serious efforts should be made to prevent mumps in children, since the disease is usually mild with few complications. However, a highly effective vaccine is available. It may be given at 1 year of age or thereafter. A delay may postpone the infection until adolescence or adulthood, when serious complications or permanent damage may occur. During recent years considerable interest has developed in mumps as a cause of abortion and congenital malformations. Douglas states, "Similarly, there is evidence that the mumps virus may result in more abortions than rubella, but only rubella produces a typical syndrome of malformations in surviving offspring."† Rogers reports a study conducted in 1960 in which it was found that 22.6% of a group of women who contracted mumps during the first trimester of pregnancy either suffered abortions or produced infants with malformations.[2]

Since 40% or more of adult persons have had inapparent mumps infection and can give no history of the disease, it is suggested that if exposed to the infection, a skin test should be done using mumps antigen. As in many other viral infections, a degree of skin sensitivity follows infection with the mumps virus. If antibodies are present, indicating previous experience with the virus, the test will show an area of erythema twenty-four to thirty-six hours after administration of the test. If the test is negative, mumps vaccine may be given. Unfortunately, the dermal test cannot be depended on as an indicator of immune status.

Mass immunization for the control of mumps is not recommended, but present evidence indicates that it may be important in protecting susceptible individuals such as military personnel, pregnant women, or other adults at risk. Research studies continue in the use of the vaccine.

Most states require that all cases of mumps (infectious or contagious parotitis) be reported to the health department. Patients should be isolated, but quarantine measures are not required.

---

*Wise, P. M.: A textbook for training schools for nurses, New York, 1902, G. P. Putnam's Sons.

†Douglas, Gordon W.: Rubella in pregnancy, Am. J. Nurs. 66:2664-2666, Dec., 1966.

Immunization

A highly effective vaccine is now available. It is given at 1 year of age or later. There is a combination vaccine (measles/mumps/rubella) available that can be given at 1 year of age.

Active immunization: can be given through live attenuated vaccine or placentally transferred immunity for newborns.

Passive immunity: provided by gamma globulin, preferably from serum containing high mumps antibody titers.

REFERENCES

1. Douglas, Gordon W.: Rubella in pregnancy, Am. J. Nurs. **66**:2664-2666, Dec., 1966.
2. Rogers, Fred B.: Epidemiology and communicable disease control, New York, 1963, Grune & Stratton, Inc.
3. Wise, P. M.: A textbook for training schools for nurses, New York, 1902, G. P. Putnam's Sons.

34
SMALLPOX (VARIOLA)

Etiology

Few diseases have been so destructive of human life as smallpox. It is one of the most contagious of all diseases and is feared because of its fatality, its terrible accompaniments, and its disfiguring effects. Smallpox is caused by a filtrable virus belonging to the poxvirus group. Several forms of the disease are recognized, including variola major (classic smallpox), variola minor (alastrium,) and varioloid. The death rate for variola major (classic smallpox) is as high as 40% among unvaccinated persons; and for variola minor as little as 1%. All are smallpox and merely represent variations in the severity of the disease. The disease is characterized by an eruption that passes through successive stages of macules, papules, vesicles, pustules, and crusts. The disease is very communicable, and the smallpox virus is highly stable and, in a dried state, may remain viable for months.

Epidemiology

In October 1972, smallpox workers throughout the world began the final phase of the World Health Organization's global campaign against smallpox, one of mankind's most feared and ancient enemies.

While smallpox was, at one time, a universal scourge, exacting a fearful toll by death, blindness, and disfigurement, it has gradually been controlled. Today, the disease continues to spread in only seven countries. In 1971, less than 200,000 cases were estimated to have occurred. But vaccination programs must continue, and, in many situations, vaccination certificates are required. Until 1971, everyone entering the United States and Canada had to be vaccinated, or show proof of recent vaccination. But this protective regulation has now been relaxed by government agencies. With jet travel, an infection picked up today in Karachi, India, can mean an outbreak next week in London, New York, or Vancouver.

Control of smallpox is but a temporary and uncertain measure; its eradication is the only effective solution. When the disease is transmitted from its recognized habitat to countries from which it has long been absent, the problem changes. It happened in 1972 in Yugoslavia which had had no cases for more than four decades.

Vital Statistics of the United States recorded no cases between the years 1963 and 1972. Statistics Canada reported no cases between 1971 and 1974. The number of countries reporting smallpox fell from forty-three in 1967 to eleven in 1973, and the number where it is considered endemic from thirty to four: Ethiopia, Pakistan, Bangladesh, and India. However, owing to major epidemics in the latter two countries, and also because of improved surveillance and better case reporting, the world total of reported cases reached 130,000 as compared with 65,000 in 1972. In 1973 over 33 million doses of vaccine were distributed by the World Health Organization to meet requests from governments.

In 1973, an outbreak of the disease occurred in London, England, when a laboratory technician, infected with smallpox at work, remained for a week in an open general ward, undiagnosed. Even after the provisional diagnosis of smallpox, an additional twelve days elapsed before two visitors to the ward were trailed as contacts. By that time they were both in hospitals with suspected gastroenteritis. They died shortly afterwards. This tragedy occurred within 10 months of the date set by the World Health Organization for the complete eradication of smallpox. No deaths from smallpox had occurred in England and Wales since 1962 and few medical personnel had ever seen the disease.

Present world situation

Smallpox is an unusual disease because its presence in an area can be readily detected. Each person infected with the virus develops the characteristic rash, and can transmit the infection until the scabs disappear. There are no silent or subclinical infections, and the virus is not present in animals or insects. If the virus is to persist in an area, the infected person must transmit the virus to a second person, and he to a third person, in a continuous chain. If the infected person does not transmit the virus to anyone, the chain is broken and the outbreak stops.

With all endemic countries now engaged in eradication programs, at least one third of all cases are now believed to be notified. The actual number of cases in 1971 was thus estimated to be less than 200,000 in contrast to the 2.5 million cases that were estimated for 1967. The number of countries reporting smallpox decreased from forty-two in 1967 to sixteen in 1971. In 1972, there were 65,000 cases of smallpox reported throughout the world, but it is estimated that the actual number of cases was at least three times greater. In 1973, continuing transmission is believed to have been limited to six countries. In 1973, more than 60,000 persons contracted smallpox, and of these, one third died.

With the decrease in smallpox incidence, importation of the disease into Europe and America has become less frequent. During 1967 and 1968, smallpox was imported into Europe on six different occasions, since then it was imported twice in 1970 and once in 1972. The number of smallpox

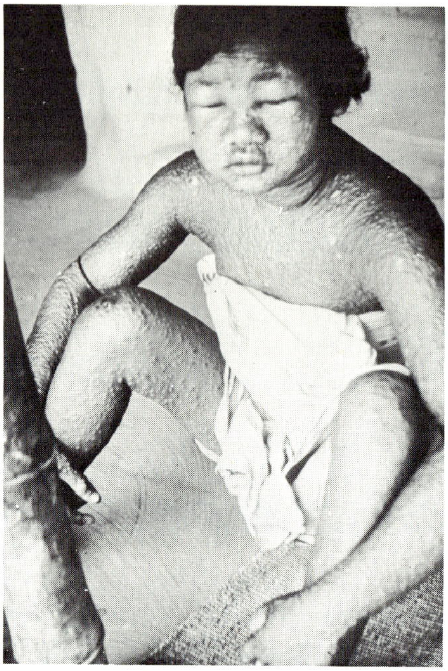

Fig. 22. Smallpox covering the body. (Courtesy National Medical Audiovisual Center, Chamblee, Ga.)

cases now occurring globally each year is comparable to the number of deaths from highway accidents annually in the United States.

Age and seasonal factors

Smallpox affects persons of all ages, and both sexes and all races are affected equally if unvaccinated. (Fig. 22). Infants from birth are susceptible, and although doubted at one time, it is now known that the fetus in utero is susceptible.

The disease occurs primarily in the colder months; however, in hot dry climates it is most likely to occur during the hottest periods. It may occur any time during the year, and in many parts of Africa and Asia it is endemic throughout the year.

Source

The virus is found in oral and respiratory secretions of patients, in lesions of the skin, mucous membranes, or anything contaminated with discharges from the pox fluid, scabs, or crusts.

Transmission

Smallpox is a highly communicable disease that is transmitted by direct contact with the infected patient and by droplet infection. It may also be transmitted by indirect contact with contaminated fomites. The disease is considered infectious from the time of the first symptoms until all crusts have dropped off. Although the virus is present in the crusts and may be found in dust, the question of airborne infection has not been completely resolved. In developing countries where sanitation is poor, the disease may be spread by insect vectors. It can be carried passively without causing disease by a person who has been vaccinated, by a sick person, or by a corpse.

Incubation period

The incubation period varies between seven and sixteen days, with an average of twelve days.

Communicability period

The communicability period lasts from one to two days before symptoms appear until the crusts all drop off, usually three to four weeks.

Clinical manifestations

Preeruptive stage. The onset of smallpox is sudden and acute, with severe headache, backache, and aching of the extremities. Prostration may be severe, malaise, chills, and vomiting occur, and the temperature may reach 105° F. The patient is toxic and appears very ill, and there is a possibility of delirium, stupor, or coma. After three or four days the temperature falls and the acute symptoms subside. Unless the patient is suspected of having been in contact with smallpox, none of these symptoms are especially characteristic of the disease and often cause confusion with a number of other diseases, such as influenza, scarlet fever, appendicitis, or leukemia.

Eruptive stage. Lesions begin to appear on the mucous membrane of the throat and mouth, and the patient complains of a sore throat. Macules appear on the face, neck, and trunk, gradually spreading to the extremities including the palms of the hands and the soles of the feet. The macules develop into papules very quickly and within a few days become vesicles. In about seven days the vesicles develop into pustules, which exhibit a depressed area in the center (umbilication), the fever returns, and facial edema and inflammation occur. The eyelids may be so edematous that the patient is unable to open the eyes, and severe pruritus is present. After approximately ten days the pustules begin to rupture, and crust formation occurs. The suppuration from the pustules and the yellow crust formation results in a very offensive odor. Although the patient may feel improved, severe pruritus continues to be very troublesome. The crusts dry and gradually begin to drop off during a period of about twenty-one days from the onset of the disease (Fig. 23).

Hemorrhage into mucous membranes and the skin (purpura variolosa or black smallpox) may occur early, before the eruptive stage of the disease, and usually is fatal, Variola pustulosa hemorrhagica, occurring during the

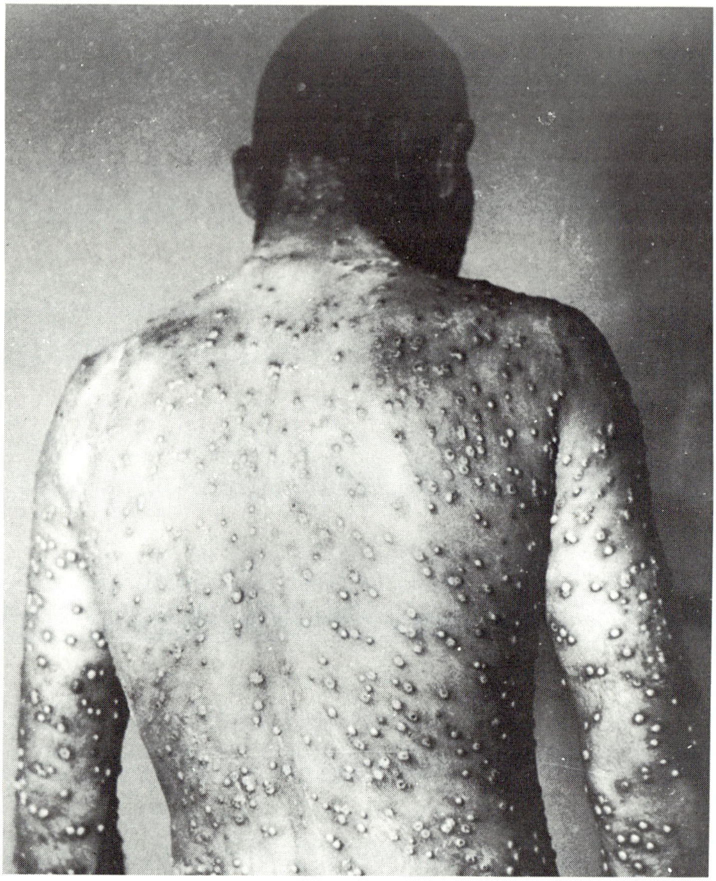

Fig. 23. Distribution of smallpox lesions on the back and arms of a man. Note the lesions on the ears and the umbilicated appearance of the lesions. (Courtesy National Medical Audiovisual Center, Chamblee, Ga.)

pustular stage of the disease, has a more favorable outcome. Varioloid is a mild form of smallpox, occurring in persons with a previous history of vaccination but whose immunity provides only partial protection.

Diagnosis

A diagnosis of smallpox can generally be made from the clinical symptoms, especially during an epidemic. The characteristic eruption is the most diagnostic feature of the disease. Diseases most commonly confused with smallpox are chickenpox, rickettsialpox, measles, impetigo, pustular acne, and drug reactions. Sulfonamide drug reaction may cause a pustular eruption that has been confused with smallpox. During the preeruptive stage of the disease, symptoms may simulate those of influenza, meningitis, or malaria.

A number of laboratory examinations are available to aid in the diagnosis of smallpox. Microscopic examination of material secured from lesions may be made to identify the virus. Other tests include the complement-fixation test, a serologic test to determine the rise in antibody titer, and tests that utilize the rabbit or chick embryo.

Treatment

There is no specific effective treatment for smallpox. Therapy is supportive and symptomatic. Adequate hydration, including electrolytes, and maintenance of nutritional requirements are necessary. Severe cases may require sedation, parenteral fluid therapy, gavage, oxygen, and blood transfusions, and digitalis therapy may be indicated. The use of analgesics or narcotics to relieve painful symptoms are usually indicated. Most authorities advise the use of antibiotic therapy such as penicillin or a tetracycline agent at the beginning of the suppurative pustular stage to aid in preventing complications.

Complications

Smallpox may complicate pregnancy, and the incidence of abortion and uterine bleeding may be high. Early mortality from smallpox is frequently caused by pulmonary edema, heart failure, or nonbacterial pneumonia.[3] Complications occurring later are usually caused by bacterial invasion. Skin infections such as impetigo and furuncles are not uncommon, and they may lead to septicemia, pneumonia, and other infections of the lower respiratory tract. Lesions in the eyes may lead to corneal ulcers.

Nursing care

All patients with smallpox should be isolated, preferably in the hospital, from the earliest symptoms until all crusts have dropped off. Strict medical asepsis is necessary, and all linens or articles contaminated by the patient should be autoclaved. Special care must be taken to prevent cross-infection. There is no danger to nursing personnel who have had a recent successful primary vaccination or revaccination with an immune reaction.

Preeruptive stage. During the preeruptive stage, nursing care is essentially the same as that for any febrile toxic patient. The comfort of the patient is important. Aching of the back is often intense, and measures for the relief of pain should be taken. An antipyretic such as aspirin may be ordered, but frequently a narcotic may be required. Before the rash appears sponges may be used to reduce temperature.

Eruptive stage. With the onset of the rash the throat becomes sore and swallowing may be difficult. The patient feels much discomfort. Not only is he generally apathetic, but he may be quite unable to move, as his muscles are incapable of being used. He may be completely unable to sleep. In some cases, the face is bloated and completely covered with lesions, the lips are swollen and covered with sores, and the mouth hangs open. Frequent mouth care with an antiseptic mouthwash and throat irrigations with warm physiologic saline solution will contribute to the patient's comfort. A water-soluble jelly such as petroleum jelly may be applied to the nose and lips to prevent drying. Efforts to maintain hydration and nutrition by the oral route should be made, but the patient will need considerable encouragement. When the eruption is extensive, the administration of intravenous fluids may also be difficult, and frequently fluids and high-calorie feedings are given by gavage.

Mild conjunctivitis and photophobia may be present, and bright lights should be avoided. The eyelids may be so swollen that it is impossible for the patient to open his eyes for days at a time. Lesions and secretions about the eyelids should be carefully cleansed by irrigation with physiologic saline solution or 2% boric acid solution. Bleeding is a common occurrence, either spontaneously or because of rough or careless handling, and so the bed linen and sleepware may be very damp from both blood and pus. The rash is provoked by irritations, and so there are more lesions on those parts of the body exposed to irritation.

There is severe pruritus and burning of the skin, and bathing with soap and water should be avoided. Sponging with a 1:10,000 solution of potassium permanganate will help to relieve pruritus and to lessen the disagreeable odor. The anogenital areas should be cleansed with physiologic saline solution to prevent infection.

During the suppurative pustular stage, turning and moving the patient may be difficult and he may be too ill to render much assistance. Carefully rolling the patient from side to side with a sheet will facilitate placement of clean linen under him. The bed should be kept as clean as possible to prevent odor and discomfort for the patient. Since warmth increases pruritus, upper bedding should be light. The patient should be turned frequently to avoid pulmonary complications and pressure areas that may break down and become infected. The room should be comfortable, free from drafts, and well ventilated, and an aerosol air freshener may be used to dispel odors.

If there is delirium, bedrails should be used and precautions taken to prevent injury to the patient. Restraints should not be used because of the skin lesions. Efforts should be made to prevent premature removal of the crusts, which may result in infection and scarring. Warm oil applied to the crusts will relieve itching.

The skin should be observed for evidence of infection such as furuncles. If smallpox complicates pregnancy, the patient must be observed for onset of labor and uterine hemorrhage. Vital signs should be monitored regularly and any change indicating the onset of complications reported promptly. Intake and output records should be maintained.

The patient with variola major will need considerable emotional support. He may fear disfigurement, and prolonged hospitalization and separation from his family may cause anxiety and worries.

The nursing care of patients with variola minor and varioloid is less demanding and differs little from the care in chickenpox.

Prevention and control

Smallpox was the first disease to which immunity was intentionally obtained by artificial means. Effective vaccination, before exposure, prevents the disease. Immunity eventually wanes, but virtually complete protection is afforded by revaccination with fully potent vaccine every three to five years. Benenson indicates that 60% of the American population are not solidly immunized.[1] It has been clearly demonstrated in the past that smallpox from the reservoirs of infection in Asia and Africa may be brought close to any city by modern jet aircraft. Intensive efforts to develop eradication programs are being made by the World Health Organization in cooperation with many countries of the world where smallpox exists. In 1966 the World Health Assembly approved a worldwide smallpox eradication program to begin in 1967, with a goal of 220 million vaccinations in the first year.[2] In 1972, the final phase of the WHO global campaign against smallpox was begun. The target is no new cases. In 1972, there were 65,000 cases reported throughout the world, but it is estimated that the actual number of cases was at least three times greater. The United States should not be complacent until worldwide eradication has been achieved (Fig. 24).

Vaccination for smallpox is contraindicated for persons with eczema, leukemia, persons receiving corticosteroids or antimetabolics, and those with hypogammaglobulinemia.

All cases of smallpox are reportable to the health department, and all countries are required to make telegraphic reports to the World Health Organization according to the International Sanitary Regulations. Control

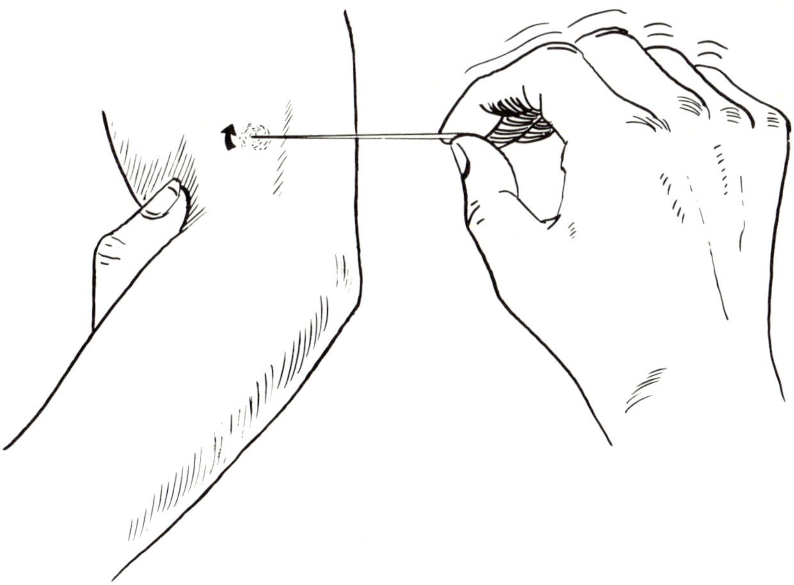

Fig. 24. Multiple pressure technic of smallpox vaccination.

requires the isolation of all patients and quarantine of all susceptible contacts for sixteen days from the last exposure and the immediate vaccination of all contacts. Epidemiologic investigation is made to determine the source of the infection.

An oral prophylactic agent N-methylisatin β-thiosemicarbazone (compound 33T57, Marboran) is currently under investigation as a prophylactic agent for all contacts, regardless of immune status.

Vaccination

Fluid or lymph containing the virus is allowed to enter the vascular layer of the skin through shallow punctures or slight scratches.

After vaccination of a previously unvaccinated person there is an incubation period of three or four days during which there are no noticeable changes. Then, if the vaccination "takes," the mild immunizing infection called "vaccinia" occurs. An eruption appears at the place of inoculation and goes through a series of characteristic changes (from papule to vesicle) for a period of about two weeks. About the seventh day, a reaction sets in that lasts several days. There is fever, loss of appetite, general discomfort, and headache. During this time specific antibodies are formed. The vaccination leaves a distinctive scar.

If a vaccinated person is "completely immune," a small red papule, sometimes with a tiny vesicle, appears within ten to seventy-two hours. The vaccination heals in five to seven days.

If the vaccinated person is "partly immune," a small, rapidly evolving "take" appears in the form of a pustule. Finally a scab develops. This reaction begins within one to five days and lasts one week to ten days.

If a person has no reaction to a vaccination it could be due to one of the following reasons: the vaccine virus is inactive, the vaccinated person is not allergic to it, or disinfectants on the skin have inactivated the virus.

The protection is complete for some time and then gradually wanes. Protection is almost completely gone in ten years.

REFERENCES

1. Benenson, Abram S.: Why does smallpox still exist? Am. J. Nurs. **62**:77-79, Sept., 1962.
2. Global program started to eradicate smallpox, Am. J. Nurs. **66**:1725, Aug., 1966.
3. Horsfall, Frank L., and Tamm, Igor, editors: Viral and rickettsial infections of man, ed. 4, Philadelphia, 1965, J. B. Lippincott Co.

35

PSITTACOSIS (ORNITHOSIS OR PARROT FEVER)

Etiology

Psittacosis is a viral disease of birds belonging to the parrot family, and it may be transmitted to man. The causative agent is *Miyagawanella psittaci* or, as it is commonly called, "Bedsonia." The disease may also be known as "parrot fever," and since it is widespread among birds and fowl other than parrots, *ornithosis* is the term generally used to cover all types of birds other than the psittacine birds.

Epidemiology

Psittacosis is worldwide, occurring as sporadic cases although in the past, serious epidemics have taken place. In 1956 confirmed reports indicated that in the United States there were 568 cases among humans.[2] In 1971, the U. S. Department of Health, Education, and Welfare reported thirty-two cases, while Statistics Canada reported three cases. In 1972, fifty-two cases were reported in the U. S., and six cases in Canada. In 1973, the number of cases in the U. S. was thirty-three, while Canada had a total of two cases reported. During the first twenty-five weeks of 1974, twenty-two cases were reported to the U. S. Communicable Disease Center, while in Canada no cases were reported to the Public Health Section, Health and Welfare Division, Statistics Canada. No deaths have been reported in the U. S. or Canada since 1963. The disease may occur as outbreaks in households where there has been contact with infected birds. Certain occupational groups are considered at risk, including laboratory workers, workers in poultry-processing plants, and persons who breed and transport parakeets and pigeons. Prior to the development of antimicrobial drugs the mortality among humans ranged from 20% to 100%, but present therapy has reduced the mortality to between 1% and 5%. It is believed that inapparent infections among high-risk groups may be relatively high.

Age and seasonal factors

Reported outbreaks of psittacosis indicate that the disease may affect all age groups. Fatal infections have been reported among children under 5 years of age. Some reports indicate a higher incidence among persons over 40 years of age, but specific confirmation may be lacking. However, it is recognized that more serious or fatal cases occur among older persons. The infection is about equally divided among the sexes.

Psittacosis may occur any time during the year. Household outbreaks have been reported during winter months, when prolonged confinement and concomitant exposure was greatest. Other outbreaks have been reported as occurring in the summer and early fall months.[1]

Transmission

The disease is readily transmitted to human beings by inhaling the dust from dried feces, feathers, and exudate from the nostrils and mouths of the sick birds. A healthy bird may also be a carrier. Rarely, but occasionally, man-to-man transfer has occurred. The nose and mouth secretions of infected human beings can also transmit the causative organism.

Incubation period

The incubation period is from four to fifteen days, but it may vary from five to twenty-eight days. The commonest interval after exposure is ten days.

Clinical manifestations

The onset of psittacosis is generally sudden, but it may be insidious. The disease is characterized by severe headache, vomiting, malaise, aching of the back, loss of appetite, sore throat, chilly feeling or frank chills, and fever varying from 100° to 105° F. It especially attacks the lungs, causing a form of bronchopneumonia. A cough may or may not be present and, if present, may or may not be productive. If the cough is productive, the sputum becomes mucopurulent but usually is not excessive in amount. The pulse rate is slow, and the respiratory rate is essentially normal. Symptoms of the disease may vary considerably. Constipation or diarrhea may be present, and abdominal distention, nausea and vomiting, and epistaxis are not uncommon. A skin rash similar to that seen in typhoid fever may occur in some cases. The disease runs a course of about ten days, with little day-to-day change, but is frequently fatal. In fatal cases cyanosis, hypotension, and circulatory collapse may occur. Recovery frequently is long and slow and marked by extreme weakness and fatigue.

Diagnosis

Differential diagnosis in psittacosis may involve typhoid fever, mononucleosis, influenza, or atypical pneumonia. A history of contact with birds, the clinical symptoms, and a roentgenogram of the chest may provide sufficient evidence for diagnosis. Laboratory examinations may be required to confirm the diagnosis or for diagnosis.

Diagnosis may be made by isolating the etiologic agent. Prior to the administration of antibiotic therapy, specimens of blood, sputum, vomitus, or throat washings are obtained and injected into mice. A complement-fixation test may be done to determine the presence of antibodies, which may appear as early as the fourth day of illness. A second blood sample should be taken two or three weeks later and should show a rise in antibody titer in a positive diagnosis of psittacosis.

Treatment

Therapy should be started early with appropriate doses of tetracycline daily. Achromycin has been used, and dramatic effects have been reported in the use of Declomycin. Although this is a departure from treatment for viral diseases, there is some evidence that the virus of psittacosis is atypical and therefore responds to antibiotic therapy. However, it should be pointed out that not all clinicians are in agreement with the value of antibiotic therapy. Supportive treatment includes bed rest and adequate fluid intake. A roentgenogram of the chest to visualize the lungs and an electrocardiogram are recommended. If cyanosis occurs, oxygen therapy is instituted, and vasopressor drugs may be administered in case of hypotension. In selected cases corticosteroid drugs have been used.

Complications

Insufficient treatment may result in relapse, which is the most frequent complication. Thrombophlebitis with pulmonary embolism and pneumonia, which may result in death, are possible. In severe cases the central nervous system may become involved.

Nursing care

The patient should be isolated and concurrent disinfection carried out. The use of a well-fitting mask is recommended if the patient is coughing. Monitoring vital signs including blood pressure, observing the patient for cardiovascular changes and cyanosis, and conserving the patient's strength should be included in the nursing care plan. Gas-forming foods should be avoided to prevent abdominal distention. During the febrile period, diet should be liquid with a gradual return to a normal diet. The appetite may be poor, and the patient may need encouragement to eat. The nursing care of the patient with psittacosis is the same as that for all patients during the febrile period of the disease.

Prevention and control

The prevention and control of human psittacosis depends on control of the disease among birds. This is best accomplished through international regulations with respect to the importation of birds. Specific regulations have been established by the Public Health Service of the United States and Canada concerning the conditions under which certain birds may be brought into these countries. In addition, when the disease occurs in pet shops, infected birds should be destroyed and the establishment placed under quarantine. The cages should be burned, or soaked in a saponated solution of cresol or some other disinfectant solution.

All cases of psittacosis should be reported to the health department. Investigation to determine the source of the infection and to identify the origin of infected or suspected birds should be made.

There is no agent at the present time that will assure active immunity to psittacosis, and although it is believed that an attack of the disease may confer immunity indefinitely, absolute proof has not been forthcoming.

REFERENCES

1. Horsfall, Frank L., and Tamm, Igor, editors: Viral and rickettsial infections of man, ed. 4, Philadelphia, 1965, J. B. Lippincott Co.
2. Top, Franklin H., and Wehrle, Paul F.: Communicable and infectious diseases, ed. 7, St. Louis, 1972, The C. V. Mosby Co.

36

VIRAL PNEUMONIA (ATYPICAL PNEUMONIA)

Etiology

Viral pneumonia may be caused by strains of several groups of viruses, which include Coxsackie virus, ECHO virus, adenovirus, and respiratory syncytial virus. It may be caused by influenza and parainfluenza viruses from the myxovirus group; however, there has been some question concerning influenza viruses causing atypical pneumonia.[2] It has been estimated that as many as twenty different serotypes causing febrile respiratory illness probably exist. It has also been reported that the cause of pneumonic conditions that are designated viral is unknown in nearly half of the cases.[1] There are a number of diseases, including Q fever and psittacosis, in which similar pneumonic conditions occur. Viral pneumonia may also complicate some communicable diseases such as measles and chickenpox.

"Primary atypical pneumonia" was originally applied to pneumonia believed to be caused by a virus. It is now recognized that this type of pneumonia is nonviral but is caused by the "Eaton agent," a pleuropneumonia-like organism (PPLO) and currently known as Eaton pneumonia, or *Mycoplasma pneumoniae*. Clinically, pneumonia caused by the Eaton agent and that caused by viruses appear very similar.

Epidemiology

Viral pneumonia is endemic throughout the world. Respiratory syncytial (RS) virus is most likely to cause viral pneumonia in infants and young children. The respiratory syncytial virus is considered the most important pathogen to invade the respiratory tract during the first 6 months of life, and it accounts for 23% to 36% of pneumonia during early infancy.[3] Outbreaks of viral pneumonia reported among servicemen have been caused by the adenovirus, whereas at the same time the Eaton agent pneumonia may be endemic among the same population with no apparent clinical differences.[2]

Most viral pneumonia occurs during the winter months; however, seasonal patterns vary. Epidemics may occur any time during the year, depending on the type of virus prevalent at the time and the susceptibility of the population. There are no differences as to age, sex, or race, although viral pneumonia may be more severe in infants and young children or when superimposed on chronic conditions in elderly persons.

Transmission

Transmission is by direct contact and droplet infection. Indirect contact with contaminated articles may be possible. Communicability is considered low.

Incubation period

The incubation period varies widely, depending on the specific virus. It may be from a few days to a week or longer. The incubation period for Eaton agent pneumonia may be as long as three weeks. Little is known concerning the period of communicability.

Clinical manifestations

Viral pneumonia, regardless of the specific etiologic agent, produces similar symptoms, but variation of symptoms may exist among cases. The disease may begin abruptly or it may be insidious. The acute phase may be preceded by a mild upper respiratory infection, which is followed by chilliness, frank chills rarely, malaise, headache, anorexia, cough, and fever. Vital signs may be normal, and the cough may be productive or nonproductive. The leukocyte count may be normal or only slightly elevated. When fever is present, it may follow a remittant course and usually falls by lysis. The febrile period will vary from one to three weeks. The disease is self-limiting and rarely fatal.

Diagnosis

Diagnosis of viral pneumonia is made from the clinical signs and roentgenogram of the lungs. Frequently diagnosis is presumptive with fluorescent antibody staining and improved cultural methods. This type of pneumonia is being recognized more frequently. In Eaton agent pneumonia, cold agglutinins develop in about half of the patients but may not be of diagnostic value, since they also develop in some other diseases.

Treatment

There is no specific drug at the present time that is effective in the treatment of viral pneumonia. Supportive therapy such as bed rest and adequate hydration may be all that is required. If the illness is severe with dyspnea and cyanosis, oxygen therapy may be required. Codeine may be used to relieve the cough if necessary. In case of bacterial invasion the appropriate antibiotic is administered.

Complications

Complications are rare in patients with viral pneumonia. Recovery usually occurs within three weeks, but a longer period for convalescence may be required.

Nursing care

Isolation of the patient and concurrent disinfection are unnecessary, but respiratory secretions should be properly disposed of. Other care is the same as that for bacterial pneumonia.

Prevention and control

There are no specific control measures available for viral pneumonia. A vaccine containing killed adenovirus has been administered to military recruits, but it is not recommended for the general population.

Epidemics should be reported to the health department, but case reports are not required.

REFERENCES

1. Conn, Howard F.: Current therapy 1968, Philadelphia, 1968, W. B. Saunders Co.
2. Harris, C. H. Stewart: Influenza and other viral infections of the respiratory tract, Baltimore, 1965, The Williams & Wilkins Co.
3. Horsfall, Frank L., and Tamm, Igor, editors: Viral and rickettsial infections of man, ed. 4, Philadelphia, 1965, J. B. Lippincott Co.

37

DIARRHEA (VIRAL)

Etiology

Viral diarrhea may be defined as the "passage of excessively frequent or liquid stools." It is a symptom of some disorder of intestinal motility.

For a long time nonbacterial summer diarrhea occurring in infants and young children has been believed to be of viral origin. In fact, there is some belief that it may be more prevalent than generally supposed. Numerous studies have provided some information concerning the role of enteroviruses in outbreaks of infantile summer diarrhea. Although it is known that enteroviruses, including poliovirus, Coxsackie virus, and ECHO virus, are present in the human intestinal tract at various times, many of the studies support evidence of ECHO viruses as having a causal relationship to summer diarrhea.

There are more than fifty enteroviruses known to be present in the human intestinal tract at various times, all of which have been known to be involved in epidemics of diarrheal disease. The same viruses have also been isolated from apparently well children. In most cases the rate has been higher for sick children than for well children in the control groups.

Epidemiology

ECHO viruses are present throughout the world, and apparently the presence of bacteria in the intestinal tract plays no part in infections caused by viruses. Examination of healthy children to detect the presence of ECHO virus has received considerable attention. The results of such investigations indicate that the presence of ECHO viruses varies with age, time of year, and socioeconomic conditions.[2] Examination of healthy adults has failed to show the presence of ECHO viruses, although similar studies showed a substantial number among children under 4 years of age. However, not all studies have found similar results.[2]

Infantile diarrheal disease occurs most commonly during the summer and early fall months.

Transmission

The precise methods of transmission are not clearly understood, but the present evidence indicates that the anal-oral route is the most likely method of transmission.

Incubation period

The incubation period is three to five days.

Clinical manifestations

Available information concerning infantile diarrhea of viral origin indicates that it may be less severe than diarrheas caused by bacterial microorganisms. The primary symptoms are vomiting and diarrhea. In adults, the onset is sudden, with severe vomiting, profuse watery stools containing no blood or pus, chilliness, malaise, abdominal pain, and occasional aching. The illness is brief and recovery occurs rapidly.

Diagnosis

There are no practical measures for the diagnosis of viral diarrhea.

Treatment

There is no specific treatment for viral diarrhea. Therapy is symptomatic. Reduction of feedings in infants and young children is indicated when there is vomiting, and adequate hydration with replacement of electrolytes as may be necessary.

Nursing care

Nursing responsibilities for infantile diarrhea that is presumed to be of viral origin are essentially the same as those for other enteric infections. The frequency and characteristics of all stools should be noted and recorded. Records of all intake and output, including vomitus, should be maintained.

Prevention and control

There are no specific preventive or control measures available for viral diarrhea. However, enteroviruses are responsible for a variety of clinical syndromes, and there is evidence of nosocomial enterovirus infections on pediatric services. Strict isolation and medical asepsis are recommended for all children with enteric infections to prevent spread from one patient to another or to hospital personnel.[1]

REFERENCES

1. Artenstein, Malcolm S., and Weinstein, Louis: Hospital-acquired enterovirus infections, N. Eng. J. Med. **267**:1005-1010, Nov. 15, 1962.
2. Horsfall, Frank L., and Tamm, Igor, editors: Viral and rickettsial infections of man, Philadelphia, 1965, J. B. Lippincott Co.

38

HEPATITIS (INFECTIOUS OR EPIDEMIC HEPATITIS, VIRUS A; SERUM HEPATITIS, VIRUS B)

Etiology

The term "hepatitis" means "inflammation of the liver due to any cause—mechanical, chemical, or biological. The specific etiologic agent responsible for hepatitis remains a matter of speculation. Present evidence incriminates a filterable virus or viruses as the probable cause. It is believed that several variants of one family of viruses are capable of causing the disease. Further evidence points to two major groups of viruses from the same family, one group causing infectious hepatitis (epidemic jaundice) and the other group causing serum hepatitis (hemologous serum jaundice). Viral hepatitis is now classified as virus A (IH) to denote infectious hepatitis and virus B (SH) to indicate serum hepatitis.

Epidemiology

Hepatitis occurs in all parts of the world. It results in fever, regional pain, gastrointestinal distress, and sometimes jaundice. The virus of epidemic or infectious hepatitis or epidemic jaundice (hepatitis virus A), once gaining entrance to the host usually does not remain unnoticed—it causes overt disease. It invades the blood and the liver and often produces prolonged inflammation of that organ for weeks or months.

In 1971, the U. S. Department of Health, Education, and Welfare reported 59,606 cases of infectious hepatitis. During the same period in Canada, Statistics Canada reported 8682 cases. In 1972, the number of cases of infectious hepatitis recorded by Vital Statistics of the United States had dropped to 54,074. In 1973, the number again decreased with a total of 50,-749 cases reported. Similarly in Canada during 1972, 7344 cases of infectious hepatitis were reported, while in 1973 the number had decreased to 6664. During 1974 Statistics Canada recorded 5316 cases, while the Vital Statistics of the U. S. reported 47,908 cases. In the U. S., between 1960 and 1969 there has been a total of 8618 deaths from infectious hepatitis. In 1971, Statistics Canada reported ninety-two deaths.

Serum hepatitis has lower statistics. In 1971, 9556 people in the U. S. contracted serum hepatitis. During the same period Statistics Canada reported a total of 102 cases. In 1972, 9402 cases were reported in the U. S., while Canada had 467. In 1973, Vital Statistics of the U. S. reported 8451 cases, while Canada recorded 541 cases. During 1974, 328 cases were recorded in Canada and 9574 in the U. S. In 1971, the deaths from serum hepatitis in Canada numbered three. No statistics are available on the death rate in the U. S. for serum hepatitis.

Limited investigation offers some evidence that hepatitis virus B, serum hepatitis, may cross the placental barrier during pregnancy and infect the fetus.

Most outbreaks of viral hepatitis occur among military forces, in institutions, and as family epidemics.

Age, sex, and seasonal factors

All age groups and races and both sexes are susceptible to hepatitis. The disease caused by virus A is most characteristic in children under 15 years of age and declines sharply after 30 years of age. However, variations may be noted among epidemics. It is believed that many inapparent infections occur in infants and young children. Virus B hepatitis may occur more frequently among older adults because of a greater use of transfusion therapy, and although susceptibility to virus A hepatitis decreases in persons after 30 years of age, susceptibility to virus B hepatitis does not decrease with age.

There are no sex differences in the overall susceptibility and attack rates. However, there is some evidence to support the belief that unknown factors may operate to affect the severity and higher mortality rate among females. The disease is usually mild in children, but may be serious in the elderly for the same reasons that all infectious diseases are likely to be more dangerous in this age group.

Virus A hepatitis may occur at any time during the year, with the seasonal incidence varying in different parts of the world. In general, epidemics begin in the fall, continuing through the winter into the spring. Virus B hepatitis may occur at any time and is not affected by seasonal factors. Once a person has had an attack, he is not likely to have a recurrence.

Socioeconomic factors

Information concerning socioeconomic factors in relation to viral hepatitis has received limited attention. Poor personal hygiene has been cited as being responsible for epidemics over the years. The fact that environmental sanitation plays an important part is documented in reports of food-borne outbreaks caused by infectious food handlers and of water-borne epidemics.

In reviewing the worldwide hepatitis situation the World Health Organization indicates that crowding, poor sanitation, and poor personal hygiene are factors that need improvement.[2]

Transmission

Man is the only reservoir of infection, which is spread from person to person. The present evidence indicates that spread is by the anal-oral route and by blood and certain blood fractions. Both viruses A and B may be transmitted by blood and serum through transfusions, or through any skin punctures, but only virus A is present in the feces. Respiratory spread has been considered possible, but there is no proved evidence to substantiate respiratory transmission. The possibility of transmission by vectors has never been resolved. Reported outbreaks caused by contaminated food, water, and milk have been documented, and transmission by contaminated syringes has occurred.

Incubation period

The incubation period for infectious hepatitis ranges from fifteen to fifty days after contact with an infectious person, whereas that for serum hepatitis is characterized by an exceedingly long incubation period, varying from two to six months.

Communicability period

The communicability period lasts from a few days before to one month or more after the onset of symptoms.

Clinical manifestations

Before jaundice occurs, hepatitis causes early extensive destruction of liver cells. However, during convalescence, regeneration and restoration of the tissues takes place in most cases. In fatal cases necropsy has demonstrated extensive involvement of other viscera and complete destruction of the liver without evidence of regeneration.

The course of hepatitis is classified into three phases, namely, preicteric, icteric, and posticteric. Hepatitis caused by virus A and that of virus B are almost indistinguishable in symptomatology. The preicteric phase of hepatitis A may begin abruptly or insidiously, with loss of appetite, an unpleasant taste in the mouth, chills, nausea, vomiting, abdominal discomfort, diarrhea, and fever ranging from 100° to 104° F. The liver is enlarged and tender. There may be some enlargement of the posterior cervical lymph nodes and the spleen. In young children the symptoms may be milder and of shorter duration, and the fever may be absent. Virus B hepatitis is likely to be more insidious in onset, but the preicteric phase is essentially the same. The duration of the preicteric stage is variable and may be as short as twenty-four hours or as long as three weeks. Prior to the onset of the icteric phase the urine becomes dark because of the presence of bile pigments. The patient may appear improved and feels better for a couple of days, but with the onset of the jaundice there may be a return of the original symptoms, accompanied by pruritus and enlargement of the liver. Early leukopenia is seen. Bile may be detected in the urine, and bowel movements are clay-colored. In adults the icteric phase lasts for an average of four weeks, but it may vary from one to ten weeks and is usually shorter in children. Considerable weight loss, irritability, loss of sleep, various forms of urticaria, and central nervous system symptoms may occur in adults. After a peak in the jaundice it begins to fade, and the patient enters the posticteric stage, during which appetite returns and the patient is convalescent. Most patients have an uneventful recovery, although a small number suffer relapse. Virus B hepatitis in elderly patients may be more severe, and the mortality is usually greater.

Diagnosis

There are no immunologic tests to assist in the diagnosis of viral hepatitis during the preicteric phase. Liver function tests provide the most reliable information to aid in the diagnosis and management of the patient. Among the laboratory tests used are urine bilirubin, urine urobilirubin, Bromsulphalein, thymol turbidity, and cephalin flocculation tests. The serum transaminase determinations, including glutamic-oxalacetic transaminase (GOT) and serum glutamic-pyruvic transaminase (GPT), are elevated in hepatitis. Prior to the icteric phase leukopenia is present, and atypical lymphocytes may be found.

Before the onset of the icteric stage of the disease, viral hepatitis may be confused with a number of other diseases, including influenza, various bacterial enteric infections, and infectious mononucleosis. In the presence of jaundice, diseases involving the liver and gallbladder or various diseases of benign or malignant etiology may have to be ruled out.

Treatment

There is no specific treatment for viral hepatitis, and treatment is symptomatic. Bed rest and a nourishing diet are indicated for all patients and constitute the basic treatment. The diet should be high in protein, calories, carbohydrates, and low in fat. During the acute phase the diet is liquid and the patient is encouraged to take sufficient fluids to maintain hydration. Since treatment is nonspecific, there are differences of opinion concerning the length of time that the patient should be kept in bed as well as the specific nutritional requirements. Drug therapy is based on symptoms, and planned for the individual patient as required. Large doses of adrenal steroids may reverse the disease process if irreversible hepatitis obstruction has not occurred.

Complications

Complications in viral hepatitis are rare. The commonest complication is relapse, the frequency of which varies from 0.6% to 14 or 18%, followed by recovery. A small number of patients may have a continuous liver dysfunction with or without symptoms. Postmenopausal women may develop chronic hepatitis, which progresses to a fatal outcome. Recently it has been observed that hepatitis may be a source of chromosomal damage.

Nursing care

It is generally believed that all patients with viral hepatitis should be isolated for seven days from the onset of the disease. Patients with serum hepatitis do not need to be isolated, but differentiation between virus A and virus B hepatitis may be difficult.

A major responsibility of the nurse is to prevent spread of the infectious agent to other patients or to hospital personnel. There should be thorough handwashing with soap and running water following each contact with the patient. Individual bedpans should be available, and the greatest precaution should be exercised in caring for bowel discharges. Rubber gloves should be worn when giving enemas or taking rectal temperatures. The sanitary disposal of nose and throat secretions is advised, although evidence supporting respiratory transmission is not convincing.

Disposable equipment is available in a wide variety of items and should be used if possible, especially syringes and needles. Laboratory personnel or nurses should wear rubber gloves when performing venipunctures for blood specimens, and care should be taken when starting intravenous infusions or when changing dressings in which there is oozing of blood or serum.[1] Needles should be removed from infusion sets before disposal, and if cartridge type injections are used, as with the Tubex, the needle should be securely bent before disposal. It is recommended that equipment be washed in the patient's room and that all nondisposable equipment be autoclaved. If nondisposable syringes and needles are used for any purpose or for any patient, autoclaving should be required.

Disposable, plastic thermometers should be used and oral temperatures taken when possible. After the patient's recovery the thermometer should be destroyed. The nurse should remember that the hepatitis virus is resistant to chemical disinfection, and the use of antiseptic solutions for rinsing the hands or soaking equipment provides only a false sense of security. If autoclaving is not possible, boiling for at least thirty minutes is recommended.

During the acute phase of the disease, nursing care is the same as that given all febrile patients. Bed rest constitutes the basic care. Alcohol or tepid sponges may be given to control temperature. Because of anorexia, the patient maly refuse food and fluids. Food should be served in small, attractive, frequent feedings. Fluids should be encouraged and should approximate 3000 to 4000 ml. daily. Since weight loss may be severe, diet during convalescence is usually high calorie, high carbohydrate, and high protein, and vitamin supplements may be ordered. Severe pruritus is uncommon in hepatitis, but some itching may occur and may be relieved by sponging with water containing starch and sodium bicarbonate, or an antipruritic agent may be ordered by the physician.

Since management of the patient is, to a large extent, dependent on laboratory studies, all specimens of blood, urine, or feces should be collected promptly as ordered, properly labeled, and sent to the laboratory.

The patient should be observed for any change in color of stools and urine, mental confusion, restlessness, hyperirritability, unusual somnalence, extreme anorexia, or coma, and prompt reports should be made to the physician. All health workers must keep these viruses constantly in mind when dealing with any materials likely to be contaminated with human blood, blood derivatives, or feces.

Prevention and control

Prevention of infectious hepatitis (virus A) requires measures to improve sanitation and to prevent fecal contamination of food and water supplies. The high incidence of inapparent infections and asymptomatic carriers increases the problem of control, since there is no reliable method to detect such individuals. There must be thorough washing of hands after bowel movements, adequate cleansing of toilets, and decontamination of food and water before use.

The use of immune globulin for protection of household contacts or institutional contacts is recommended. Immune globulin does not prevent the disease, but it may have a modifying effect. Active immunization with gamma globulin with the subclinical level of the disease may provide active immunity. Passive immunization with pooled gamma globulin may be used after known exposure.

In serum hepatitis the problem is somewhat different. The increased use of blood and blood products during the past two decades and the prolonged duration of the carrier state increases the problem of prevention and control. At the present time there are no tests to detect the carrier and no chemical agent that is effective in treating blood to ensure its safety. Methods have been devised whereby gamma globulin and serum albumen have been rendered safe for parenteral administration. Opinions vary concerning the efficacy of administering immune globulin to persons being transfused with whole blood.

The practice of using multiple-dose syringes should be discarded and emphasis placed on adequate sterilization of syringes and needles. One point that must be stressed and remembered is that hepatitis viruses are exceptionally resistant to heat. They can resist baking for ten minutes, probably longer. They are also somewhat resistant to chemical disinfectants.

A breakthrough in the prevention of serum hepatitis was reported in Washington in March, 1975. A serum has proved to be successful on animals and is ready to be tried on humans.

Regulations vary among countries, but reporting of all hepatitis is considered advisable. Epidemiologic investigation should be made during epidemics to locate possible source of contamination.

REFERENCES

1. Top, Franklin H., and Wehrle, Paul F.: Communicable and infectious diseases, ed. 7, St. Louis, 1972, The C. V. Mosby Co.
2. WHO Expert Committee on Hepatitis, Second Report, Technical Report Series no. 285, Geneva, 1964, World Health Organization.

39

HERPES SIMPLEX (COLD SORE OR FEVER BLISTER)

Etiology

The herpesvirus group is responsible for infections in man, some animals, and some fowl. Herpesviruses that are known to be pathogenic for man include herpesvirus hominis, which is the cause of herpes simplex, often referred to as a "cold sore" or a "fever blister," which occurs around the mouth, face, and mucous membranes.

Herpes simplex occurs in two forms. The first is a primary infection, which generally occurs during infancy or early childhood before neutralizing antibodies are present in the serum. The second form occurs after recovery from the primary infection, when the individual becomes a carrier of the virus and may have recurrent infection throughout life. It is probable that the virus is continually present as a latent infection in the facial tissues of some people. The existence of neutralizing antibodies in the bloodstream does not protect against recurrent infections, but it does protect against any occurrence of another primary infection.

Epidemiology

Man is the natural reservoir of herpes simplex virus and herpes zoster virus. Herpes simplex is worldwide in distribution and is regarded as the most widely disseminated parasitic agent to infect man. The disease occurs at all ages and in all races and both sexes, and there are no seasonal variations in the rate of infection. The incidence is greatest among low socioeconomic groups.[1] Eruptions occur when extreme changes in temperature, either hot or cold, or fever, from whatever cause, are encountered. Exposure to ultraviolet irradiation, menstruation, or emotional stress may also cause fever blisters to form.

Neutralizing antibodies cross the placental barrier during pregnancy, resulting in a passive immunity of the offspring; however, the titer may be quite low. Infants under 1 year of age seem to be relatively resistant to the infection, with most primary infections occurring after the first year of age. However, infants of nonimmune mothers are susceptible and may become infected any time after birth. Disseminated herpes simplex may occur during the neonatal period and is highly fatal. Rarely, but occasionally, the disease may occur without dissemination during this period.[3]

Transmission

The herpes simplex virus is spread by close contact. The infectious lesions are present on the skin and mucous membrane of the lips, mouth, and genitalia, and the virus has been recovered from urine and feces. It may be present in the saliva for seven weeks after recovery from stomatitis. Transmission among adults may occur from kissing or from coitus when genital lesions are present.[1]

Incubation period

The incubation period is variable but may be between two and twelve days, with an average of four days.

Clinical manifestations

It is estimated that about 90% of primary infections are inapparent. Symptoms of primary herpes simplex depend on numerous factors, including the patient's age and the portal of entry of the viral agent. In infantile eczema the virus may enter the eczematous lesions, resulting in a severe cutaneous infection. Acute herpetic gingivostomatitis, also known as infectious gingivostomatitis, ulcerative stomatitis, and Vincent's stomatitis, is the commonest type of primary infection. The infectious process is characterized by both local and constitutional symptoms. In about two thirds of the cases the infection begins abruptly. The temperature is elevated from 103° to 105° F., the gums are edematous, red, and may bleed, vesicular lesions of varying size appear on the mucous membrane of the oral cavity, and regional lymph nodes are enlarged and tender.

Acute herpetic gingivostomatitis may occur as a primary infection at any age but occurs most commonly in children between 1 and 4 years of age. The disease varies in severity, and patients with a mild case may be expected to recover in about one week, whereas severe cases may require two weeks. After healing of the vesicular lesions in the mouth the lymph nodes may remain swollen for several days longer.

Primary infections with herpesvirus may be manifest by other clinical conditions, including vulvovaginitis, keratoconjunctivitis, and meningoencephalitis. It may also follow traumatic cutaneous injuries such as burns or abrasions; however, these manifestations are considered rare.

After the patient has recovered from the primary infection, the viral agent probably remains latent throughout life, with neutralizing antibodies in the serum. There is no recurrence of the primary infection with constitutional symptoms, but recurrent vesicular manifestations (cold sore or fever blister) may follow a variety of stimuli, which include exposure to sun, fever, and menstruation and may occur with trigeminal neuralgia. The vesicular lesions characteristically occur about the lips and nares.

Diagnosis

Diagnosis of primary herpes simplex includes both the clinical manifestations and laboratory examinations. As evidenced by the variety of clinical manifestations that may occur, the question of differential diagnosis has to be considered. In these situations laboratory examinations are helpful. Laboratory examinations in use include the following: (1) isolation of the viral agent from a vesicular lesion or the blood, (2) a demonstrated rise in the neutralizing antibody titer between early and convalescent serum, and (3) isolation of specific types of cells by a fluorescent technic. An intradermal skin test similar to the tuberculin test has been used successfully among age groups between 4 and 50 years.[1]

Treatment

There is no specific drug or treatment for herpes simplex. Treatment is largely symptomatic and directed toward relieving pain and discomfort. When lesions are in the mouth, oral intake of food and fluids may be painful and may be refused. Preventing dehydration may require the administration of intravenous infusion of fluids and electrolytes.

Herpetic keratitis is treated by the ophthalmologist, and 5-iodo-2-deoxyuridine (IDU) has been used effectively in treatment.[2]

In recurrent herpes a drying agent such as 70% alcohol is applied to the vesicles, and as the vesicles dry a lubricant may be applied. The use of IDU in recurrent herpes is inconclusive at this time.

Complications

Complications in herpes simplex include bacterial infection, which may accompany herpetic gingivostomatitis, dehydration, and acidosis. In recurrent infection in children, impetigo may infect vesicular lesions.

Nursing care

The nursing care of patients with herpetic infections should be directed toward providing as much comfort as possible. Special care should be taken to prevent infants and young children with eczema from exposure to herpesvirus infection. In acute herpetic gingivostomatitis, secretions from the mouth should be collected in tissues and properly disposed of. Patients should be carefully observed for evidence of dehydration, and intake and output records should be maintained during the acute stage of the disease.

Horsfall describes an infection occurring on the fingers of nurses that results from minor unnoticed injuries becoming infected from exposure to contaminated secretions.[1] Based on such possibilities nurses should be especially careful in collecting and handling secretions and in proper handwashing after patient care.

Prevention and control

There are no effective preventive or control measures for herpes simplex.

REFERENCES

1. Horsfall, Frank L., and Tamm, Igor, editors: Viral and rickettsial infections of man, Philadelphia, 1965, J. B. Lippincott Co.
2. Modell, Walter, editor: Drugs of choice 1974-1975, St. Louis, 1974, The C. V. Mosby Co.
3. Wilson, Miriam G., and Martini, Michael M.: Primary nondisseminated herpes-simplex infection in a newborn infant, N. Eng. J. Med. **267**:708-710, Oct. 4, 1962.

40

HERPES ZOSTER (SHINGLES)

Etiology

Herpes zoster, a painful disease, commonly called "shingles," is caused by a virus identical to the chickenpox virus. The agent is called varicella zoster (V-Z) virus. The virus isolated from vesicles of varicella and those from herpes zoster indicate that the viruses are indistinguishable. The dermal lesions are often very similar. Patients with herpes zoster, commonly persons over 40 years of age, usually have a history of clinical childhood varicella.

Epidemiology

Herpes zoster is a disease of adults, with the greatest incidence after 40 years of age. The disease is considered rare in children; however, some believe that it may be more common in children than generally believed but may not be recognized, since in children it is milder and shorter in duration.[2] Herpes zoster occurs as sporadic cases rather than in epidemics. The disease may occur in apparently well persons but is often seen in persons with chronic debilitating disease or with toxic diseases. It has been observed in patients with tuberculosis, lymphoma, and disseminated cancer. The incidence of the disease is believed to be fairly frequent, and although most cases have been reported in the spring and fall, investigators report no specific seasonal pattern.

Transmission

The way in which herpes zoster is transmitted appears to be like that of chicken pox and measles. An adult with herpes zoster can infect a child who in turn will usually develop chickenpox. Children with chickenpox can infect adults who may develop herpes zoster.

Incubation period

The incubation period for herpes zoster is thought to be four to twenty-four days. Often the average is four days.

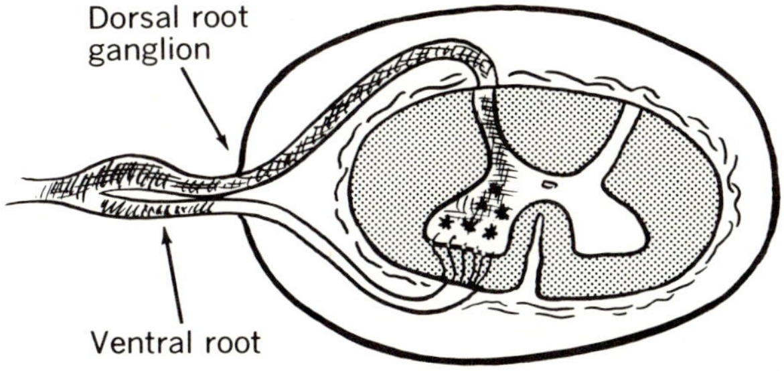

Fig. 25. Herpes zoster. Lesions are located in the posterior spinal ganglia and adjacent parts.

Clinical manifestations

The virus of herpes zoster affects the ganglion of the posterior nerve roots or the extramedullary cranial nerve ganglion and areas of the skin to which the corresponding sensory nerves extend. (Fig. 25). The cutaneous manifestation occurs along the corresponding course of the sensory nerves. Any part of the trunk may be affected, but the thoracic segment is most commonly involved. Other areas that may be affected are the extremities and branches of the fifth and seventh cranial nerves. There also seems to be a tendency for the skin lesions to occur where there exists continuous irritation, such as caused by restricting clothing.

The varicelliform eruption is unilateral and never crosses the midline of the body. An old idea once held by lay people, that if the rash encircled the body death would occur, is, of course, untrue.

Although herpes zoster is a localized disease, symptoms of systemic involvement may occur in some patients. There may be a prodromal period of one or more days with fever, malaise, anorexia, and headache. Pain of varying intensity is a presenting symptom in about two thirds of the patients. The pain occurs from one to five days prior to the development of the rash and is neuraligc and paroxysmal in type. It may be described as stabbing or burning, and the patient may complain of pruritus. The pain is usually worse at night and may be intensified on movement.

The skin rash is the most characteristic feature of the disease. The erythematous base of the skin lesion appears first but is followed within twenty-four hours by the appearance of the vesicle. Clusters of vesicles appear to form patches, which coalesce to form an irregular bandlike distribution. The vesicles become pustular, break down, and form crusts. Brownish spots may remain after healing. The regional lymph nodes are involved early in the disease (Fig. 26). The disease is rarely fatal, but can cause much intense discomfort.

Diagnosis

The characteristic skin rash may be diagnostic, but the preeruption pain may be referred and be similar to that experienced in myocardial infarc-

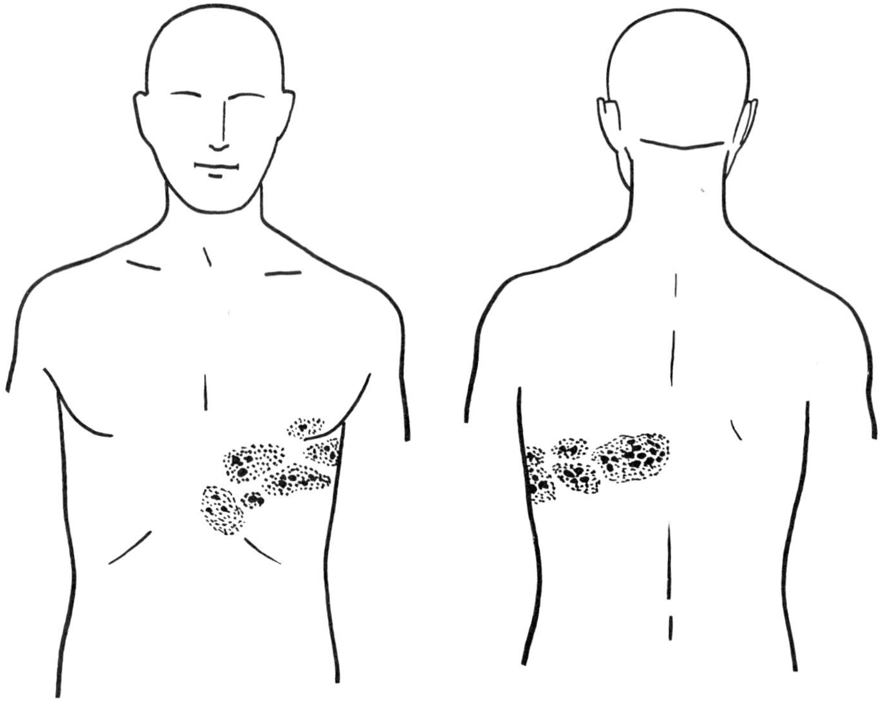

Fig. 26. Herpes zoster. Distribution of varicelliform cutaneous rash in the thoracic area.

tion, renal colic, or peritonitis. Other conditions that require differentiation are chickenpox, herpes simplex, and rickettsialpox. One attack of herpes zoster produces active immunity, and second attacks should be confirmed by laboratory studies.

By tissue culture technic the virus of herpes zoster may be isolated from fluid taken from newly developing vesicles. The neutralizing antibody titer may not be significant, since considerable antibody may be present at the onset of the disease; however, there are some patients in whom the convalescent antibody titers may be significant.

Treatment

Herpes zoster is a self-limiting disease, and there is no specific drug or therapy that will alter the course of the disease. However, it can be prevented by zoster-immune gamma globulin. Treatment is palliative and is directed toward relief of the pruritus and pain. An antipruritic agent such as calamine lotion, Cetaphil lotion, basic shake lotion, or 1:20 solution of Burrow's solution may be used as cool compresses.[1] Analgesics are usually necessary to relieve the pain, and aspirin or dextropropoxyphene (Darvon) may be adequate, but in some instances narcotics may be required. Every effort should be made to prevent infection, provide rest, and maintain nutrition and fluid balance. Most patients recover in about two to four weeks.

Complications

Complications are very rare; however, encephalitis may occur. Paralysis resulting from motor damage when the cranial nerve is affected and involvement of sacral areas may cause urinary retention.

Nursing care

There is no specific nursing care. Most patients will be seen in the physician's office. Hospitalized patients may have herpes zoster superimposed on an already-existing debilitating disease. The patient should be kept as comfortable as possible and the environment controlled to provide for rest. Efforts should be made to prevent secondary infection. Sterile dressings may be required in some cases.

Prevention and control

At the present time zoster-immune gamma globulins prevents the disease.

REFERENCES

1. Modell, Walter, editor: Drugs of choice 1974-75, St. Louis, 1974, The C. V. Mosby Co.
2. Winkelmann, Richard K., and Perry, Harold O.: Herpes zoster in children, J. Am. Med. Assoc. **171**:876-880, July, 1959.

41

POLIOMYELITIS (INFANTILE PARALYSIS)

Etiology

Poliomyelitis is caused by one of the three serotypes of the poliovirus group belonging to the larger family of enteroviruses. In 1949, the three serotypes were identified and are presently classified as types 1 (Brunhilde), 2 (Lansing), and 3 (Leon). All strains that have been isolated subsequently have been found to belong to one of these serotypes. A large proportion of urban adults have antibodies to all three types in their serum, yet have never had any disease recognizable as polio. They undoubtedly have had subclinical immunizing infections. Type 1 is responsible for most epidemics, and although one attack usually produces lasting immunity, a second attack by a different type is possible. In such cases present evidence indicates that types 1 and 3 are involved.

Classification of forms of poliomyelitis has sometimes been made on the basis of the muscle groups involved, but in general, the disease is classified as abortive, paralytic, and nonparalytic. In addition, paralytic poliomyelitis may be designated as acute anterior, bulbar, or bulbospinal.

Epidemiology

Most cases of poliomyelitis occurring at the present time in the United States and Canada are among children with no or incomplete immunization. However, it is believed that the incidence of inapparent infections may remain high and that many young children acquire neutralizing antibodies early in life as a result of contact with subclinical infections.[1] In 1971, the Vital Statistics of the United States reported a total of twenty-one poliomyelitis cases with seventeen of these classified as paralytic. During the same period in Canada, six cases were reported. In 1972, the Vital Statistics reported an increase to thirty-one cases, twenty-nine of these being paralytic in nature. However, the number of cases reported in Canada had decreased to two. In 1973, the U. S. had eight cases, while Canada reported five cases. During 1974, the Vital Statistics recorded five cases of poliomyelitis while Canada reported three cases. During the 10-year period between 1960 and 1969, the U. S. recorded 516 deaths. According to available statistics no deaths from poliomyelitis have been reported in Canada since 1971.

Age, sex, and seasonal factors

Poliomyelitis has been called a disease of children, thus the old name "infantile paralysis." Most cases occur in the first thirty years of life, and a large proportion before adolescence. However, it may occur in persons of all ages. Older persons appear to be more likely to develop severe paralysis. Among children the incidence is highest for boys, but for adults attack rates are about the same for males and females. All races are susceptible, but rates are higher for white persons than for persons of other races. Poliomyelitis may occur any time during the year, but it commonly occurs as epidemics during the summer and early fall months.

Transmission

The precise method of transmission of the poliovirus has been the subject of intensive study, and is found to be through oral contamination by pharyngeal and intestinal excretions, by direct contact, and by droplet infection. The viral agent enters mainly by way of the mouth and travels through the intestinal tract, from which it may be recovered from the feces. Exactly how the virus reaches the nervous system remains controversial. A current belief is that the virus enters the bloodstream by way of regional lymph nodes in the intestinal tract, resulting in viremia. Another theory holds that the virus travels along nerve fibers from the intestinal tract to the central nervous system. Once the virus reaches the central nervous system, it spreads along neural pathways.

Incubation period

The incubation period is from seven to fourteen days.

Communicability period

The communicability period occurs during the latter part of the incubation period and the first week of acute illness.

Predisposing factors

Considerable evidence has been accumulated to indicate some degree of relationship between paralytic poliomyelitis and certain physiologic factors other than those of the infecting agent. One of these factors that has received considerable attention is the increased incidence of poliomyelitis occurring among children after tonsillectomy. Among 2446 cases of poliomyelitis that occurred in New York City in 1949, there was an increase of 29.5% more cases among children with tonsillectomy than would have been normally expected.[3] Although the increase is generally evidenced within one month after surgery, it may extend to three or four months. It has also been shown that the virus finds entrance through the tissues around the gums, especially if there is injury as would result from tooth extraction. It is therefore recommended that surgical procedures involving the gums, tonsils, and pharynx not be done during seasons of prevalence of polio.

Poliomyelitis may occur within one month after diphtheria, pertussis, and tetanus (DPT) injections and that a positive correlation exists between the injection site and that of paralysis. Other types of injections do not appear to have the same relationship.

A higher incidence of poliomyelitis has been found among pregnant women than among an equated group. It has been postulated that endocrine factors related to normal physiologic changes occurring with pregnancy may influence susceptibility to the disease.

Other factors including heredity, dietary deficiency, physical exertion, and certain environmental conditions have been investigated by various researchers.

Clinical manifestations

Symptoms vary little during the prodromal period for all forms of poliomyelitis. *Abortive poliomyelitis* may be undiagnosed, since clinical evidence does not support a confirmed diagnosis. There is headache, slight elevation of temperature, nausea, vomiting, and loss of appetite. The symptoms appear abruptly and subside within twenty-four to forty-eight hours.

In *nonparalytic poliomyelitis* the same symptoms as those in the abortive form are present, but they may be intensified and in addition, central nervous system involvement is evidenced by stiffness of the neck and back, and some pain may be present on movement. Headache, chills, nausea, fever, and extreme irritability occur. Characteristically, the muscles of the neck are held rigid. There may be no further progression of the disease, and in the absence of known exposure to poliomyelitis or epidemic conditions it may be necessary to rule out infection caused by other enteroviruses.

Paralytic poliomyelitis (spinal and bulbar) begins in much the same way as the nonparalytic form, but the patient appears more acutely ill. A lapse of several days may occur between an abortive form and the onset of a paralytic form, with the individual apparently well during the intervening period. In some cases the paralytic condition may be the first indication of illness. The extent of the paralysis depends on the location and concentration of the affected neurons.

In the spinal form the motor neurons in the cervical or lumbar cord may be involved. When the cervical cord is affected, the intercostal muscles and the diaphragm may be paralyzed, creating a serious respiratory situation. Involvement of the motor neurons in the lumbar cord may produce flaccid paralysis of the lower extremities, abdomen, and back and may affect the urinary bladder.

The medulla oblongata is affected in bulbar poliomyelitis, causing a disturbance of respiration, circulation, and pharyngeal paralysis. Any of the cranial nerves may be affected, and muscle groups served by specific nerves may be weakened or paralyzed; for example, involvement of the tenth cranial nerve (vagus nerve) may result in paralysis of the pharynx, vocal cords, and soft palate.

Bulbar poliomyelitis is the most serious form of the disease because of the possibility of respiratory failure. Approaching failure is characterized by changes in the rate and depth of respirations, rapid pulse rate, rise in blood pressure, anxiety, insomnia, and cyanosis. When the vasomotor center is involved, the pulse rate becomes very rapid, the blood pressure is elevated, the pulse pressure is decreased, the lips are very red, and shock and pulmonary edema occur.

Diagnosis

A clinical diagnosis of poliomyelitis in abortive and nonparalytic cases is extremely difficult. Although paralytic poliomyelitis may provide more conclusive evidence for diagnosis, it is also noted that poliomyelitis-like illness caused by other enteroviruses may bear a close resemblance to true poliomyelitis.[1] Illnesses occurring during an epidemic or when seasonal incidence is expected may provide clues to diagnosis.

Abortive and nonparalytic cases can be diagnosed by laboratory methods. The tissue culture is widely used to isolate the viruses from feces, oral secretions, and similar sources. The poliovirus is present in the throat during the acute stage of illness and may be recovered from feces for several weeks. Isolation of the poliovirus will confirm diagnosis. Stool specimens taken during the first ten days of illness provide the most reliable source for virus isolation. Spinal fluid examination reveals slight changes in pressure; an elevated cell count and increased protein are considered diagnostic. The complement-fixation test may show a rise in antibody titer between the acute and convalescent stages of the disease.

Numerous diseases or disorders may be confused with poliomyelitis, among which are aseptic meningitis, meningoencephalitis, acute infective polyneuritis (Guillain-Barré's syndrome), osteomyelitis, transverse myelitis, and hysteria.

Treatment

There is no specific treatment for poliomyelitis. Each patient is handled according to his individual needs. Patients with abortive and nonparalytic poliomyelitis may require bed rest, reduced physical activity, and mild analgesics. Hospitalization may or may not be required, depending on the severity of the symptoms. Antibacterial prophylaxis may be ordered. Both adults and children need support and reassurance for they are fearful of the diagnosis "polio." The treatment of paralytic poliomyelitis requires a team of specialists, and treatment begins with the first indication of the disease and continues until complete recovery or until the individual has received maximum benefit from restorative and rehabilitative care.

Complications

The most important complications that may arise include emotional disturbances, respiratory failure, circulatory collapse, electrolyte imbalance, bacterial infection, urinary problems related to retention or paralysis of the urinary bladder, and abdominal distention.

Nursing care

The nursing care is symptomatic. The hospitalized patient with poliomyelitis is isolated for seven days and medical aseptic technic carried out. All respiratory secretions and bowel discharges must be carefully disposed of. The room should be warm and free from drafts and extraneous noise. The patient must avoid fatigue. The bed should be prepared with fracture boards and a firm mattress, protected with a rubber or plastic cover. A footboard should be provided that extends 4 inches beyond the mattress. The bed is made with a blanket on the bottom to absorb moisture and prevent chilling, which may increase muscle spasm. A cotton sheet may be placed under the buttocks and head. No pillow should be used, but a small sponge-rubber ring may be substituted. The bedding should be arranged over the footboard or over a bed cradle. When the patient is lying on the abdomen, prevent pressure on the toes by pulling the mattress away from the foot of the bed and let the feet hang over the edge of the mattress.

Personal hygiene. During the acute stage of illness, bathing should be omitted and rubs with alcohol or lotion avoided. During convalescence a warm daily bath with the skin patted dry may be given. Especially in the bulbar type of poliomyelitis, meticulous oral care should be given, using glycerin and lemon juice, with a water-soluble jelly applied to the lips. In the acute stage, therapy consists of suctioning the pharynx and postural drainage to prevent aspiration of secretions.

Impaired muscle tone in the alimentary tract is common, and abdominal distention should be watched for and prevented if possible. Feces may be removed by a small enema, but repeated enemas are generally avoided. Since the feces contain the virus they should be considered infectious. A rectal tube may be inserted for short periods to relieve flatus. Opinions differ concerning the use of neostigmine, bethanechol chloride, or vasopressin to relieve alimentary tract disturbances. Some physicians believe that a nasogastric tube connected to the Wangensteen suction is preferable to the use of drugs.

Urinary retention may occur early, and catheterization every six to eight hours may be necessary, or the physician may order a retention catheter inserted and connected to sterile closed drainage. In placing the patient on a warmed bedpan, pillows should be used above and below the pan to prevent arching of the back. Intake and output records are maintained throughout the period of acute illness.

Positioning. During the acute stage of illness there should be as little unnecessary handling of the patient as possible because of the severe muscle pain. When moving the patient, joints must be supported, but handling or pressure on muscles must be avoided. The position should be changed frequently to prevent pulmonary congestion and to relieve aching of dependent parts of the body. Placing the patient in the prone position relieves pressure on sensitive back muscles and promotes lymphatic and venous drainage. In positioning the patient all body parts should be supported to prevent muscle spasm and to maintain good body alignment. A sufficient number of persons should be available to move the patient with as little discomfort to him as possible.

Hot packing. The use of moist hot packs to relieve pain and relax muscle spasm and discomfort may be ordered by the physician who will determine the muscles to be packed, the duration, and the interval for treatment. Packs are wrung completely dry and applied at a temperature of 115° to 120° F. and allowed to cool gradually. No oil or lubricant is used on the skin being packed, and packs should not be placed over joints. No heating devices such as hot-water bottles, heat lamps, or light cradles should be used over packs.[3] Hot packing is discontinued as soon as the pain is relieved, and the patient is placed in the Hubbard tank for treatment.

Diet. During the acute stage of the disease, liquids are given. As the patient convalesces, a gradual return to a nourishing regular diet is indicated. Nurses must be alert to any difficulty in swallowing and should withhold oral feeding in such instances until ordered by the physician. When swallowing is affected, as in bulbar poliomyelitis, feeding by gavage and intravenous infusion may be necessary.

Respirator care. Respirator care may be lifesaving when paralysis of intercostal muscles or the diaphragm occurs. The objective of such care is to provide adequate ventilation to support life. The patient in a respirator requires continuous nursing care and should never be left alone. Oxygen therapy may be required, and a tracheotomy may be performed. Several types of respirators are available and the type used will vary. Operation of the respirator will not be reviewed here, but nurses should be completely familiar with the operation of the equipment in each particular situation.

Physiotherapy. Therapy is required to prevent contracture from muscle shortening and to lessen residual disability. Manipulation of affected extremities within the normal range of motion may be done by the nurse or physiotherapist with permission of the doctor.

Convalescence and rehabilitation

Convalescence begins with the end of the acute stage of the illness, but rehabilitation begins with the onset of the initial symptoms. During the acute phase, intelligent positioning and support of muscles must receive conscientious attention. An important principle during convalescence is rest. A program of gradual graded activity with a view to muscle reeducation is started. Weak muscles may be supported by various methods, such as braces, splints, or surgery. Stress must be placed on preventing deformity and disability. Rusk believes that muscle function that is likely to return will do so within nine months and that further improvement is unlikely after about eighteen months after the onset of the disease.[4] Depending on the extent and type of disability a program planned for each individual, which may include activities of daily living, education, vocational training, and placement, should be instituted as soon as possible.

Prevention and control

When a case of polio is diagnosed, care is centered on proper disposal of respiratory secretions during the first two or three weeks of the disease and adequate disposal and disinfection of stools for blood four weeks from onset. The disinfection of feces from infected persons is not an acceptable practice in all hospitals. There is, however, every indication that feces and objects contaminated with feces are important vectors of the infection. Dishes and other objects used by the patient should be thoroughly disinfected. It is known that the polio virus is inactivated by boiling and by adequate exposure to chlorine (chloride of lime, laundry bleach). Disinfection of hands must be placed high on the list of prevention controls.

The Salk vaccine. Dr. Jonas Salk first demonstrated his vaccine, an inactivated polio vaccine, in 1954. Since then various schedules of inoculation with the Salk polio vaccine have been recommended. The one most commonly used advises four doses of the vaccine—three doses four to six weeks apart, and the fourth dose about seven months later. Booster doses are recommended at intervals of three or more years. Persons of all ages may be vaccinated. The Salk vaccine does not necessarily prevent "infection" by the polio virus, but it does prevent serious paralytic polio, especially the crippling and often fatal spinal or bulbar polio. The vaccine appears to be at least 90% effective in preventing paralytic polio. The side effect of vaccination with the Salk vaccine is a gastrointestinal infection caused by "wild" active polio strains. The mild infection appears to have the beneficial, immunizing effect of booster doses of vaccine. The Salk vaccine may also be administered as a quadruple vaccine with diphtheria, pertussis, and tetanus (D.P.T.).

The Sabin oral polio vaccine. The Sabin vaccine, a live attenuated poliovirus vaccine, was approved for general use in 1961. The vaccine is administered orally to children and adults in a small amount of prepared culture fluid in candy, food, and beverages. It is usually dropped on the tongue of infants over 3 months of age; this avoids hindering the action of the vaccine by residual maternal antibodies in the bloodstream of infants. Many physicians, however, feel it is advisable to have the vaccine administered within the first few hours or days of life because newborns have not yet been infected with extraneous enteric viruses.

The vaccine is administered at intervals of three to six weeks. Following the oral administration, multiplication of the virus occurs in the gastrointestinal tract and the virus is expelled in the feces. No perceptible symptoms occur.

With the widespread use of this vaccine, polio is being forgotten, as is the preventive measure of immunization. Control of polio requires reporting of all cases to the local health department. Persons travelling to countries where polio is prevalent are advised to be immunized. Outbreaks still occur and will continue to occur as long as the one method of control is ignored.

Triple active polio vaccine (Trivalent vaccine). A second type of oral vaccine (Orimune) was licensed by the United States Department of Health in 1963. This vaccine contains all three types of active, attenuated polio viruses. It yields a high degree of immunity if given in two doses, two months apart, instead of in the three or four doses required by the other vaccines. It is very effective as a supplement to other immunizing processes.

Because the incidence of polio in adults in the United States and Canada is at present negligible, authorities have advised that vaccine should be given only to those under 18 years of age, except in outbreaks or in other circumstances, such as travel, in which adults might be exposed to unusually high risk.

REFERENCES

1. Horsfall, Frank L., and Tamm, Igor, editors: Viral and rickettsial infections of man, Philadelphia, 1965, J. B. Lippincott Co.
2. Larson, Carroll B., and Gould, Marjorie: Calderwood's orthopedic nursing, ed. 6, St. Louis, 1965, The C. V. Mosby Co.
3. Rogers, Fred B., editor: Studies in epidemiology, selected papers of Morris Greenberg, New York, 1965, G. P. Putnam's Sons.
4. Rusk, Howard A.: Rehabilitative medicine—a textbook of physical medicine and rehabilitation, ed. 3, St. Louis, 1971, The C. V. Mosby Co.

42

RABIES (HYDROPHOBIA)

Etiology

Rabies is caused by a neurotropic virus as yet unclassified, but observation with the electron microscope indicates that it has some properties common to the myxovirus group. Although the virus may be filterable, it is not readily accomplished. The Negri body found in the cytoplasm of the neurons is the characteristic lesion of rabies. The isolation of the Negri body is important in the laboratory diagnosis of the disease. By indirect fluorescent antibody tests it is possible to see rabies antigen in masses smaller than the Negri body distributed throughout the cell cytoplasm (Fig. 27).[2]

The virus is readily destroyed when exposed to the natural elements of sunlight, heat, and air. It is also inactivated by ultraviolet irradiation, bichloride of mercury, and strong acids and bases.

Epidemiology

Rabies is primarily a disease of mammals that is transmitted to man in the same way as mumps. The respiratory secretions in the saliva of rabid animals gain entrance to wounds caused by bites or scratches from these animals. The disease may be transmitted to and by a great many species of biting mammals, such as dogs, cats, skunks, foxes, rodents, cattle, pigs. Dogs have been considered the principal reservoir of infection in urban areas. (Fig. 28). Vampire bats and other species of bats are important vectors in certain parts of Europe, South America, and the United States. Certain persons including veterinarians, laboratory workers, animal handlers, sportsmen, and campers have been designated as high risk groups. In 1972, twenty states reported a total of 180,019 animal bites. In 1973, eighteen states reported a total of 174,325. As animal bites are only optionally reported, no accurate statistics are available.

In 1967, two cases of rabies were reported in the U. S., with the subsequent death of both persons. In 1968, Vital Statistics of the United States reported one case of rabies in man, which ended in death. In 1969, again one case was reported by the U. S. Department of Public Health, and again one death was recorded. Vital Statistics Canada has reported no cases of rabies in man between 1971 and 1974. Vital Statistics of the United States has recorded four cases of rabies since 1971, one in 1971, two in 1972, and one in 1973. The case reported in 1971, a small child, recovered.

Age and seasonal factors

Persons of any age may contract rabies if exposed under favorable conditions. Children are most likely to be infected because of their attraction

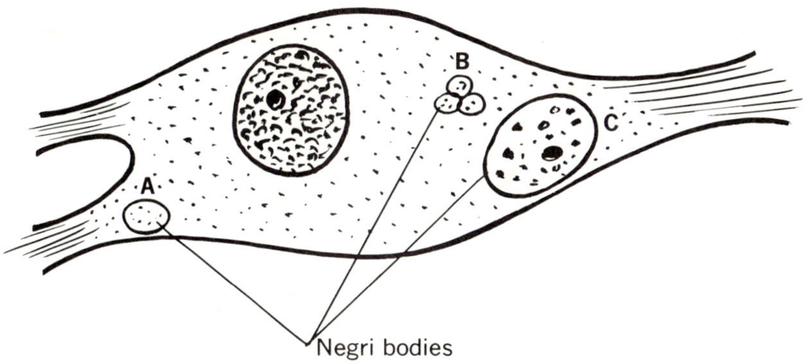

Fig. 27. Negri bodies. **A** to **C**, Lesions are present in the brain in rabies.

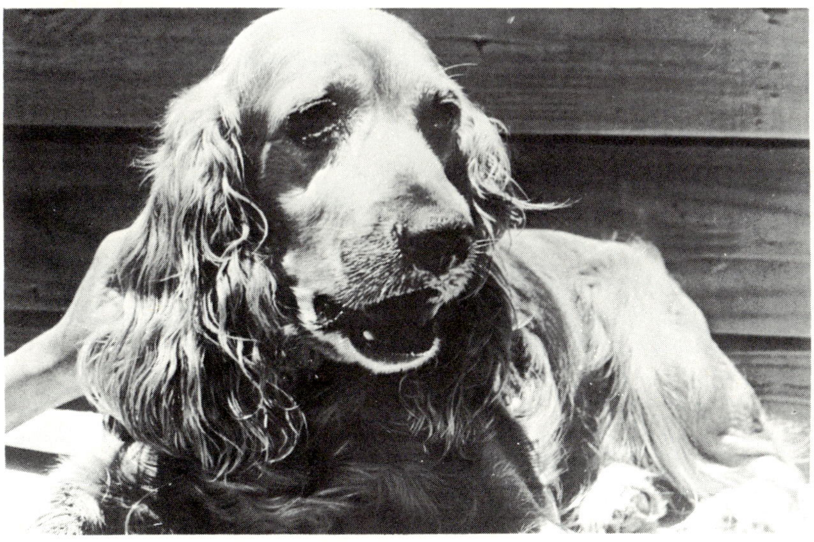

Fig. 28. Early paralytic rabies in a dog. Note the paralysis of the jaw. (Courtesy National Medical Audiovisual Center, Chamblee, Ga.)

to small animals such as dogs and cats. Children have a tendency to pick up small animals or birds found on the ground, and these may be sick and infected with the disease.

Rabies may occur at any time during the year. The incidence may tend to be greater in temperate climates and in countries where legal control of dogs is not enforced.

Transmission

Rabies is transmitted by the bite of an infected animal in which the saliva of the animal is introduced into the wound. However, the bite of a rabid animal does not necessarily mean that rabies will develop, since the virus may not be in the saliva at the time of the biting, or if present, it may not be in effective concentrations. Also, the presence of thick clothing over the site of the bite may prevent the entrance of the virus into the tissues. The severity and location of the wound must also be considered. Bites on the hands, arms, or face are more dangerous than those on the legs and feet because the virus is then inoculated closer to the brain. Transmission by the virus entering a scratch or cutaneous abrasion is possible. Man-to-man transmission has never been confirmed. Several studies have been made of infected bats that roost in caves in various parts of the United States to determine the possibility of airborne transmission. The results of these studies support the theory that airborne transmission is possible.[1] Such studies have involved only transmission to animals. Compared with animals, humans appear to be fairly resistant to the disease, even though they may be untreated.

Incubation period

There is a wide variation in the incubation period and between that in man and in animals. In dogs the period ranges from three to eight weeks, whereas in man it may vary from ten days to two years with an average of two to six weeks; however, factors cited earlier may influence the length of the incubation period.

Clinical manifestations

The rabies virus is conveyed from the wound, chiefly by the path of the nerve trunks, to the central nervous system, which it particularly affects.

In human rabies the neurotropic virus attacks and results in damage to the pons, medulla, brainstem, and thalamus. The disease is characterized by three phases or stages: (1) prodromal period, (2) excitement phase, and (3) paralytic phase. The disease is terrifying, as the patient usually passes through all stages with clear consciousness.

The *prodromal period* lasts for two to four days and is characterized by headache, malaise, nausea, sore throat, mental depression, temperature of 100° to 103° F., and rapid pulse rate. In about 80% of patients there will be numbness and tingling about the site of the wound. This symptom is of diagnostic significance during the prodromal stage of the disease. The patient may be especially sensitive to bright lights, noise, drafts, and the weight of bed covering. There may be increased salivation, perspiration, and lacrimation.

The *excitation phase* develops gradually and lasts from one to three days, with increasing nervous irritability, restlessness, anxiety, and apprehension. A significant symptom is the severe spasm of the muscles of swallowing. During this period the sight of food or liquids or the sound of running water may cause severe spasm of the muscles of swallowing. This symptom gave rise to the name "hydrophobia" (*hydro-*, meaning water and *phobia,* meaning morbid fear). During the period of excitement there is drooling, spitting, maniacal behavior, convulsions, and thrashing about. There may be spasms of the muscles of respiration, resulting in dyspnea, apnea, and cyanosis. These periods of extreme excitement alternate with periods of relative calm and quiet. Most patients die during the excitation period.

If the patient survives the excitation phase and progresses to the *paralytic stage* of the disease, the muscle spasms cease. The patient may be able to swallow but gradually progresses to stupor and coma, with progressive paralysis and death. Death occurring during this stage is usually caused by cardiac failure.

The duration and differentiation between stages of the disease are not uniform among patients.

Until 1971, once the symptoms of rabies appeared, death was considered inevitable. In 1971, a small boy was bitten by a bat believed to be infected with rabies. The child was treated with many specific drugs to prevent each symptom before it had a chance to develop. The child survived due to the fact that careful attention was paid to all disease details.

Diagnosis

Diagnosis can usually be made on the basis of clinical symptoms with a history of exposure. When there is a long incubation period and failure to recall a minor wound, the diagnosis may be missed. Some cases of rabies may be confused with poliomyelitis, encephalitis, or tetanus.

At the present time the most reliable laboratory test is the fluorescent rabies antibody staining test for detection of rabies antibody in blood serum.

If possible, the animal should be caught and held for observation for ten days, but not killed unless it is diagnosed rabid by a competent veterinarian. If the animal has rabies it will rarely survive ten days after the development of symptoms. If the animal shows unmistakable symptoms before this time, it is killed and an examination of the brain is made.

If the animal has been killed prior to an observation period, send the head, packed in ice, immediately to the Department of Health or a competent veterinarian for examination.

Treatment

The onset of the disease must be prevented because there is no definitive treatment and the mortality rate is close to 100%.

Bites of animals suspected of being rabid should be thoroughly cleansed immediately with soap and water. A soft syringe may be used to force soapy water into the depths of the wound. The wound should be allowed to bleed freely. If it seems reasonably certain that the biting animal was rabid, the treatments should be started without delay.

In the case of severe bites by known rabid animals, especially when the bite is near the head, face, or on the upper extremities, the use of antirabies hyperimmune serum, containing ready-formed antirabies antibodies is of great value and can prevent the terrible death from rabies. The serum should be given immediately, but no later than seventy-two hours after the bite. It is injected into the tissues around the wound. The serum injection is followed by a course of vaccine treatments. The results obtained are excellent.

For persons frequently exposed to rabies an initial series of several immunizing doses of the duck embryo vaccine or Semple vaccine, prepared from rabbit brains, should be given, followed by booster doses repeated at two to three year intervals. They give perfect protection. Duck embryo vaccine should not be administered to persons who are allergic to the protein of chicken or duck eggs, or to those receiving adrenocorticotropin or corticosteroids.

The Pasteur treatment (avianized vaccine). The Pasteur treatment is given to all persons who might have been infected by the virus through bites. This method, based on principles established by Pasteur results in active immunity. It is not a cure. The treatment must be started as soon as possible after the bite has occurred so that the patient has time to develop antibodies before the disease has time to establish itself. The treatment consists of fourteen injections. These are very painful and consist of injecting the vaccine under the skin of the abdomen, alternating sides. Although the method of preparing antirabic vaccine differs greatly from the original method of Pasteur, the administration of the vaccine is still referred to as the Pasteur treatment.

Rabies can be eradicated from civilized communities by measures designed for intensive control of stray dogs, immunization of house pets, and elimination of any wild animals acting as reservoirs for the infection.

New anti-rabies vaccine. An anti-rabies vaccine that has many advantages over the types used at present promises to be available soon. Three to four inoculations of the new vaccine give better protection than does a course of fourteen to twenty-one inoculations with the vaccines now in use. First trials on exposed volunteers have been initiated by the World Health Organization.

Nursing care

Transmission of rabies from one human being to another is very rare. Continuous nursing care must be provided. The patient should be isolated in a slightly darkened private room, and all extraneous noise must be controlled. The use of a mask is probably indicated. A gown and gloves should be worn as a prevention against saliva entering any cuts or scratches on the nurse's body. Concurrent disinfection of all articles contaminated by secretions from the mouth and nose must be carried out. The patient should not be bathed, and there must not be any running of water in the room or within hearing distance of the patient. If intravenous infusions are given, they should be placed away from the patient's visibility. Needles should be securely anchored in the vein to prevent dislodging during periods of restlessness. Padded bedrails should be used, and restraints may be necessary in some cases. During periods of consciousness the patient should be reassured, and the patient's family should be given emotional support.

Prevention and control

The eradication of rabies should be on a global scale and should include measures to prevent and control the disease in animals and wildlife. These measures may include the following:

1. Legislation should provide for the following:
   a. Vaccination of all dogs
   b. Registration, licensing, and taxation of all dogs

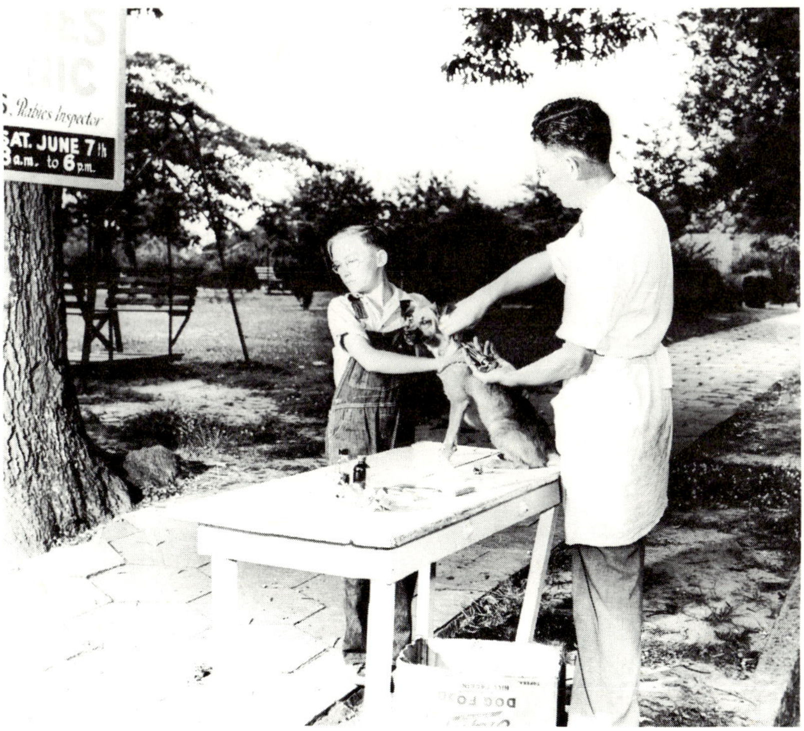

Fig. 29. Outdoor rabies clinic. Veterinarian inoculating a dog. (Courtesy National Medical Audiovisual Center, Chamblee, Ga.)

c. Enforcement of regulations for pickup and destruction of stray dogs
d. Enforcement of leash laws and pickup of dogs when found loose and off the owner's property
e. Confinement for seven days or longer of any dog that has bitten a person
f. Laboratory facilities for observation and diagnosis

2. Educational programs to train wildlife personnel in control activities of seeking, trapping, or poisoning animals in epidemic areas
3. Public education, especially of children, in avoiding and reporting all animals that appear sick
4. An understanding of legal authorities and willingness to prosecute violations by persons who seek to circumvent the law

Reporting of rabies is mandatory in most countries (Fig. 29).

REFERENCES

1. Constantine, Denny G.: Rabies transmission by nonbite route, Public Health Reports 77:287-289, April, 1962.
2. Larsh, Susanne E.: Indirect fluorescent antibody and serum neutralization response in pre-exposure prophylaxis against rabies, Ann. Int. Med. 63:955-964, June, 1966.

SECTION FOUR

Arthropod-borne diseases

43

ENCEPHALITIS

Encephalitis is an inflammatory disease involving part or all of the central nervous system. It may be caused by a variety of pathologic agents, including bacteria, viruses, fungi, rickettsiae, toxins, chemical substances, or trauma. It may occur as a complication secondary to a disease, as in measles or as postvaccinal encephalitis after vaccination for smallpox or rabies. It may occur as a primary infection caused by viral agents having a predilection for the central nervous system. Whatever the cause, the clinical syndrome is much the same.

In this chapter the discussion will be limited to four types of viral encephalitis transmitted to man by an arthropod vector and the ones that are most commonly encountered in the United States. The four types are (1) eastern equine encephalitis, (2) western equine encephalitis, (3) St. Louis encephalitis, and (4) Japanese B encephalitis.

Etiology

The virus of arthropod-borne viral encephalitis belongs to the group of arborviruses. The viruses of eastern and western encephalitis are classified in group A, whereas the viruses of St. Louis and Japanese encephalitis are in group B. The natural habitat of the filterable virus appears to be many species of wild birds and some domestic birds that live in a symbiotic relationship with several known species of mosquitoes, many of which belong to the *Culex* group. The virus of eastern and western viral encephalitis may also cause encephalitis in horses.

Epidemiology

The virus of *eastern* encephalitis was established as the cause of encephalitis in humans in 1938 during an epidemic in Massachusetts, where thirty-four cases with twenty-five deaths were reported. Mortality from this disease may run as high as 55% or even 80% in older persons and children. Most cases of eastern encephalitis occur as small outbreaks or as sporadic cases.

Western encephalitis, first discovered in California in 1930, primarily affects young persons, particularly infants. Outbreaks of the disease among humans usually coincide with the occurrence of encephalomyelitis among horses. It appears to be present in nearly all areas of the United States, western Canada, and some Central and South American countries. Mortality rates are considerably lower among persons with western encephalitis than with the eastern type.

In 1971, Vital Statistics of the United States reported 1580 cases of Western encephalitis, while in 1972 the number dropped slightly to 1524. During 1971, Statistics Canada reported no cases. In Canada during 1972, eight cases were reported. In 1973 Vital Statistics recorded 1509 cases; no cases were reported in Canada. The death rate for acute infectious encephalitis has remained, according to Vital Statistics, fairly consistent throughout the ten-year span between 1960 and 1969 with an average death rate of 493 persons.

St. Louis encephalitis is the most prevalent of the encephalitides. It has its greatest incidence in persons of middle age or older.

Japanese encephalitis occurs in areas of Asia, Korea, islands of the western Pacific, Japan, and India.

Age, sex, and seasonal factors

Epidemic encephalitis affects persons of all ages. However, attack rates vary quite widely. In recent outbreaks both morbidity and mortality has been greater in the very young and elderly persons.

In western encephalitis the incidence is considerably greater among males than among females, whereas in other types of encephalitis the sex distribution is about equal. All races appear to be equally susceptible.

Epidemic encephalitis is a disease of the hot summer months, usually beginning in late June or early July and continuing until early fall.

Transmission

Each type of epidemic viral encephalitis is caused by its own specific virus, which is transmitted to humans by the bite of an infected mosquito. A mosquito becomes infected by biting an infected bird, and after incubating the virus in its own body for five to seven days, the mosquito carries the virus to healthy birds, horses, and humans. Infection of man is the end of the cycle, since the infection is not transmitted from man to man and mosquitoes do not carry the virus from humans. In epidemic areas the incidence of inapparent infections is reported to be very high.

Incubation period

The incubation period is five to fifteen days, with a range from four to twenty-one days. It varies as to the type.

Clinical manifestations

The symptoms of epidemic encephalitis appear to follow a similar pattern in all types. The onset is abrupt, with fever in all cases. The temperature may be 104° to 105° F., with a rapid pulse rate. Headache occurs in 90% of the patients and remains severe for three or four days, and slight relief is obtained from analgesics. There is nausea and vomiting in about 50% of the cases. Neurologic signs include tremor of the hands, tongue, and lips in two thirds of the patients; speech difficulty, stiff neck, drowsiness, and an altered level of consciousness occurs in nearly all patients. In severe cases convulsions, coma, and death may occur. Leukocytosis is present, with counts from 10,000 to 25,000 leukocytes.[3]

Western encephalitis in infants results in convulsions in about 90% of the cases, and convulsions are common in all children under 4 years of age. In eastern encephalitis, in which mortality rates are higher among young children and elderly persons, severe symptoms with convulsions occur early, with progressive neurologic symptoms and death within three to five days. Young children who survive may suffer permanent residual damage to the nervous system.[1] In most cases a continued high fever and convulsions indicate a poor prognosis.

Diagnosis

Arthropod-borne encephalitis cannot be positively diagnosed on the basis of clinical signs because of the variety of diseases presenting similar neurologic symptoms. Mild cases, especially in children, often resemble febrile disorders occurring during the summer months. Positive diagnosis can be made only by serologic tests or isolation of the viral agent on autopsy examination. Serologic tests in common use include the complement-fixation test and the hemagglutination-inhibition antibody test.[2]

Treatment

There is no specific treatment for viral arthropod-borne encephalitis. In general, treatment is symptomatic and similar to that of poliomyelitis.

Complications

Complications as such are probably limited, but sequelae after attacks may result from the disease. Among such sequelae are recurring convulsions, mental retardation, and paralysis, all of which occur primarily among children.

Nursing care

Patients with arthropod-borne viral encephalitis do not need to be isolated. The patient should be in a private well-ventilated room, and all noise should be effectively controlled. There should be sanitary disposal of nose and throat secretions, but concurrent disinfection as such is unnecessary, since the infectious agent is not present in the secretions. Tepid or alcohol sponges may be given if the temperature is excessively high. Unless the patient is comatose, oral fluids should be encouraged. If stupor or coma is present, intravenous fluids and gavage feeding may be ordered. Expert oral care at regular intervals must be given to the comatose patient. A mouth gag and protective devices such as bedrails should be available in case convulsions occur. Intake and output records are maintained, and temperature, pulse, and respiration rates are taken at four-hour intervals or oftener if indicated. Patients should be observed for neurologic signs involving speech, swallowing difficulty, twitching, eye movements, and indication of paralysis. The beginning, duration, and frequency of all convulsions should be carefully observed and recorded. There is no danger to nursing personnel who are caring for patients with encephalitis.

Prevention and control

Preventive measures are directed toward the identification of mosquito vectors, elimination of breeding places, destruction of larvae, screening of homes, use of repellents, and avoidance of mosquitoes during their biting hours. A broad public education program is an important phase of all preventive programs.

Formalin-inactivated chick embryo vaccine has been used to immunize animals against western and eastern equine encephalitis. Vaccines suitable for use in human beings are still in the experimental stages.

All types of viral encephalitis are reportable to the health department in most states and foreign countries. All aircraft arriving from countries where the disease is prevalent are carefully inspected and sprayed for the presence of mosquitoes.

REFERENCES

1. Horsfall, Frank L., Jr., and Tamm, Igor, editors: Viral and rickettsial infections of man, ed. 4, Philadelphia, 1965, J. B. Lippincott Co.
2. Quick, Donald T., Serfling, Robert E., Sherman, Ida L., and Casey, Helen L.: The 1962 epidemic of St. Louis encephalitis in Florida. Part III. A survey for inapparent infections in an epidemic area, Am. J. Epidem. **81**:405-414, March, 1965.
3. Quick, Donald T., Thompson, John M., and Bond, James O.: The 1962 epidemic of St. Louis encephalitis in Florida. Part IV. Clinical features of cases occurring in the Tampa Bay area, Am. J. Epidem. **81**:415-427, March, 1965.

44

MALARIA

Etiology

Malaria is caused by a protozoan parasite of the genus *Plasmodium.* Four species are responsible for malaria in man: (1) *P. vivax,* (2) *P. malariae,* (3) *P. falciparum,* and (4) *P. ovale. P. vivax* is the most widely distributed, whereas *P. ovale* is considered rare.

Epidemiology

Malaria has plagued countries of the world for centuries, and its total eradication, even in the most developed countries, remains to be completed. The World Health Organization reported in 1967 that 334 million people now live in areas of the world where malaria is no longer a problem but that 638 million people still live where malaria transmission takes place.[4] More than 180 million people in Africa live under the destructive influence of malaria, and it is estimated that 200,000 to 500,000 infants and young children die annually as the result of malaria.[1]

Most cases of malaria occurring in the United States, and Canada are the result of persons traveling to countries where the disease exists. Peace Corps volunteers, missionaries, and military personnel account for most of the cases. In 1971, Vital Statistics of the United States reported 2375 cases of malaria. During the same period Statistics Canada recorded seven cases. In 1972, 742 cases appeared in the U. S., while again in Canada seven cases were reported. In 1973, there were 237 cases in the U. S. and twenty-four in Canada. During 1974, 255 cases were reported by the U. S. Communicable Disease Center, while in Canada thirty-six cases were reported. Between 1960 and 1969, sixty-four deaths were reported from malaria in the U. S.; no deaths have been reported in Canada since 1971.

Age, sex, and seasonal factors

All ages, races, and both sexes are susceptible to malaria. A significant exception occurs among African Negroes who carry the genetic trait of sickle cell anemia—they appear to have a resistance to malaria. Climate plays an important part in the incidence of the disease. In tropical and subtropical countries malaria may be endemic throughout the year. In colder climates it occurs during the warm months, when the prevalence of mosquitoes is greatest.

Transmission

Man is the reservoir of malaria infection, and the disease is transmitted by species of female mosquitoes called anopheles. After an incubation period and with the onset of symptoms in the victim, the noninfected mosquito becomes infected by biting the human, and the cycle begins over again. Thus the disease is carried from man to man by the vector and from man to vector. The disease is not transmitted from man to man except through blood transfusions or contaminated syringes and needles, as in the case of drug addicts.

Incubation period

The incubation period in the human varies with the particular species of *Plasmodium* and varies from *twelve* to *fourteen* days for *P. vivax* to as long as thirty days for *P. malariae.* Some strains of *P. vivax* may have a delayed incubation period of eight to ten months. Malaria resulting from blood transfusion has a shorter incubation period.

Clinical manifestations

Malaria may be acute and is often a chronic disease. The clinical manifestations vary little among the species of *Plasmodium.* Attacks coincide with the completion of the asexual cycle of the parasite in the human body, and the regularity of attacks in untreated individuals is predictable with a high degree of accuracy. In *P. vivax* attacks occur in a cycle of forty-two to forty-eight hours; in *P. malariae,* 72 hours; in *P. falciparum,* 48 hours; and in *P. ovale* 50 hours. Characteristically each episode has three stages: (1) chill, (2) fever, and (3) profuse sweating.

The attack begins with slight malaise and a feeling of chilliness, which develops into a severe shaking chill, usually lasting for ten to fifteen minutes but may last longer, and nothing will relieve it. The temperature begins to rise rapidly, reaching 103° to 106° F. The skin is hot, dry, and flushed, headache is present, and occasionally nausea and vomiting may occur. There may be generalized aching and abdominal pain. The fever lasts for four to six hours and falls rapidly, followed by profuse sweating of the entire body and a feeling of weakness.

Most deaths from malaria are caused by *P. falciparum,* in which the symptoms occur suddenly with great severity. The disease may progress to electrolyte depletion because of severe and prolonged vomiting and diarrhea. Neurologic symptoms develop, including delirium, convulsions, and coma in untreated or inadequately treated persons.

Diagnosis

An accurate diagnosis of malaria can be made only by laboratory examination. A film of blood is placed on a slide, stained, and examined microscopically. The species of *Plasmodium,* the number, and a positive diagnosis may be made in this way.

Treatment

The oldest drug specific for malaria is quinine sulfate. However, in recent years a number of new synthetic antimalarial agents have been developed. During World War II quinacrine (Atabrine) was used extensively, but like quinine its use has diminished.

Synthetic agents in current use include chloroquine phosphate, chloroguanide, amodiaquin, pyrimethamine, and primaquine. There have been reports of alleged resistance of some strains of *Plasmodium* to these antimalarial agents. The World Health Organization urges that very careful studies of such reports should be made. The apparent failure to cure the disease may result from (1) a poor quality of drug, (2) inadequate dosage, and (3) actual failure to take the drug. It further points out that resistance to the synthetic antimalarial agents would be a serious obstacle to the eradication of the disease.[3]

Recently, work has been done in using diaminodiphenylsulfone (DDS), a drug used in the treatment of leprosy. It has been used both as a chemoprophylactic and chemotherapeutic agent in malaria.

In 1961 a program was initiated of placing 4% chloroquine diphosphate in salt. According to the World Health Organization this technic has almost eliminated malaria in British Guiana. However, it believes that widespread use of this method of treatment needs further evaluation.[4]

Nursing care

The nursing care of the patient during the febrile period may include the application of external heat and hot drinks during the chill stage. It will probably do little to relieve the chill but will provide comfort and psychologic support for the patient. During the fever stage, tepid sponges, alcohol rubs, an ice cap to the head, and analgesics for headache may be ordered. The patient should be encouraged to take plenty of fluids. As the temperature falls and sweating begins, warm sponge baths may be given, and the bed and clothing should be kept dry to prevent chilling. When the sweating ceases, most patients feel relatively well and often go about their regular activities until the next attack occurs.

Prevention and control

Prevention depends on stopping the transfer of infection from person to person by mosquitoes.

The present program of prevention and control of malaria is based on the concept of global eradication. In the attainment of this goal the World

Health Organization believes that the problems to be encountered are (1) epidemiologic, (2) climatic, (3) geographic, (4) social, and (5) economic and that each must be dealt with and treated accordingly.[3]

Numerous factors operate to make eradication difficult, among which are the mobility of certain population groups who live a nomadic life, the resistance of mosquitoes to insecticides and pesticides, and the parasitic resistance to therapeutic drugs. Other problems encountered are the inertia of some countries and their incapacity to develop effective programs. In some areas of the world the people and the vector are inaccessible.[2]

In the United States and Canada case reporting of malaria is mandatory. Isolation of patients is unnecessary, but screening of homes is important. Control measures require the destruction of mosquito breeding places, the spraying of homes, and the use of insect repellents when indicated. The development of a vaccine for malaria is still experimental.

REFERENCES

1. Hinman, E. Harold: World eradication of infectious diseases, Springfield, Ill., 1966, Charles C Thomas, Publisher.
2. MacDonald, George: Eradication of malaria, Public Health Reports **80**:870-879, Oct., 1965.
3. Resistance of malaria parasites to drugs, WHO Chronicle **19**:181-183, May, Geneva, 1965, World Health Organization.
4. WHO Expert Committee on Malaria, Tenth Report, no. 272, Geneva, 1964, World Health Organization.

45

PLAGUE (PASTEURELLA PESTIS)

Etiology

Plague, caused by the plague bacillus *(Pasteurella pestis)*, occurs among wild and domestic rodents, primarily the rat. The principal reservoir of infection is among the more than 200 different animals known to host the infection. The rat flea *(Xenopsylla cheopis)* carries the infectious agent from rat to rat, thus maintaining the chain of infection. The disease is transmitted to man through the bite of the flea or from handling an infected rodent.

Epidemiology

Plague is one of the oldest diseases known, and its destructive epidemics have been well documented in history. The following three forms of the disease are recognized:

1. Bubonic plague is the commonest form of the disease, whereas septicemic plague is a type of bubonic plague with bloodstream involvement, which develops prior to the development of the characteristic bubo or pulmonary manifestations.
2. Pneumonic plague may occur as a primary infection with extensive involvement of the lungs.
3. Sylvatic plague affects rodents and animals and may occur in epizootics.

Plague is endemic in many parts of the world, occurring in epidemics and as sporadic cases. The World Health Organization reported 1256 cases in 1962. In 1963 it reported 864 cases with 142 deaths, and in 1964, 1457 cases with 121 deaths. Between 1971 and 1974 Statistics Canada reported no cases of plague. Vital Statistics of the United States reported thirteen cases in 1970, two cases in 1971, one case in 1972, and two cases in 1973. These cases occurred in Arizona and New Mexico. All but one case recovered.

Sylvatic plague is widely distributed in the western third of the United

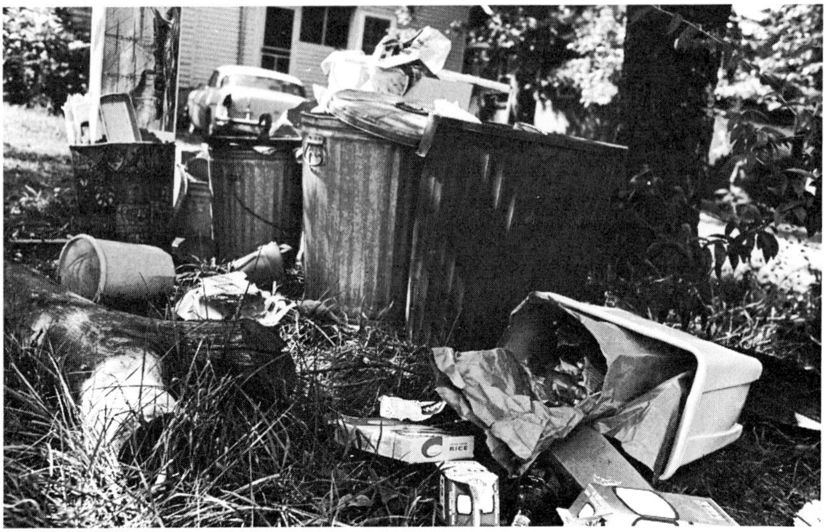

Fig. 30. Uncollected trash and garbage provide the optimum haven for rats.

States. More than 200 species of wild rodents and animals are known to harbor the infectious organism and to create a reservoir of infection. Periodic epizootics occur among ground squirrels, chipmunks, prairie dogs, rats, and mice. Because of the large number of persons traveling abroad today, the increasing incidence of plague is more probable. There has been a steady increase in the disease from 1963, when 115 cases and seventeen deaths were reported, to 1966, when 2755 cases and 145 deaths occurred.

Problems exist in large urban centers where there are uncovered garbage containers that are allowed to remain, unsanitary crowded conditions in slums and ghettos, open dumping grounds for trash and garbage, and litter in wayside parks and camping grounds, all of which provide a haven for rodents. Persons living in or near these areas may be at risk to possible exposure to the plague bacillus (Fig. 30).

Age, sex, and seasonal factors

There are essentially no human differences in susceptibility to plague with respect to biologic factors of age, sex, and race. Although the disease may occur less frequently in very young children, both bubonic and septicemic cases have been reported in children under 2 years of age.[1] Men who work around docks loading and unloading ships' cargo may be at risk from infected rats that hitchhike aboard ships from countries where the disease is endemic. Laboratory workers who handle plague bacillus are also at risk.

In tropical and subtropical countries the disease increases during the spring months when the humidity is high, whereas in colder climates the disease is most prevalent during the summer months.[1]

Transmission

Bubonic plague is transmitted to man by the vector *X. cheopis* (rat flea). Transmission by other species of flea is not very effective. Primary pneumonic plague is spread from man to man by droplet infection. Bubonic plague with pulmonary complications may also be spread from person to person by droplet infection.

Incubation period

The incubation period of plague is short, varying from two to six days for bubonic plague and about two to four days for pneumonic plague.

Clinical manifestations

Symptoms develop suddenly with fever ranging from 102° to 105° F., but it may be much lower in septicemic plague. The pulse is rapid and irregular, there is malaise, restlessness, and development of neurologic symptoms that affect speech and gait, mental confusion, delirium, and coma. Painful buboes appear in the groin, axilla, and neck. Pneumonic plague begins abruptly with fever, chills, headache, nausea, vomiting, and productive cough with thin, frothy, blood-tinged sputum that is teeming with the causative organism. If untreated, mortality rates are high, but if diagnosed early and with prompt treatment, death rates have been greatly reduced. An attack of plague usually brings about a state of permanent immunity.

Diagnosis

Early diagnosis of sporadic cases of plague may be difficult, but in epidemics clinical diagnosis may be made on the basis of the characteristic symptoms. However, accurate diagnosis requires the assistance of the laboratory. Specimens for laboratory examination should be secured prior to beginning therapy and should be handled aseptically.

Laboratory examinations include smears and cultures made from sputum and fluid aspirated from a bubo. Extreme care and familiarity with the technic of bubo aspiration is necessary to avoid exposure to the infection. Agglutination tests and fluorescent antibody stains will confirm diagnosis. Final confirmation may include animal inoculation, usually of the guinea pig.

Treatment

The treatment for all forms of plague is with broad spectrum antibiotics and sulfonamides. Streptomycin is extremely valuable in therapy. Other agents that may be used are chloramphenicol and the tetracyclines. Penicillin has no effect on the plague bacillus, but it may be administered if infection by other bacteria occurs.

Nursing care

Patients with plague in all forms should be isolated—in the hospital, if possible. Medical aseptic technic must be carried out. On admission to the hospital the patient's clothing must be thoroughly disinfected. Physicians and nurses who work with epidemic pneumonic plague victims wear hooded masks with goggles, overalls rather than gowns, and gloves.[1] Bubonic plague is not transmissable, but draining buboes may release the plague bacillus into the air. Therefore, a well-fitting and properly constructed mask, a gown with long sleeves, a cap, and gloves should be worn by the nurse when dressing draining buboes. In pneumonic plague the causative organism will disappear from the sputum in about twelve hours after initiating drug therapy. Sputum and dressings from draining wounds should be carefully collected and disposed of immediately by burning. All urine and feces should be disinfected prior to disposal.

Supportive care during the febrile period is essentially the same as that for any febrile patient. Tepid or alcohol sponges may be given to control the temperature, fluids should be encouraged, and intravenous fluids may be ordered by the physician. Liquid diet is offered during the febrile period, with a gradual return to a nourishing regular diet.

Prevention and control

The prevention and control of plague is primarily a problem of ecology and requires persons trained in several disciplines, including entomology, mammalogy, laboratory technics, sanitation, and medicine. Control requires the destruction of the reservoir of infection, namely rats and rat fleas.

Contacts are quarantined for six days, and sulfadiazine is administered daily for six days. All cases of plague or suspected plague are reportable in the United States, Canada, and other countries. In the United States autopsy is mandatory if plague is suspected as the cause of death. Bodies of plague victims must be handled aseptically.

The International Sanitary Regulations of the World Health Organization outline specific measures that apply to all ships, aircraft, or other transport arriving from areas where plague exists. Although plague immunization is not required for foreign travel, persons with or suspected of having the disease are not permitted to leave the country.

Active immunization with a live, avirulent vaccine has been administered in countries where the disease has been epidemic; however, it is not recommended for general use. It has been suggested that persons among high-risk groups such as laboratory workers might consider such protection.

REFERENCE

1. Dubos, Rene, and Hirsch, James G., editors: Bacterial and mycotic infections of man, ed. 4, Philadelphia, 1965, J. B. Lippincott Co.

46

ROCKY MOUNTAIN SPOTTED FEVER (TICK FEVER)

Etiology

Rocky Mountain spotted fever, one of the most severe of all infectious diseases, is caused by the *Rickettsia rickettsii*. The acute febrile illness is transmitted to man by the bite of certain ticks, such as the sheep, wood, and dog ticks (Fig. 31).

Epidemiology

Rocky Mountain spotted fever was once believed to exist only in the far West, but it is now known to be widespread in the United States, Canada, Mexico, Colombia, and Brazil. Since the introduction of antibiotics, the incidence and deaths caused by the disease have been cut by about 50%. The number of cases reported in the United States in 1963 was 216; in 1964, 227; in 1965, 281; and in 1966, 249. In 1971, the U. S. Department of Health, Education, and Welfare reported 432 cases, while no cases were

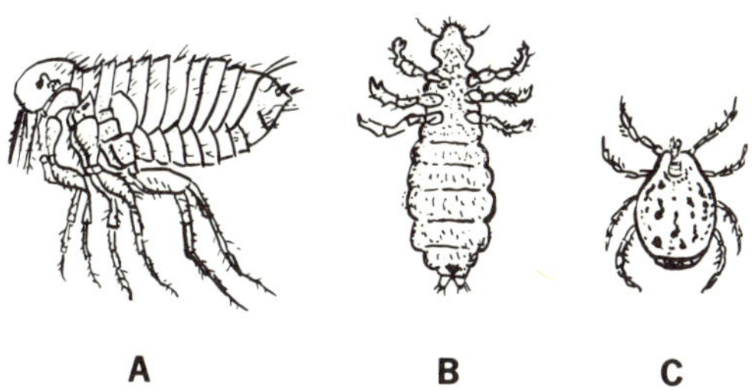

Fig. 31. Arthropod vectors. **A,** *Xenopsylla cheopis* (rat flea), vector of plague. **B,** *Pediculus humanus corporis* (human body louse), vector of typhus. **C,** *Dermacentor andersoni* (Rocky Mountain wood tick), vector of Rocky Mountain spotted fever.

reported in Canada. In 1972, 523 cases were contracted in the U. S. During this same period, Statistics Canada reported one case. During 1973 and 1974, no cases have appeared in Canada. In 1973, 668 cases were reported by Vital Statistics of the United States, and during 1974, 765 cases were contracted. During the ten-year period between 1960 and 1969, 184 deaths have occurred in the U. S. No deaths have been reported in Canada since 1971.

The ecologic distribution of ticks shows that the wood tick is responsible for most of the infections in the Rocky Mountain states, whereas the dog tick is the vector in the eastern and southern states, and the Lone Star tick is the vector in the southwest part of the country.

The reservoir of infection is maintained by a variety of rodents and both small and large animals, including the domestic dog and cat. The infection may be maintained by the tick, since the infected male infects the female, who passes the infection on to its offspring.

Age, sex, and seasonal factors

Persons of all ages are susceptible to Rocky Mountain spotted fever; however, there has been some indication of geographic differences with reference to age and sex. More adult males in the western states contract the disease than females, whereas in the eastern states the attack rates have been higher for women and children.

Seasonal factors are related to attack rates for the disease. The tick season begins in the late spring, continuing through the summer. However, in the South the season may be longer, and cases have been reported during all months of the year. Domestic cats and dogs may harbor infected ticks throughout the year unless the ticks are removed.

Transmission

The disease is transmitted to humans by the bite of an infected tick or by contamination of the skin with tick feces or tissues. The infection is not transmitted from man to man. The longer ticks remain on the skin the greater the danger of their transmitting the disease. Caution should be exercised in removing ticks so as not to crush them, and gloves should be worn when removing ticks from animals. In the past, large animals were frequently dipped in a solution designed to kill the ticks.

Incubation period

The incubation period varies from two to twelve days, but it may be as long as fourteen days, with an average of about seven days.

Clinical manifestations

Rocky Mountain spotted fever may vary in severity from mild to severe. A prodromal period of malaise, headache, and loss of appetite usually precedes a sudden onset of temperature, ranging from 103° to 104° F., chills, generalized aching, possibly severe pain in joints and muscles, and nausea and vomiting. In severe cases the temperature may remain high for two weeks or longer, with remission in the morning and elevation in the afternoon. The temperature falls by lysis after about two weeks.

The characteristic maculopapular cutaneous eruption appears in about two to five days after the onset of fever. Typically, the rash is confined to the arms and legs, but it may cover the entire body, beginning on the flexor areas of the wrists, ankles, forearms, and palms of the hands and soles of the feet. After three or four days the cutaneous lesions may vary from petechial to confluent ecchymotic areas, where necrosis and sloughing may occur. After the disappearance of the purpuric skin lesions, pigmentation with desquamation follows. In mild cases the rash may not reach a hemorrhagic stage.

In severe cases the pulse is weak and rapid, the respiratory rate is increased, and hypotension, a nonproductive cough, photophobia, constipation, abdominal distention, oliguria or anuria, and azotemia may occur. Splenomegaly and severe anemia are not uncommon. Neurologic symptoms include continuation of the severe headache, restlessness, deafness, stiffness of the neck, delirium, convulsions, and coma.[2]

Diagnosis

During the prodromal period before the appearance of the rash, diagnosis may be difficult. When illness follows, the history of a tick bite, especially in regions where a tick reservoir is known to exist, may form the best evidence for clinical diagnosis.

The complement-fixation test is probably the most reliable laboratory test for Rocky Mountain spotted fever. The Weil-Felix reaction is an agglutination test, which, if positive, may suggest a presumptive diagnosis. Attempts to isolate the causative agent are usually not advised except in research studies.

The preeruptive stage of the disease may be confused with a number of other illnesses. With the appearance of the rash, differential diagnosis includes murine typhus fever, meningococcemia, measles, and rickettsialpox.

Treatment

Therapy for Rocky Mountain spotted fever is both specific antibiotic and supportive care. When treatment is started early, antibiotics produce dramatic results and reduce the febrile period. The therapeutic agents of choice are chloramphenicol, chloretetracycline, and oxytetracycline.

Supportive therapy is based on altered physiologic conditions and the clinical syndrome. Frequent laboratory studies of hemoglobin, electrolytes, hematocrit, and protein will guide the physician in the management of the patient. Fluid balance is maintained to provide at least 1500 ml. of urinary output daily. Parenteral administration of 3000 to 4000 ml. of fluid may be necessary.[1]

Complications

Complications with Rocky Mountain spotted fever are rare, and if they do occur, they are usually the result of bacterial infection. Pneumonia occasionally occurs as a secondary infection. Cardiac failure is rare, and its occurrence may result from too rapid administration of parenteral infusions.

Nursing care

Patients admitted to the hospital with Rocky Mountain spotted fever do not need to be isolated, but they should be in a quiet, well-ventilated, slightly darkened room. The body should be carefully inspected for the presence of ticks that may be attached to the skin. Various methods have been suggested to make tick removal easier, including touching the tick with an applicator dipped in gasoline or whiskey[2] or touching the tick with a lighted match. Forceps should be used, placing them close to the mouth of the tick. The wound should then be washed with soap and water or an antiseptic solution. On admission, the patient's clothing should be disinfected, preferably by autoclaving.

Patients with Rocky Mountain spotted fever who have not been previously immunized are very sick, and everything possible should be done to provide comfort. The patient's position should be changed frequently to prevent pulmonary complications and to relieve pressure on bony prominences, where necrosis resulting from the ecchymotic skin rash is most likely to occur. Procedures to control fever and oral care are the same as those for other febrile patients. Constipation and flatus may be relieved by small enemas or a well-lubricated rectal tube for short periods.

If intravenous fluids are administered, they must be regulated to drip slowly to prevent edema or myocardial failure. Because of the hypoproteinemia that is often present, the diet should be high in calories and planned to include 3 to 5 Gm. daily of protein per kilogram of body weight. Small frequent feedings may be tolerated better than a regular three-meal regimen.

Vital signs must be closely monitored and urinary output observed for any evidence of anuria. Intake and output records should be maintained. Although convulsions are rare, a mouth gag and bedrails should be available, and neurologic conditions may require the use of restraints. Oxygen may be given if pneumonia develops or in case of circulatory failure. During the acute stage of illness, continuous nursing care is required.

Prevention and control

Persons should avoid tick-infested areas if possible. If they cannot, protective white clothing including boots should be worn, an insect repellant should be used, careful inspection of the body and clothes should be made at three-hour intervals and ticks should be removed using care not to crush them. White clothes make the ticks highly visible.

Persons whose occupation requires them to be in areas infected with ticks should secure immunization with *R. rickettsii* vaccine. If continued exposure is likely, a booster dose each year is recommended. An attack renders a person immune for life.

All cases of Rocky Mountain spotted fever are reportable in the United States and Canada.

REFERENCES

1. Conn, Howard F., editor: Current therapy 1968, Philadelphia, 1968, W. B. Saunders Co.
2. Horsfall, Frank L., Jr., and Tamm, Igor, editors: Viral and rickettsial infections of man, ed. 4, Philadelphia, 1965, J. B. Lippincott Co.

47

TYPHUS FEVER

Etiology

The word typhus translated from Greek means "stupor," and refers to the stuporous, confused mental state of typhus patients. Typhus fever occurs in three forms, all of which are caused by *Rickettsia*. Epidemic typhus (classic typhus) is caused by *R. prowazekii* and is transmitted by the vector *Pediculus humanus corporis* (human body louse). Brill-Zinsser disease is caused by the same organism as epidemic typhus, but it occurs in the absence of louse infestation; however, there is a history of prior infection with epidemic typhus. Murine typhus is caused by *R. mooseri* and is transmitted to humans by *Xenopsylla cheopis* (rat flea). The different types of typhus fever resemble each other but vary in severity.

Epidemiology

Throughout several centuries, classic typhus was epidemic in Europe, Africa, and Asia, and millions of persons succumbed to its ravages. Severe epidemics have occurred during war, famine, and crowding. World Wars I and II were no exception. During World War II an immunizing vaccine (Cox type) became available and was administered to both military forces and civilians in areas where the disease was epidemic. In 1960 less than 700 cases were reported, whereas in 1959, 5800 cases were reported.[2]

The disease remains endemic in many areas. The largest number of cases reported by the World Health Organization in 1966 were in Ethiopia, where 3557 cases occurred.

Brill-Zinsser disease has been identified in many countries, including the United States. The disease occurs in persons who have had epidemic typhus, although the infection may have been inapparent. Many persons who recovered from typhus during World War II subsequently migrated to various parts of the world, including the United States. Studies have indicated that a person with the disease may infect lice who feed on them. The results of these studies provide a clue to sporadic cases and epidemics of typhus that occur in nontyphus areas.[5] However, the disease may also occur in typhus zones.

The occurrence of murine typhus is worldwide and is closely related to the prevalence of rats that harbor the vector. No cases have been reported by Statistics Canada between 1971 and 1974. Vital Statistics of the United States reported twenty-three cases in 1971, eighteen cases in 1972, and thirty-two cases in 1973. No deaths have been reported in the U. S. from this disease since 1960.

Age, sex, and seasonal factors

Persons of all ages are susceptible to all forms of typhus, including Brill-Zinsser disease, although the incidence of epidemic typhus is greatest between 3 and 36 years of age. Males and females are affected equally, but the disease is milder in children and fatality rates increase with age. The mortality rate of epidemic typhus is as high as 10% to 40%. Murine typhus is usually much milder than epidemic typhus, and most of the fatalities are in persons over 50 years of age.

Epidemic typhus is a disease of cold climates and occurs during the winter months, whereas murine typhus is most prevalent during the warm months of summer and early fall. There are no specific seasonal factors related to Brill-Zinsser disease.

Transmission

Epidemic typhus is transmitted from man to man by an infected body louse, *P. humanus corporis.* The causative organism is excreted in the feces of the louse, and when it bites, the person scratches or otherwise infects the wound with the feces. Transmission by inhalation of dust containing dried louse feces, principally from dirty contaminated clothing, may occur. Lice become infected by feeding on the blood of infected persons.

Brill-Zinsser disease is not transmitted from man to man, but lice may become infected by feeding on the patient early during the febrile period.

Murine typhus is transmitted to man by the bite of an infected rat flea, *X. cheopis,* and infection occurs in the same way as in epidemic typhus. The reservoir of infection is maintained by the rat-flea-rat cycle.

Incubation period

The incubation period for epidemic typhus is about ten to fourteen days, with some variation depending on the size of the dose of the infecting organisms. The period is essentially the same for murine typhus, with an average of about twelve days. The incubation period for Brill-Zinsser disease is unknown.

Clinical manifestations

The onset of epidemic typhus is abrupt with malaise, headache, chills, nausea, dizziness, and generalized muscle tenderness and pain during the first two days. There is a gradual increase in fever until it reaches 104° to

105° F. by the third day, where it remains without remission until recovery or fatal termination. The pulse and respiratory rates are rapid, and there is hypotension, nonproductive cough, photophobia, constipation, and deafness.

Between the fourth and seventh days the characteristic rash appears, first on the trunk and gradually spreading over the entire body, including palms of the hands and soles of the feet. The rash begins as pink or red macules or maculopapules, which change in color to reddish purple by the second week. In some cases the rash may be petechial or purpuric in character. The extent of the rash may vary with the severity of the disease and in mild cases may be absent. The patient is lethargic and delirious.

A variety of symptoms such as renal insufficiency, elevated blood urea nitrogen, anemia, and incontinence of urine and feces are present. Neurologic symptoms may vary from deafness and mental dullness to stupor, delirium, and coma.

By the third week the temperature falls by lysis and all symptoms subside rapidly, although complete recovery and convalescense may require two to three months. In fatal cases death usually occurs between the ninth and twentieth days.

Symptoms of Brill-Zinsser disease differ little from those of epidemic typhus. The disease is milder and shorter in duration. The cutaneous eruption may be absent, and fatality rates are usually lower.

Murine typhus is essentially the same as epidemic typhus. In fact, clinical symptoms are so similar that differentiation from epidemic typhus is difficult. The primary differences include a more insidious onset, the febrile period is shorter, and the cutaneous eruption is less severe. The temperature tends to fluctuate more widely than that in epidemic typhus.

Diagnosis

Clinical diagnosis of typhus may be difficult during the preeruptive stage, and it may not be possible to distinguish epidemic typhus from murine typhus. In children clinical diagnosis may be particularly difficult. In areas where Rocky Mountain spotted fever exists there may be confusion between the two diseases. During the preeruptive stage, typhus may be confused with other rickettsial diseases, smallpox, measles, yellow fever, and meningococcemia.

Laboratory diagnosis should be made by serologic tests, blood cultures, and the Weil-Felix reaction. Tests have now been developed that may be made at the bedside in three to five minutes.

Treatment

The treatment of all forms of typhus is with broad-spectrum antibiotics and supportive therapy. Antibiotics used include chlortetracycline, oxytetracycline, and chloramphenicol. If oral administration is impossible because of nausea and vomiting or if the patient is comatose, administration may be by the intravenous route. Drugs are continued until the temperature has been normal for twenty-four to forty-eight hours.[1] There are various opinions concerning administration schedules and the effectiveness of antibiotics. Most authorities agree that the use of antibiotics in typhus has been limited and that their effectiveness is based on their use in other rickettsial infections.[3]

Paraldehyde or chloral hydrate are used as sedation for restlessness and delirium, and codeine may be administered for headache. If cyanosis occurs, oxygen is given by mask or nasal catheter. Based on laboratory examinations, infusions are given to maintain fluid and electrolyte balance.

Immunity

If the patient recovers from an attack, he is permanently immune.

Complications

Invasion by bacteria may lead to bronchopneumonia, otitis media, and furunculosis. Inadequately treated patients may suffer from a relapse. Necrotic conditions of the skin, as in Rocky Mountain spotted fever, may occur, and gangrene of toes, fingers, ear lobes, and nose may result from thrombosis of small blood vessels. Cardiovascular and renal complications may occur in untreated patients.

Nursing care

Careful delousing of the patient should be done immediately on admission to the hospital. All persons should be protected by a surgical gown and rubber gloves. The patient's entire body is bathed, using a 1% solution of Lysol, followed by dusting with 10% DDT, including the bed and hospital clothing. The dusting is continued at weekly intervals until the patient is discharged. The patient's admission clothing should be autoclaved.

The nursing care of the patient is the same as that for Rocky Mountain spotted fever. The patient should be encouraged to take sufficient fluids to provide a urinary output of 1500 ml. daily. A liquid or soft diet may be given or if the patient is comatose, gastric gavage may be necessary. The diet should be high calorie, and if hypoproteinemia occurs, increased protein should be provided. Frequent turning is important to prevent pulmonary complications and necrosis of the skin. Continuous nursing care is necessary during the febrile period. No isolation of the patient is necessary after proper delousing has been done.

Prevention and control

Immunization of all persons who have had contact with epidemic typhus is advisable. The Cox-type vaccine is recommended with two subcutaneous injections of 1 ml. each at an interval of ten to fourteen days and a booster dose as advised. The vaccine should not be given to persons sensitive to egg protein.

Quarantine for fifteen days in a vermin-free room, delousing, and the application of insecticides are required for louse-infested contacts, and immunization is required for all immediate contacts.

The control of murine typhus emphasizes the control of fleas with suitable insecticides, followed by rat control through poisoning or trapping and rat-proofing buildings. Since fleas leave a dead rat, the control of fleas should precede rat destruction. Isolation, quarantine, and immunization of contacts are not required for murine typhus.

Reporting of endemic typhus is mandatory by the International Sanitary Regulations, and most countries require the reporting of murine typhus. Although typhus immunization is not required by any country as a condition of entry, it is, nevertheless, recommended to travelers when plans include visits to countries that are infected, or those in which living conditions are generally poor.

REFERENCES

1. Conn, Howard F., editor: Current therapy 1968, Philadelphia, 1968, W. B. Saunders Co.
2. Hinman, E. Harold: World eradication of infectious diseases, Springfield, Ill., 1966, Charles C Thomas, Publisher.
3. Horsfall, Frank L., Jr., and Tamm, Igor, editors: Viral and rickettsial infections of man, ed. 4, Philadelphia, 1965, J. B. Lippincott Co.

48

YELLOW FEVER

Etiology

Yellow fever is caused by a filtrable virus belonging to a group of arborviruses. It is recognized in two forms, classic yellow fever transmitted from man to man by a vector, *Aedes aegypti,* a semidomestic mosquito. Jungle yellow fever, or sylvatic yellow fever, occurs among wild animals and is transmitted to man by several genuses of mosquito vectors. However, except for the epidemiologic aspects the two diseases are identical. The jaundice the patient suffers gives the disease its name.

Epidemiology

The great epidemics of yellow fever that occurred prior to the twentieth century have been well documented in history. As early as 1901, William G. Gorgas believed that yellow fever could be eradicated from the world, but it was 1915 before attempts toward elimination were made. Since 1930 concentrated efforts have continued. Although efforts were being made in many parts of the Western Hemisphere to eradicate the vector, the United States failed to take any steps toward elimination in this country.[5] The problem of eradication of the *A. aegypti* is etiologic, and since the United States began its program in 1964, yellow fever–receptive areas have been identified in South Carolina, Florida, Georgia, Alabama, Mississippi, Tennessee, Arkansas, Louisiana, and southeastern Texas, where the *A. aegypti* is widely distributed in both urban and rural areas. Parts of the Virgin Islands, Puerto Rico, and some counties of Florida and southern Texas show heavy infestation and breeding occurring throughout the year.[4] Statistics Canada reports that Canada has been free of the disease from 1960 to the present time. Vital Statistics of the United States similarly reports that no cases of yellow fever have been reported in the United States since 1964.

Although some countries of South America have been reported free of the disease, in some of the countries yellow fever remained endemic throughout 1965 and 1966.[1]

Age, sex, and seasonal factors

All age groups and both sexes are susceptible to yellow fever. The adult male may be the victim of jungle yellow fever more often than the female since his work brings him closer to the natural habitat of the vector; however, in some areas women and children are also affected because the *A. aegypti* mosquito is a household pest, breeding in most artificial water deposits such as cisterns, rain gutters, and flower vases. There has been some evidence that the disease may be less severe in children and Negroes. Present evidence seems to support the belief that in enzootic areas of the world the virus may be maintained and transmitted by man to mosquito to man at any time of the year. Although the principal vectors of sylvatic yellow fever are found in the tropical rain forest, the virus has been known to survive for prolonged dry seasons.[2]

Transmission

The virus of yellow fever is transmitted to man by the bite of an infected mosquito, the cycle of transmission being man-mosquito-man.

Incubation period

The usual incubation period for yellow fever is three to six days.

Clinical manifestations

Yellow fever may be mild or severe, and it is now known that a large number of inapparent infections occur. The onset is abrupt, with a rapid rise of fever to 104° F. or more with bradycardia, myalgia, headache, dizziness nausea, vomiting, and prostration. By forty-eight hours after the onset, mild jaundice and hemorrhagic manifestations appear. There is bleeding from the gastric system, the so-called "black vomit" that was diagnostic at the beginning of the century. Hemorrhage from other body orifices occurs. Urinary output may become scanty, and hypotension, weak pulse, collapse, and death may result. Neurologic symptoms such as delirium and extreme restlessness may or may not occur. In cases that terminate fatally, albuminuria and leukopenia are commonly present with significant changes in blood chemistry.

Diagnosis

In the absence of an epidemic, clinical diagnosis may be missed. The most reliable diagnostic procedure is isolation of the virus from the blood during the first three or four days of illness. Serologic diagnosis may be made in primary infections to determine specific antibody titer. In fatal cases a pathologic diagnosis can be made by finding the characteristic liver lesions. Specimens of liver tissue may be secured on necropsy or by using a viscerotome without necropsy.

Treatment

There is no specific treatment for yellow fever. Therapy is symptomatic and may include blood transfusions, fluid and electrolyte maintenance, analgesics for pain, and methods to control fever.

Nursing care

Isolation and concurrent disinfection are unnecessary, but whether in the home or in the hospital the patient's room should be well screened. In the absence of screens the room should be sprayed with an insecticide having a residual effect. The patient should be in a quiet room with maximum provision for rest. Continuous nursing care is necessary, and bedrails and restraints should be available to prevent the patient from self-injury in case of severe delirium. Personal care is the same as that for all febrile patients. Needles for intravenous infusion should be well anchored to prevent their being dislodged during periods of intense restlessness. As soon as vomiting ceases, oral fluids should be encouraged. There should be careful observation to determine blood loss from hemorrhages. Specific dietary requirements will be ordered by the physician. Prognosis depends on the severity of the disease, and mild cases may recover within a week, whereas severe cases may terminate fatally in three or four days. If the patient recovers, convalescence is generally prolonged.

Prevention and control

Yellow fever is preventable by vaccination with 0.5 ml. of 17 D strain yellow fever virus vaccine. Indications are that antibodies persist for as long as seventeen to nineteen years after immunization. Further control measures require the destruction of the *A. aegypti* mosquito and its breeding places.

Reporting of all cases is required by all countries, and vaccination should be given to all international travelers over 6 months of age when their destination is yellow fever–receptive areas of the United States.[3]

REFERENCES

1. Epidemiological and Vital Statistics Report 20, no. 4, Geneva, 1967, World Health Organization.
2. Horsfall, Frank L., Jr., and Tamm, Igor, editors: Viral and rickettsial infections of man, ed. 4, Philadelphia, 1965, J. B. Lippincott Co.
3. Immunization information for international travel 1967-1968, Public Health Service Publication no. 384, Washington, D. C., 1967, U. S. Government Printing Office.
4. Schliessmann, Harold J.: Aedes aegypti eradication program of the United States —progress report 1965, Am. J. Public Health **57**:460-465, March, 1967.
5. Soper, Fred L.: The eradication of urban yellow fever in the Americas through the eradication of Aedes aegypti, Am. J. Public Health **53**:7-16, Jan., 1963.

SECTION FIVE

Diseases caused by fungi

Fungi are a group of organisms belonging to the plant kingdom. Many fungi are known to be beneficial to man, such as those from which many of our antibiotics are derived. Some, such as molds, may be helpful under certain circumstances but under others may be found associated with inflammatory conditions of the skin. Mycotic infections of man are primarily caused by "true fungi" and largely by Fungi Imperfecti. Infections caused by these fungi are classified as superficial mycoses that involve the skin, as in ringworm infection, and other forms of tinea that cause infection of the beard, smooth skin, feet, and nails. Collectively these superficial fungus infections are known as dermatophytoses. A second group of fungi infections are deep mycoses, or systemic infections. In recent years considerable attention has been given to the deep mycotic diseases because some of them cause morbidity and mortality in man. In this section discussion will be limited to three that occur most commonly, blastomycosis, coccidioidomycosis, and histoplasmosis.

49
BLASTOMYCOSIS

Etiology

A number of forms of blastomycosis caused by different organisms have been recognized, all of which have certain commonalities. North American blastomycosis (Gilchrist's disease) is caused by *Blastomyces dermatitidis;* South American blastomycosis *(paracoccidioidal granuloma)* is caused by *B. brasiliensis;* and keloidal blastomycosis has also been called South American blastomycosis and is frequently confused with it. However, it is caused by *Loboa loboi.* A fungus disease known as cryptococcosis is also called European blastomycosis, and the etiologic agent is *Cryptococcus neoformans.*[1]

Epidemiology

In general, blastomycosis is an uncommon disease and the exact incidence is unknown. North American blastomycosis occurs as sporadic cases in the southeastern United States, Canada, Africa, and Central America. The disease has also occurred in some animals, particularly horses and dogs. South American blastomycosis is endemic in Central America, where most of the cases are reported from Brazil. Cryptococcosis (European blastomycosis) occurs throughout the world as sporadic cases. Between 1960 and 1969, 153 deaths occurred from the disease. In the United States this disease is only "optionally" reported so accurate statistics are not available. However, in 1972, eleven states reported forty-five cases and in 1973, thirty-nine cases were reported by eleven states. No statistics are available for Canada as it is not a notifiable disease.

Age, sex, and race

All ages are probably susceptible to blastomycosis; however, with the exception of cryptococcosis the extent of susceptibility and resistance is unknown. Most cases of the disease occur among persons from 15 years of age to between 30 and 45 years of age. In all forms the incidence is considerably greater among males than females. In South American blastomycosis the ratio is ten males to one female. Apparently there are no significant racial factors in the incidence of the disease.

Transmission

The exact methods of transmission have not been clearly established. It is believed that the etiologic agent is present in the soil and dust and that the spores are inhaled. There is no evidence that blastomycosis is transmitted from person to person.

Incubation period

The incubation period of blastomycosis is unknown.

Clinical manifestations

North American blastomycosis is a systemic disease, chronic in character, that involves the lungs. The disease may begin with upper respiratory symptoms similar to those of influenza that become progressively worse with a productive cough and involvement of bones, central nervous system, body organs, and tissues. Although only about 50% of persons have clinically apparent infection, unless treated the fatality rate is high.

The disease may begin with cutaneous manifestations characterized by a papule that progresses to a wartlike lesion, which ulcerates and spreads outward. The lesion may continue to spread over a period of months or years. The lesions are usually on the hands, wrists, and feet. Systemic involvement is usually present, and the cutaneous lesion is simply a manifestation of the general infection.

Symptoms associated with South American blastomycosis include ulcerative lesions of the buccal cavity. Lesions occurring about the teeth may cause loosening and loss of the teeth. The disease may involve the lymphatics in the neck and infect internal viscera. The disease is considered highly fatal.

Diagnosis

The most satisfactory method of diagnosis is the isolation of the *B. dermatitidis* from cultures. Specimens for microscopic examination may be secured from sputum, urine, or pus from cutaneous lesions. Although serology tests and the intradermal skin test using blastomycin have been used, they have been shown to be less reliable than in some of the other deep mycotic infection.[2]

For treatment and nursing care see the section entitled Nursing care of patients with systemic mycoses in Chapter 51.

REFERENCES

1. Gordon, John E., editor: Control of communicable diseases in man, ed. 10, New York, 1965, American Public Health Assn., Inc.
2. Kaufman, Leo: Serology of systemic fungus diseases, Public Health Reports **81:** 177-185, Feb., 1966.

50

COCCIDIOIDOMYCOSIS (VALLEY FEVER)

Etiology

Coccidioidomycosis (valley fever), one of the most infectious of the fungus diseases, is a systemic fungus infection caused by the *Coccidioides immitis*. Two clinical forms of the disease are recognized: (1) primary coccidioidomycosis, a self-limited pulmonary or extrapulmonary cutaneous infection; and (2) progressive disseminated coccidioidomycosis (coccidioidal granuloma), a highly fatal form of the disease. If the disease has been present for less than six months, it is considered acute, whereas if its duration is more than six months, it is regarded as chronic. It may have a single or multiple focus of infection, and only about 0.5% of cases become disseminated.[1]

Epidemiology

This highly infectious fungus disease is endemic in southern California, Arizona, New Mexico, Utah, Nevada, and western Texas. It also occurs in Mexico, southeastern Europe, and Central America. The infection rate is so high that most persons who live in the endemic area for any length of time will become infected. However, only about 50% to 60% of infections produce clinical symptoms, and less than 1% develops serious disease. In 1972, 951 cases were reported in the United States by thirteen states. This disease is only optionally reported. The two states reporting the greatest incidence were Arizona with 517 cases and California with 415 cases. In 1973, twelve states reported 436 cases. No statistics are available for Canada. Between 1960 and 1969, 553 deaths were recorded in the United States as a result of this disease.

Age, sex, race, and seasonal factors

Persons of all ages and races and both sexes are susceptible to coccidioidomycosis. It is believed that in permanent populations, children acquire a primary infection during early childhood that is demonstrated only by sensitivity to the coccidioidin skin test. The disease occurs most frequently among males between 15 and 25 years of age, and dark-skinned races are infected ten times more frequently than white persons. In primary nondisseminated coccidioidomycosis, erythema nodosum occurs most frequently in white females, whereas the dark-skinned races develop the disseminated form of the disease from 30% to 40% more often than white persons.

Seasonal factors are important in the incidence of the disease. During rainy periods the incidence decreases, but during warm dry periods, particularly when there is wind, the spores are blown about on air currents causing an increased incidence of the disease.

Transmission

The source of the disease is the spore-laden soil and dust, and the infection is the result of inhaling the spores. Laboratory workers are at risk while working with cultures containing the organism. Although it is believed rare, extrapulmonary cutaneous infection through open wounds or abrasions is a possibility. Indirect transmission through respiratory secretions and contaminated clothing is considered rare.

Incubation period

The incubation period for coccidioidomycosis varies between seven and twenty-one days.

Clinical manifestations

In primary coccidioidomycosis the clinical syndrome varies in severity. Fever is usually about 101° F., but it may be higher, and chills, headache, backache, loss of appetite, malaise, and a nonproductive cough are commonly observed. Pleural pain is an outstanding sign, and a mild nonproductive pharyngitis and a fine toxic erythematous skin rash may occur in some patients. X-ray examination of the lungs may reveal pneumonitis, which is usually resolved leaving only calcified scars, or small lesions called coccidioidomas may remain and often tend to break down later causing cavities. Although these cavities may increase in size, they do not spread and develop new pulmonary lesions. However, if they become extensive in size, hemorrhage may occur or the lesions may be invaded by bacteria or rupture into the pleural space.[2]

About 5% of persons exhibit a hypersensitivity characterized by erythema nodosum, joint pain, and conjunctivitis, commonly referred to as valley fever because of the high incidence in the San Joaquin valley in California. Persons who recover from primary coccidioidomycosis develop an immunity that protects against progressive disseminated disease.

Progressive disseminated coccidioidomycosis is characterized by extrapulmonary spread of the disease and usually has its beginning during the primary stage of the disease. It is believed to be caused by some defect in the individual's immune mechanism that permits the infection to spread.

It is estimated that less than 1% of persons infected develop this serious complication. The clinical syndrome depends on the site and extent of the lesions and may vary from a single lesion presenting no symptoms to widely disseminated infection with septic fever and severe toxicity. In disseminated infections lesions may occur in bones, lymph nodes, viscera, meninges, brain, and heart. The spread is not unlike that found in extrapulmonary tuberculosis.

Diagnosis

Diagnosis of coccidioidomycosis begins with the cutaneous intradermal skin test with coccidioidin. The test is similar to the tuberculin test in that it is simply an indication of recent or remote infection, but it does not indicate the stage of the disease or its activity. The test consists of 0.1 ml. of 1:100 dilution of coccidioidin in sterile saline solution, which is injected into the skin of the flexor surface of the forearm. The test is read and graded the same as the Mantoux tuberculin test.

The complement-fixation test is widely used and may be indicative of the severity of the infection. If the serology test is negative even though the skin test may be positive, the prognosis is considered good. However, a negative skin test with a positive complement-fixation test may indicate widespread dissemination of the disease and a poor prognosis.[3] Taken together, the coccidioidin skin test and the complement-fixation test provide valuable diagnostic and prognostic information.

Two new laboratory tests are being used, including (1) the immunodiffusion test, a rapid test used for screening, and reported to be 95% effective for identifying the disease; (2) the microcomplement-fixation test, which is also a rapid test.

Positive proof of the disease may be obtained by isolation of the specific fungus in cultures or stained sections of tissue.

For treatment and nursing care see the section entitled Nursing care of patients with systemic mycoses in Chapter 51.

REFERENCES

1. Conn, Howard F., editor: Current therapy 1968, Philadelphia, 1968, W. B. Saunders Co.
2. Samter, Max, editor: Immunological diseases, Boston, 1965, Little, Brown & Co., chap. 31.

51

HISTOPLASMOSIS (DARLING'S DISEASE)

Etiology

Histoplasmosis is caused by *Histoplasma capsulatum,* once believed to be a protozoan but now identified as a fungus that grows in moist, fertile soil in many parts of the world. Infection caused by *H. capsulatum* is very much like that caused by *Coccidioides immitis.* The disease has many striking similarities to tuberculosis, and evidence seems to indicate that the disease, as in tuberculosis, depends on developing a hypersensitivity to the organism rather than the multiplication and spread of the infectious agent throughout the body.[7]

In addition to man, histoplasmosis affects at least seventeen species of wild and domestic animals.[3]

Epidemiology

Histoplasmosis has been found in thirty-one countries, where it is endemic in all of the major river valleys of the United States, Canada, Africa, Southeast Asia, Burma, India, Thailand, and Pakistan. It is estimated that 30 million persons are infected, with 500,000 new infections annually. No exact figures are available, but it is estimated that in the United States between 2000 and 3000 persons are admitted each year to tuberculosis sanatoria with active histoplasmosis.[5] Between 1960 and 1969, 719 deaths were reported in the United States. In some areas of the mideastern and midwestern United States 80% of the population have evidence of past or present infection as shown by the histoplasmin skin test.[7] In 1972, sixteen states reported a total of 226 cases. In 1973, twenty-two states reported a total of 284 cases. This is an optionally reported communicable disease in the United States, but is not notifiable in Canada.

H. capsulatum is found in the soil, where it manifests a preference for warm, humid, and moist temperature. Although the fungus has been found primarily in rural areas, epidemics have occurred in urban areas. In the past, birds, particularly the starling, have been linked to epidemics of the disease. Soil about chicken houses and manure used as fertilizer on gardens and yards have also been incriminated as the cause of infection. Present evidence appears to indicate that the only relationship is that bird droppings and fertilizer provide the media for the fungus to grow as a saprophyte. When the soil is disturbed, the infectious particles from the fungus (spores-conidia) are released into the air, where they may be inhaled.[3]

Age, sex, and race

Histoplasmosis may occur in a serious form at any age, but 30% of the progressive forms occur in children under 10 years of age. Chronic pulmonary histoplasmosis is commonest in persons past 40 years of age. Persons with some degree of immunity after a primary infection have a greater danger of an endogenous reinfection after 50 years of age, and the danger increases with age.

The distribution between sexes is equal in persons under 10 years of age, but in adults, males with histoplasmosis outnumber females 3:1.

From various studies the rate of infection is essentially the same for white and Negro races. Persons who contract the disease tend to be those spending much time outdoors such as construction workers, farmers, and spelunkers.

Transmission

Histoplasmosis is contracted by inhaling the airborne spores from *H. capsulatum* into the lungs. The disease is not transmitted from person to person, and there is no evidence that the disease is transmitted from animals to humans or from animals to animals. There has been some speculation that the disease may be contracted by ingestion of the spores. Christie states that histoplasmin complement-fixing antibodies may be transferred from the mother to the infant in the same manner as syphilis is transferred.[1]

Incubation period

The incubation period for histoplasmosis varies between five and eighteen days, with an average of ten days.

Clinical manifestations

The onset of the disease occurs about ten to fourteen days after the inhalation of the spores. The dust-laden spore lodges in the lung, and from 50% to 60% of persons thus infected recover spontaneously with no symptoms. Apparently the healthy body is able to destroy the fungus before much lung tissue is involved. The only evidence of a primary infection may be a positive histoplasmin skin test and the presence of complement-fixing antibodies, which develop two to three weeks after onset of the disease. These infections are generally referred to as benign asymptomatic histoplasmosis.

The disease may also be benign and symptomatic, in which symptoms similar to influenza develop. There may be fever, malaise, cough that may or may not be productive, and intermittent chest pains. These patients are usually weak and have prostration, which confines them to bed for as long as four to six weeks. In many of these patients calcified lesions in the lungs may be observed on x-ray examination. In some persons enlarged lymph nodes, splenomegaly, and ulcerative lesions of the mucous membranes may occur. Although convalescence may be protracted, recovery is spontaneous.

Generalized disseminated histoplasmosis may be acute or chronic, with the infection spread to various parts of the body by the bloodstream or through lymphatic channels. In disseminated progressive disease there are oral and gastrointestinal ulcerations, endocarditis, pericarditis, meningitis, splenomegaly, and adrenal insufficiency.[7] About one third of the disseminated cases occur in children under 10 years of age, and they are uniformly fatal. In a study made by Furcolow and co-workers of 108 patients with disseminated disease, 83% died within one year after diagnosis.[4]

Chronic pulmonary histoplasmosis is commonest in persons 40 years of age and older. The disease is slowly progressive, with cavitary infiltration and fibrosis of the lungs. There is moderate fever, blood-streaked sputum, and loss of weight. The disease is so similar to pulmonary tuberculosis that it is clinically indistinguishable. The disease is ultimately fatal but somewhat more protracted than disseminated infection. In the study by Furcolow and co-workers previously cited, among eighty-five patients with chronic pulmonary histoplasmosis the average length of life was 3.6 years. Among two thirds of the patients at the time of the study one half were disabled.[4]

Diagnosis

The only positive proof of histoplasmosis is recovery and identification of *H. capsulatum* by the culture technic. Specimens for cultures may be obtained from blood and bone marrow, scrapings may be made from ulcerated lesions, and biopsy tissue may be obtained from the spleen, liver, and lymph nodes.[6]

The histoplasmin skin test is performed using 0.1 ml. of the antigen administered intradermally and read the same as the tuberculin test. Sensitivity to the antigen develops in about two weeks after exposure, and as in tuberculosis, the histoplasmin test tends to remain positive. However, the test merely indicates experience with the organism and does not indicate the presence of disease.

Work has been done with five serology tests. Serology tests may be diagnostic by indicating activity of the disease and may also be prognostic by showing a progressively or consistently high antibody titer.

Differential diagnosis

Among the commonest diseases confused with primary histoplasmosis are influenza and atypical pneumonia. Progressive histoplasmosis may need to be differentiated from various malignant conditions such as the leukemia-lymphoma group of diseases and Hodgkin's disease. From the number of patients with histoplasmosis in tuberculosis sanatoria it would appear that tuberculosis is a frequent diagnosis, although both diseases may be found in the same person. Evidence supports the view that when tuberculosis and histoplasmosis occur in the same person, it is by chance rather than cause and effect. Ulcerative lesions of the skin and mucous membranes may be suggestive of syphilis, tuberculosis, or other fungous diseases that affect the skin and mucous membranes.

Treatment of deep mycoses

Most authorities agree that the perfect drug for treatment of systemic mycosis has not been found. The three diseases reviewed in this section are treated with amphotericin B (Fungizone). The drug is relatively toxic and may produce toxic reactions.

Patients with blastomycosis frequently respond well to amphotericin B in the beginning, but a high relapse rate occurs. However, high relapse rates have occurred with other agents used to treat the disease. Amphotericin B is administered intravenously, beginning with an initial dose of 1 to 5 mg. in 5% dextrose in water and administered over a two- to six-hour period. The drug is increased daily by 5 to 10 mg., until a total of 1 to 2 Gm. has been given. The total amount given may be increased for lung cavitation or in bone disease. Another drug that has been used is 2-hydroxystilbamidine isethionate, which is administered intravenously daily for a total of 7 to 10 Gm.

Coccidioidomycosis is treated with amphotericin B but is more resistant to the drug than blastomycosis or histoplasmosis. In some instances a total of 10 Gm. has been administered over a one- to three-year period. The infusion is started with 10 mg. of the drug in 5% dextrose in water and administered over a four-hour period. The amount of drug is increased daily until 1 mg. per kilogram of body weight has been attained. The infusion then may be given every other day. It is recommended that patients who are to undergo surgery should be treated with amphotericin B for two or three weeks prior to surgery, and in some cases the treatment may be continued after surgery.[2]

Persons with mild histoplasmosis do not usually require treatment. However, consideration is being given to short periods of treatment in primary symptomatic histoplasmosis aimed toward preventing dissemination. Chronic pulmonary histoplasmosis and severe disseminated histoplasmosis are treated initially with amphotericin B administered intravenously over a two- to six-hour period. Treatment may be given daily or every other day, depending on the patient's tolerance for the drug. Treatment is usually continued for approximately four months. Sulfonamides and a new antibiotic agent have been used on an experimental basis, and no information is available at this time concerning their potential therapeutic value.[7]

Nursing care of patients with systemic mycoses

The nursing care of patients with systemic mycoses requires a broad range of knowledge, understanding, and skills. Patients on treatment schedules require hospitalization for weeks or months, often away from their home and family. Diagnostic examinations may be painful and lengthy, as well as time consuming. The patient may feel socially isolated and rejected because of extensive skin lesions and worried and anxious because of the economic aspects of prolonged treatment, all of which combine to make him irritable and unhappy. The patient may be acutely or chronically ill with a variety of painful symptoms, and the skills and knowledge of good medical nursing care will be required. Some patients will be prepared for surgical procedures such as lobectomy, which requires good preoperative preparation and postoperative nursing care. Two-way protection from infection may be necessary for patients with open skin lesions. The patient must be protected from nosocomial infection, although the environment may need to be protected from spores that may be disseminated from the patient. In some situations isolation and medical aseptic technic will be required.

The long tedious treatments will be more acceptable to the patient if

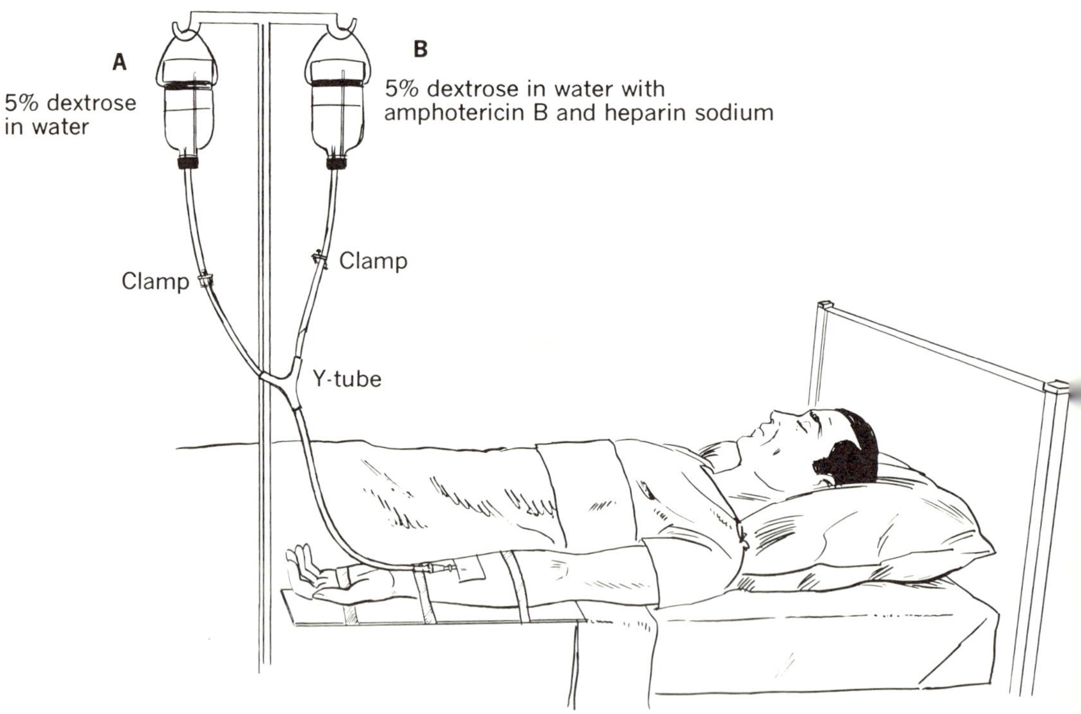

Fig. 32. Intravenous setup to minimize side effects and avoid phlebitis resulting from the administration of amphotericin B. Begin the infusion with 5% dextrose in water, leaving **B** clamped. Alternate, releasing the clamps on **A** and **B** for two to three minutes at twenty-minute intervals. If the reaction occurs, clamp **B** and open **A**, allowing only dextrose in water to run until the reaction subsides, then continue with solution **B.** Keep **B** bottle agitated to prevent the drug from settling in the neck of the bottle.

he knows what to expect, if he has the emotional support of the nurse, and if he believes that the nurse is interested, understands his disease and his problems, and does everything possible for his comfort.

Amphotericin B is a moderately toxic drug, and many patients will experience side effects, including nausea, vomiting, chills, fever, headache, and loss of appetite. Occasionally more severe reactions occur such as cyanosis and changes in the pulse and respiratory rates. Frequently pretreatment medication will reduce the incidence of side effects. Antihistaminics, aspirin, sedative drugs, and corticosteroids may be used for this purpose. The patient should understand that side effects may occur, and if continuous nursing care is provided for several days, it will help him to adjust to treatment and relieve his anxiety.

In the absence of nausea and vomiting, the taking of fluids orally should be encouraged, especially those high in potassium such as orange juice, since diminished potassium in the body may occur as a side effect of the drug. Phlebitis is a possible complication and should be cared for according to the physician's directions. However, the danger of phlebitis can be minimized by using a small-gauge needle and the infusion administered as shown in Fig. 32.

Nurses assisting with the administration of amphotericin B need to be familiar with the behavior of the drug. It is unstable in powder form, should be protected from light, and stored in the refrigerator. It should not be used beyond the expiration date indicated on the vial. It is also relatively insoluble, and the powder should be dissolved in 5% dextrose in water or in sterile water. Saline solution should not be used. The drug should be prepared immediately prior to its addition to 500 or 1000 ml. of 5% dextrose in water for the infusion. During the administration the infusion bottle should be agitated every fifteen to twenty minutes to ensure an even distribution of the drug in solution and to provide a uniform rate of administration.[7]

REFERENCES

1. Christie, Amos: The disease spectrum of human histoplasmosis, Ann. Int. Med. **49**:544-555, March, 1958.
2. Conn, Howard F., editor: Current therapy 1968, Philadelphia, 1968, W. B. Saunders Co.
3. Emmons, Chester W.: Histoplasmosis, Public Health Reports **72**:981-988, Nov., 1957.
4. Furcolow, Michael L., Doto, I. L., Tosh, F. E., and Lynch, H. J., Jr.: Course and prognosis of untreated histoplasmosis; USPH cooperative mycosis study, J. Am. Med. Assoc. **177**:292-296, Aug. 5, 1961.
5. Samter, Max, editor: Immunological diseases, Boston, 1965, Little, Brown & Co., chap. 31.
6. Top, Franklin H., and Wehrle, Paul F.: Communicable and infectious diseases, ed. 7, St. Louis, 1972, The C. V. Mosby Co.
7. Utz, John P., and Benson, Margaret E.: The systemic mycoses, Am. J. Nurs. **65**: 103-110, Sept., 1965.

52

SUPERFICIAL MYCOSES (DERMATOPHYTOSES; RINGWORM OR TINEA)

Etiology

Superficial mycoses are highly communicable fungous infections involving the skin, hair, and nails. The commonest type of infection is ringworm or tinea. These diseases are classified as tinea capitis (ringworm of the scalp), tinea barbae (ringworm of the beard), tinea corporis (ringworm of the smooth skin), and tinea pedis (ringworm of the feet, or "athlete's foot"). The etiologic agents in these infections are various species of *Microsporum* and *Trichophyton.*

Microsporum is responsible for most infections of the scalp, and *Trichophyton* may cause infection of the scalp, beard, skin, and nails, whereas *Epidermophyton* may be the etiologic agent in ringworm of the hands, feet, nails, and skin on the body but does not cause ringworm of the scalp.

Epidemiology

Tinea is one of the oldest and most prevalent skin infections to affect man. In the past, treatment was long and tedious and posed a significant public health problem, especially among school children. With the development of new effective drugs the problem has been ameliorated to a considerable extent. However, all forms of tinea occur worldwide and in frequent epidemics. Tinea capitis is widespread in many urban areas of the United States and Canada. Certain species of the organism cause infections in domestic and wild animals, especially in dogs and cats, which maintain a reservoir of infection that is transmissible to man. In 1971, Vital Statistics, of the United States reported 103 cases. In 1972, 1226 cases were reported by eighteen states and in 1973, 953 cases were reported by fourteen states. Statistics Canada reported sixteen cases in 1972, forty-three cases in 1973, and seven cases during the first twenty-five weeks of 1974.

Persons of all ages and races and both sexes are susceptible to all forms of tinea, but there are differences in infection rates among different age groups and between sexes. Tinea capitis is more common among prepubertal children than among adults, and infection rates are higher among males than females. There are no age differences with tinea corporis, but infection occurs more often among males than among females. The greatest incidence of tinea pedis is among adult males, whereas tinea barbae occurs on bearded areas of the face and neck of adolescent and adult males.

Transmission

The disease is transmitted by both direct and indirect contact. The causative organism may be transmitted through barbershops, clippers, brushes, and combs. In homes common toilet articles, towels, and clothing may be a source of infection. It has been generally believed that tinea pedis was contracted from areas about swimming pools and locker, shower, and dressing rooms. Opinions vary concerning this source of infection. The fungus is widespread in the environment, and there is some belief that certain individuals have a decreased resistance to the fungus, and when the feet come in contact with it, regardless of its location, the infection may be acquired.

Characteristics of tinea infections

The fungi causing tinea capitis produce several types of lesions, which vary from a single round patch on the scalp to inflammatory pustular lesions. Some infections give rise to numerous patches in which complete alopecia results, whereas another type called black dot ringworm is characterized by a small black dot at the site where the hair breaks off. In all cases of tinea of the scalp the hairs become dry, dull, and lusterless and either fall out or may be easily pulled out, leaving a scaly denuded area.

Tinea corporis occurs on nonhairy smooth skin, forming a circular lesion that is slightly raised and erythematous about the periphery. The lesion gradually increases in size and exhibits a scaly appearance. As the lesion increases, small vesicles or pustules may be noted about its periphery.

Tinea barbae, or "barber's itch," results in a nodular type of lesion with infiltration and abscess formation. The regional lymph nodes are enlarged and tender, and the hairs of the beard become loose and fall out.

Tinea pedis, or athlete's foot, may be mild or severe and is a common form of dermatophytosis. There is cracking and scaling of the skin between the toes, with vesicular lesions that contain a thin watery fluid. The infection may spread to the soles of the feet, where severe itching occurs. It is not uncommon for the infection to be spread to the hands, especially around the nails. The infection is most prevalent in warm weather, and any condition, including certain occupations, that causes sweating of the feet may predispose to the disease. If untreated, the disease may become chronic and very resistant to therapy.

Diagnosis

Clinical diagnosis of tinea is relatively simple, but for most effective treatment laboratory confirmation is recommended. Infections caused by *Microsporum* are diagnosed by using Wood light (filtered ultraviolet light). Hairs placed under the light will fluoresce and aid in determining the extent of the disease and in following the progress of therapy. Infections caused by *Trichophyton* fungus do not fluoresce, and diagnosis depends on microscopic examination of hairs or scrapings from lesions. Cultures are made from the fungus in order to classify the specific etiologic agent.

Treatment

There may be some variation in treatment, depending on the extent of the disease. In minor infections caused by *Microsporum* and *Trichophyton,* topical application of benzoic and salicylic acid ointment rubbed into the skin twice daily may clear the lesion. If the infection is extensive, the treatment of choice is griseofulvin. The drug is for oral administration, and the dosage varies with the weight of the patient and the extent of the infection. Treatment of tinea pedis includes a number of preparations such as the following: propionate-propionic acid and undecylenate-undecylenic acid, ointments, and griseofulvin. Publicity of products in newspapers and magazines should be viewed with considerable reservation, since such claims about products rarely achieve the desired results.

In some infections a combination of topical and systemic therapy is used. All treatment is continued until complete cure has been achieved, otherwise recurrences may occur.

Prevention and control

Patients with superficial fungous infections are rarely admitted to the hospital. Public health nurses will frequently encounter infected children in schools or among families that are visited. All children with tinea should be under medical care and treatment, and in some places they are allowed to remain in school if the head is covered with a cap. It should be pointed out that enforcement of this may be difficult, since it creates an embarrassing situation for the child and sets him apart from other children. The psychologic damage to the child may be as bad as the infection. Epidemics in schools should be reported to the local health department, and follow-up of home contacts and regular inspection with biweekly shampoo for contacts are recommended.

Persons with tinea corporis should be excluded from swimming pools and showers or any activities where exposure of others may occur. The same applies to persons with epidermophytosis. Tinea pedis can often be prevented by careful drying, especially between the toes, after daily bathing and the use of a medicated dusting powder with daily airing of shoes.

Clothing, caps, socks, and bedding of persons with superficial fungous infections should be thoroughly washed and boiled if possible. Socks should be changed twice daily and shoes disinfected with formaldehyde fumes or destroyed. Showers, tubs, and the like should be thoroughly scrubbed and disinfected after use by infected persons.

SECTION SIX

Helminth infections

Helminths are Metazoa that belong to the animal kingdom and represent a subdivision of parasites. There are three phyla of Metazoa of particular importance because they affect the health and welfare of man. These include (1) Platyhelminthes, (2) Nematoda, and (3) Arthropoda. The Platyhelminthes are flatworms, which include flukes and tapeworms, and the Nematoda are roundworms, which include *Ascaris*, hookworms, pinworms, and *Trichinella*. The Arthropoda include a number of parasites that are primarily vectors transmitting diseases. Some of these, such as the tick that transmits Rocky Mountain spotted fever, have been discussed in previous chapters. In this section, discussion will be limited to certain of the flatworms and roundworms. When these worms invade man, they may cause serious changes in the human organism. Some of these changes include the following:

1. They may feed on the host's blood, causing severe anemia.
2. Some utilize nutrient materials, depriving the host of essential nutritive elements.
3. They may cause irritation and damage to the host's tissue.
4. Some may undergo abnormal growth or increase in number so as to block vital ducts and passageways.
5. It appears that some may produce poisons and toxins that injure the host.
6. Some cause severe allergic tissue reactions.

Public education and chemotherapeutic agents have done much to reduce the incidence of some of the helminth infections in the United States; however, in many parts of the world where countries are underdeveloped, infection remains as a serious problem.

53
FLATWORM INFECTIONS

FLUKES (TREMATODA)

Flukes are not naturally found in North America, but in some countries of the world more than half of the population are infected, and there is evidence of increasing infection.

Flukes are flat, nonsegmented parasites whose complicated life cycle requires an intermediate host. Two species are pathogenic for man: (1) *Distoma,* which include various genera of flukes, and (2) *Schistoma,* a genus of blood flukes, some species of which are pathogenic for man and some of which cause disease in animals.

The *Distoma* cause distomiasis, which affects the digestive tract (fasciolopsiasis), the lungs (pulmonary distomiasis), and the bile ducts (clonorchiasis). Three species of the *Schistoma* are pathogenic for man: (1) *S. mansoni,* (2) *S. haematobium,* and (3) *S. japonicum,* all of which cause schistosomiasis.

Fasciolopsiasis

Fasciolopsiasis is a disease affecting the small intestine. The larvae of the parasite attach themselves to plants growing in water, and people who eat the uncooked plants become infected. The larvae hatch in the intestine and the small worms, which are about 1 by 1½ inches, attach themselves to the intestinal mucosa by two suckers. About three months after ingestion of the larvae, eggs will be produced by the adult worm and will be passed in the human feces. The infection produces a severe form of diarrhea alternating with constipation and edema of the face, abdominal wall, and extremities. Vomiting, ascites, and an abnormal increase in the number of eosinophils in the blood are characteristic of the disease. In countries where malnutrition is a problem, heavy infection of flukes may result in death.

Drugs used in treating the infection are tetrachloroethylene and hexylresorcinol; however, their effectiveness is variable.

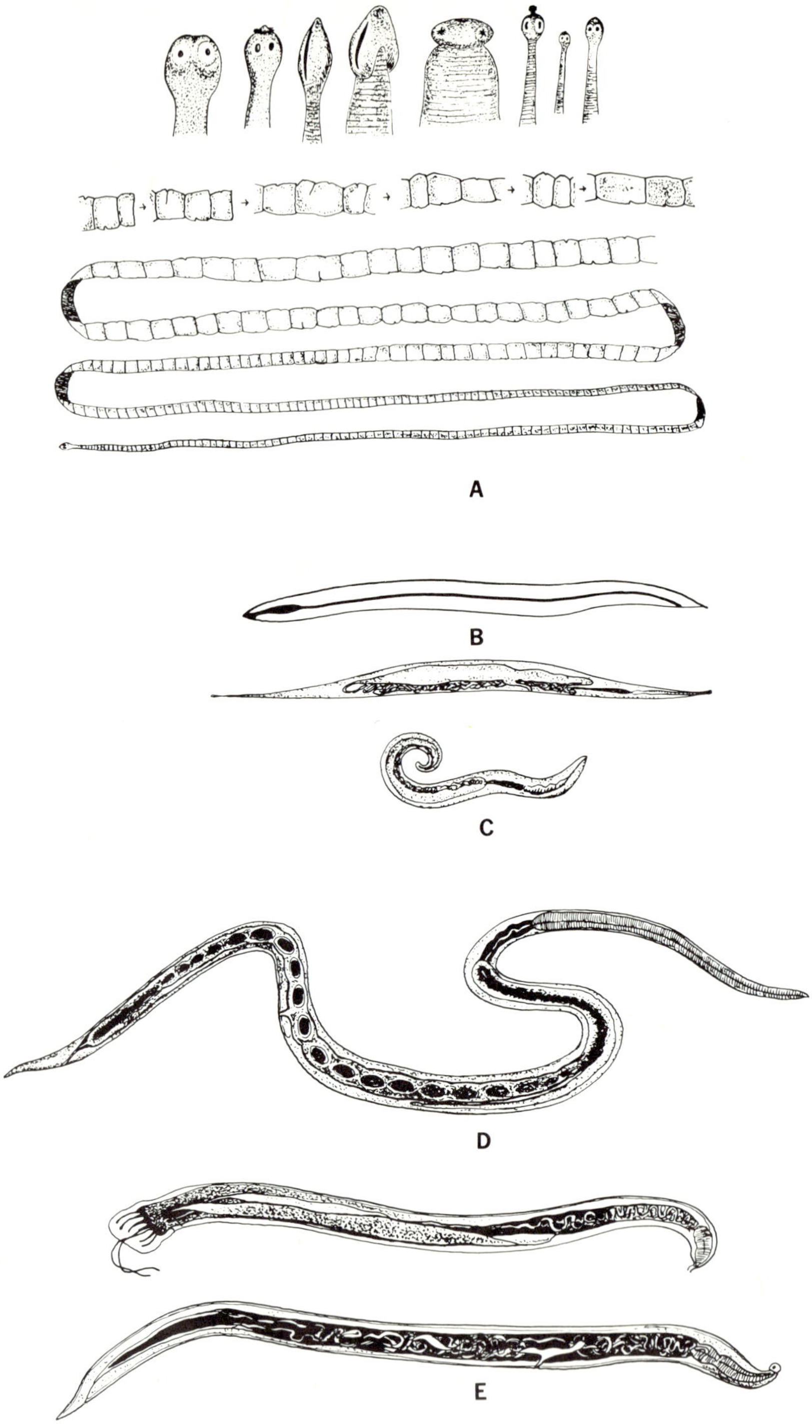

Fig. 33. Helminths that cause serious infections in humans. **A,** Tapeworm. **B,** Roundworm. **C,** Pinworm. **D,** Roundworm. **E,** Filaria. (From Johnston, Dorothy F.: Total patient care–foundations and practice, ed. 2, St. Louis, 1968, The C. V. Mosby Co.)

Paragonimiasis (pulmonary distomiasis)

Paragonimiasis is an infection of the lungs caused by a fluke called *Paragonimus westermani.* After an intermediate stage cycle the larvae penetrate freshwater crabs or crayfish, where they become encysted. Infection of man results from ingestion of raw or insufficiently cooked crab or crayfish containing the larvae. The larvae penetrate the duodenal wall of man, passing through the diaphragm, and enter the lungs, where the adult worms develop and eggs are produced. The infected areas of the lungs develop an inflammatory condition, resulting in fibrous cystic lesions that may appear similar to those of pulmonary tuberculosis. The symptomatology is that of chronic pulmonary disease with chest pain, productive cough, and hemoptysis. Although the sputum may contain worm eggs, it is not directly infective for man. The eggs are also present in the feces as the result of swallowing sputum. Diagnosis may be made by microscopic examination of sputum and feces for the presence of eggs.

The larvae of *P. westermani* may infect other organs, including the brain, lymph nodes, subcutaneous tissues, and genitourinary system. Several agents are used in treatment of the disease, including emetine hydrochloride, chloroquine, and bithionol, all of which may result in improvement but not necessarily in a cure.

Clonorchiasis (hepatic distomiasis)

Clonorchiasis is an infection of the bile ducts caused by a small fluke, *Clonorchis sinensis.* The eggs of the fluke are discharged in feces and contain fully developed, free-swimming larvae, which penetrate the body of a snail. The cercariae develop within the snail and escape into water from which they enter a second intermediate host, freshwater fish, where they become encysted in the flesh of the fish. Human infection results from ingestion of uncooked or partially cooked fish. During the digestive process the larvae are released from the cysts and migrate to the common bile duct and capillaries of the gallbladder and bile ducts.

Early symptoms of the infection are diarrhea, abdominal discomfort, and loss of appetite. Later splenomegaly, cirrhosis and enlargement of the liver, ascites, and edema occur.

Clonorchiasis has been of interest to the United States because of its geographic distribution. The infection is widespread in Korea, Vietnam, and Japan. In 1958 it was estimated that 500,000 persons from Puerto Rico were in the United States, of which 10% were probably infected. During World War II several thousand American servicemen were infected while serving in Leyte and imprisoned in the Philippines and were subsequently treated in United States Veteran's Hospitals.[4] From 25% to 30% of Chinese immigrants in the United States have been found to be infected. Agents used to treat the disease include chloroquine or gentian violet medicinal.[3]

Schistosomiasis (bilharziasis)

Schistosomiasis is caused by any of the three species of blood flukes known to be pathogenic for man. S. *mansoni* and S. *japonicum* infect the intestinal tract, whereas S. *haematobium* affects the venous plexus around the urinary bladder. In addition to man, S. *japonicum* infects various farm animals and some species of rodents.

The infectious agent is present in human feces and urine, and when discharged into freshwater, the ova hatch into free-swimming larvae (miracidia). The intermediate host is certain species of freshwater snails, and the ciliated embryos enter the snail. After several weeks they emerge as free-swimming cercariae, which in turn, penetrate the skin and mucous membrane of persons who work, wade, or swim in the contaminated water. After penetrating the capillaries, the cercariae are carried to the right heart and by way of the pulmonary arteries eventually reach the portal circulation, where maturation takes place. The female worms release eggs, which reach the intestinal tract and bladder from which they are discharged in the urine and feces, and the cycle begins again.

As far as is known, all ages and races and both sexes are susceptible to schistosomiasis. Infection is generally more severe in children. Although there is some evidence of an acquired immunity after an initial infection, confirmed evidence is lacking.

Symptoms begin about four to six weeks after infection. During this period allergic manifestations often accompany the intestinal form of the disease. These may include urticaria, attacks of asthma, and increase in leukocytes and eosinophils with edema of subcutaneous tissues. In addition some patients may have diarrhea, headache, fever, loss of appetite, loss of weight, and splenomegaly. Abdominal pain, enlargement of the liver, and anemia commonly occur. Infections caused by S. *haematobium* result in irritability of the urinary bladder, dysentery, hematuria, and leukocytosis.

Serious complications may arise from chronic infection with schistosomiasis that include portal hypertension, serious liver disease, and obstruction in the urinary system, particularly in the presence of other urinary tract disease.

Schistosomiasis may be diagnosed by an intradermal skin test, which can be read in fifteen minutes. However, opinions vary concerning the reliability of the test. Serology tests have been in use for many years, and although a number of different tests have been used, the complement-fixation test is the most widely used today. The need for a rapid screening test for mass epidemiologic testing has been recognized for some time. Recently a plasma card test used with a plasma collection slide in which only a drop of blood from the finger is required had preliminary evaluation and may prove to be useful as a screening technic.[5]

Schistosomiasis is treated with a 5% solution of tartar emetic, administered intravenously. The drug is highly toxic, and hospitalization is required during the treatment.

Stibophen (Fuadin) in a 6.3% solution is administered intramuscularly every other day. Toxic symptoms may occur that require adjustment of the treatment schedule.

Astiban is another drug that has been under investigational use, and reports indicate that it is effective and shortens the treatment period.[3]

Schistosomiasis is believed to affect between 150 and 200 million persons in the world, and efforts toward control have not been strikingly effective. In fact, present evidence indicates that the incidence of infection is increasing. The need for water for agricultural purposes as well as for human consumption and the lack of understanding of the fundamental principles of sanitation are major obstacles in prevention and control. To a large extent control depends on scientific knowledge concerning the intermediate host, the snail, and the development of more effective therapy. If the same emphasis was placed on teaching hygienic disposal of human waste as is placed on vector control, mass immunization programs and eradication of schistosomiasis and similar infections might be made a little easier.[2]

TAPEWORMS (CESTODES)

True tapeworms generally have segmented bodies, but some forms do not. The segment at the anterior end contains a head and neck (scolex), which contains a specialized hold-fast mechanism by which the adult worm attaches itself to the intestinal mucosa of the host. The head is extremely small in relation to the overall size of the worm (Fig. 34), and new segments are constantly being formed by a process of separation from the sco-

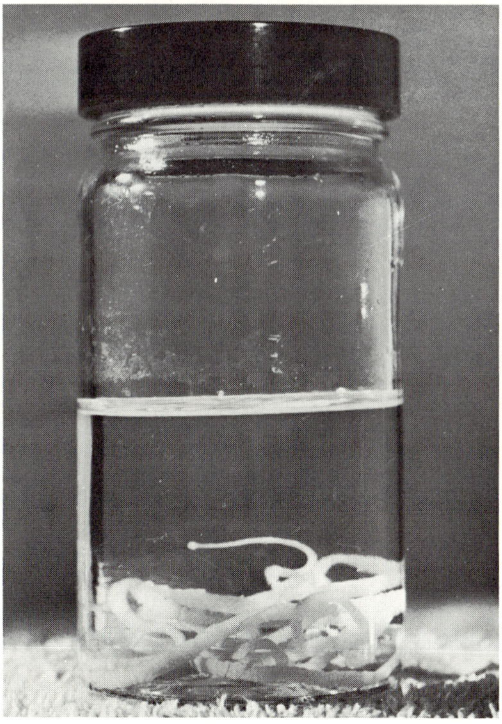

Fig. 34. Tapeworm. Notice the small head and segmented body. (Courtesy Georgia Cooperative Extension Service, University of Georgia, Athens, Ga.)

lex. Several genera of tapeworms are known to cause infection in humans. The three chief forms that infect people in the United States and Canada are the dwarf, beef, and fish tapeworms.

Dwarf tapeworm (Hymenolepis nana)

The dwarf tapeworm is a very small worm about 1 inch long. The worm does not require an intermediate host as do the beef and fish tapeworms. The eggs of the worm are expelled in human feces and if ingested, hatch in the human intestinal tract. Persons with dwarf tapeworm may transfer the eggs to food if they do not wash their hands after using the toilet. All persons are susceptible to the infection, although children in areas where sanitation is poor are most commonly affected.

Beef tapeworm (Taenia saginata)

The beef tapeworm is found in the muscles of cattle. Humans ingest the larvae with insufficiently cooked beef, and cattle ingest the eggs while grazing on pasture contaminated with human excreta. The eggs hatch in the animal's small intestine, from which they enter the bloodstream by boring through the intestinal wall. The larvae then lodge in the animal's tissues, where a protective capsule develops giving the appearance of a cyst about ¼ inch in diameter. In the human intestine the beef tapeworm may reach a length of 25 feet, and as long as the head remains attached to the human intestine, new segments will grow and produce eggs. The eggs are then passed in the feces.[6] The beef tapeworm is the one most frequently seen in adults in the United States and Canada and in persons who live in countries where beef is eaten raw or is insufficiently cooked.

Fish tapeworm (Diphyllobothrium latum)

The fish tapeworm is less common than the beef tapeworm, but it is now believed to be more prevalent than previously thought. It occurs as the result of human feces being discharged into freshwater, where the eggs mature and embryos escape into the water. The embryos are eaten by small shellfish, and when the shellfish are eaten by larger fish, the embryos mature in the flesh of the fish. Human infection results from ingestion of raw or poorly cooked infected fish. The tapeworm has been known to live for as long as sixteen years and to grow 30 feet in length. Infection with the fish tapeworm has been found in Canada, northern Michigan, Minnesota, and Florida.[6] Infection is also endemic in many European countries, Japan, South America, Israel, and Australia. Although the infected individual may experience no symptoms, infection may cause severe toxemia and secondary anemia.

There are few symptoms related to tapeworm infection, and if present, they usually do not present a specific clinical syndrome. Evidence suggests that dwarf tapeworm infection in children may cause systemic toxemia and a great increase in eosinophils in the blood. Studies made in Finland of fish tapeworm infection indicate that the parasite has a special affinity for vitamin B_{12} and that it will absorb from ten to fifty times more than other species. In addition it causes severe anemia, which resembles primary anemia and may cause a decrease in potassium and iron levels in the blood.[1]

The diagnosis of tapeworm infection may be made by observing segments of worms in the stools. The eggs cannot be seen in the stools, and fecal specimens must be obtained for microscopic examination for the eggs.

Several drugs are used in the treatment of tapeworm, but the drug of choice is quinacrine (Atabrine). The method of treatment varies, and in a small number of patients complete success may not be obtained with one treatment. Because of the frequency of vomiting after oral administration of the drug, Modell recommends instillation directly into the duodenum by intubation. The diet may consist of clear liquids for forty-eight hours prior to the treatment; however, a light lunch and liquid supper may be allowed on the day before treatment. On the following morning, with the patient in a fasting state, a sedative is given orally and a duodenal tube inserted. One gram of quinacrine is dissolved in 20 ml. of water and administered through the tube, followed by a small amount of water to wash through any residue of the drug remaining in the tube or syringe. About two hours later a saline purgative such as 60 ml. of magnesium sulfate solution is administered orally. In case satisfactory results are not achieved, a soapsuds enema may be given. A regular diet is then resumed. All stools for seventy-two hours are collected and carefully examined for the head of the worm.[3]

If quinacrine is administered orally, doses are divided and the total dose may vary from 0.3 to 1 Gm. Preparation of the patient for oral administration is the same as for duodenal administration. If retreatment is required, it is usually not given until about two months later.

For a discussion of the prevention of helminth infections refer to Chapter 54.

REFERENCES

1. Cheng, Thomas C.: The biology of animal parasites, Philadelphia, 1964, W. B. Saunders Co.
2. Hinman, E. Harold: World eradication of infectious diseases, Springfield, Ill., 1966, Charles C Thomas, Publisher.
3. Modell, Walter, editor: Drugs of choice 1974-75, St. Louis, 1974, The C. V. Mosby Co.
4. Most, Harry: Current concepts in therapy. I. Anthelminthic therapy, New Eng. J. Med. **259**:341-342, Aug. 28, 1958.
5. Samter, Max, editor: Immunological diseases, Boston, 1965, Little, Brown & Co.
6. Tapeworm, Health Information Series no. 48, Public Health Service Publication no. 158, Washington, D. C., 1966, U. S. Government Printing Office.

54

ROUNDWORM INFECTIONS (NEMATODA)

ASCARIS LUMBRICOIDES

Ascaris lumbricoides is a large round worm ranging from 4 to 12 inches in length, and in general appearance it is similar to the common earthworm. Infection is the result of ingestion of embryonated eggs containing the larvae. After a roundabout migration through the body of the host the larvae eventually reach the small intestine, where the worms hatch and reach maturity. The female worm is a prolific egg producer, releasing as many as 27 million eggs, which are passed in human feces. These may be deposited on the ground with human feces. The eggs become mixed with the soil, and under proper conditions of temperature and moisture they develop and are eventually blown away in the dust. Thus the soil becomes the infective medium to the host, from which the infection is "dust-borne, food-borne, hand-borne, and money-borne."[9] Under proper conditions the eggs may live in the soil indefinitely.

Infection with *A. lumbricoides* is worldwide, and it is estimated that 644 million persons in the world are infected. Three million infected persons live in North America.[3] Examination of 140 fecal specimens from agricultural workers from the British West Indies showed that 4.3% were infected with *Ascaris*.[2] The World Health Organization reported that examination of 800 specimens from migrant workers in Texas showed an infection rate of 31% among Puerto Ricans and 33% among those from Mexico.[9]

Persons of all ages and races and both sexes are susceptible to infection with *Ascaris*. Males are more often infected than females, and younger persons are infected more often than older persons. Large numbers of parasites in children may cause serious complications, and deaths have been reported from such infections. Investigation indicates that only partial immunity results from an initial infection, as evidenced by reinfection of persons successively treated and cured.[10] The usual incubation period is eight to twelve weeks.

During the larva stage of the disease, allergic manifestations may include wheezing, urticaria, asthma, and an increase in the eosinophils in the blood. Other symptoms may include malaise, cough, loss of appetite, leukocytosis, and angioneurotic edema. During the pulmonary migration of the larvae there may be a mild dry cough and hemoptysis. Death may result from the presence of larvae in the lungs.

It requires two months for the worm to mature in the intestine, and during the intestinal stage of the infection, colicky abdominal pain, nausea, vomiting, and malnutrition may occur. Children with heavy infections suffer from malnutrition, dehydration, and electrolyte imbalance. The worms may crawl up the esophagus to the pharynx and be vomited or crawl from the nose and mouth, or they may find their way to the lungs, causing a fatal pneumonia.

Complications resulting from heavy infection with *Ascaris* may include intestinal obstruction or perforation of ulcers and peritonitis, obstructive jaundice, hepatic abscess, appendicitis, and bowel obstruction by twisting the intestine.[5]

It should be noted that many infected persons have few if any symptoms, and infection is observed only by observing worms in vomitus or stools.

There are no satisfactory laboratory tests available at the present time for diagnosis of *Ascaris* infection. The only method of diagnosis, other than seeing the worms, is the microscopic examination of feces for the ova.

Infection with *Ascaris* is treated with piperazine, the action of which causes paralysis of the neuromuscular junction within the worm. This in turn inhibits the worm's activity to such an extent that it is carried away in the feces. The drug is available in several preparations, and dosage varies with the particular form of drug used. If retreatment is required, one week must elapse between treatments.[1] The drug is safe, and no pretreatment, dietary restrictions, or post-treatment purgative is necessary. Side effects are limited and disappear with completion of the treatment.

HOOKWORM DISEASE

Hookworm disease is caused by two species of hookworm, *Ancylostoma duodenale* and *Necator americanus*. The latter is widely distributed in the southern United States, Central and South America, and West Africa. *A. duodenale* is most prevalent in Europe and Asia, but both species are found in Asia, Central and South America, and the British West Indies.

The two species of hookworm pathogenic for man are very similar, the chief difference being in the structure of the mouth. Although slightly different, both have hooks or a pinching mechanism by which they attach themselves to the intestinal mucosa.[11]

The source of hookworm infection is the soil contaminated by human feces that contain hookworm ova. A single hookworm may produce as many as 5000 to 10,000 eggs daily. Eggs deposited in moist soil, rich in oxygen, will develop into embryos within twenty-four to seventy-two hours.

The larvae will penetrate the unbroken skin of the feet and legs of the host, entering through the sudoriferous glands and the hair follicles. The larvae then penetrate the blood and lymph vessels, damaging them in the process, after which they migrate through the body the same as the *Ascaris*. Eventually they reach the lungs, where some may be coughed up and expectorated, whereas others are swallowed and reach the small intestine, where maturation occurs and egg production takes place. The incubation period is six weeks.

The incidence of hookworm infection varies, but it is still considered the most important helminth infection of man. It has been estimated that 1.5 million people in the world are infected. The World Health Organization reported in 1964 that 98% of the people of northern Peru were infected. Examination of 800 specimens from migrant Puerto Rican workers in Texas showed that 27% were infected.[9] British West Indian workers in the United States were examined, and of 140 fecal specimens 54.3% showed hookworm infection.[2] In other areas of the world 90% of the population may be infected. Stoll believes that hookworm is one of the most important problems in tropical countries, where it affects the health and efficiency of a large segment of the population.[12]

All persons, regardless of age, sex, or race, are susceptible to hookworm disease. However, variations are noted. In general, the greatest incidence of infection is found among persons between 15 and 25 years of age. The disease is primarily one of rural areas where sanitary disposal of human excreta is inadequate. Tropical and subtropical countries where the climate is warm and humid and where people do not wear shoes provide an environment for the infection to flourish.

Symptoms of hookworm disease depend on the number of worms present in the intestine. Few worms or even a few hundred worms may produce no symptoms; however, their effect on the host is insidious. They may engulf small bits of tissue from the intestinal mucosa, causing the development of small lesions. They feed on the host's blood and may consume 50 ml. or more of blood daily.[3] The gradual loss of blood eventually results in iron deficiency anemia, the severity of which depends on the extent of infection and the blood loss. Other symptoms may include abdominal pain, diarrhea, and allergic reactions such as urticaria. Children infected with worms are often underdeveloped mentally and physically, have a protruding abdomen, and are lethargic.

There is no skin test or serologic test to aid in the diagnosis of hookworm disease. Diagnosis is made by microscopic examination of feces for the eggs.

Several drugs are available for the treatment of hookworm infection. The most commonly used agent is tetrachloroethylene, which is administered orally for two mornings about two hours prior to breakfast. No purgative is required after treatment. Stool specimens should be examined in one week to determine the effectiveness of the treatment.

ENTEROBIASIS (PINWORM, THREADWORM, OR SEATWORM)

The *Enterobius vermicularis* is a small round worm, the female being about ¼ inch long and the male somewhat shorter. Enterobiasis, commonly called pinworms, results from anal-oral transmission of the eggs of the same host. Indirect transmission may result from eggs of the parasite that contaminate clothing, bedding, or food. Objects commonly used by other persons, such as washbowls, furniture, and doorknobs, may be a source of infection. Infected bedding or clothing that is shaken may disperse eggs into the air, from which they may be inhaled.

The life cycle of the pinworm is much simpler than that of other helminths. The ingested eggs pass into the stomach where they hatch, and the larvae proceed through the small intestine into the large intestine where the mature worms develop. The entire process takes about six weeks. When the gravid worms are ready to lay their eggs, they move downward through the rectum and anus, where the eggs are deposited in the folds of perineal skin. After releasing the eggs the worms die. In most instances the migration and deposition of eggs occur about thirty minutes after the infected person has retired for the night, but in severe infections it may occur during the day.[8]

Enterobiasis occurs worldwide, and persons of all ages and races and both sexes are susceptible. The disease is most prevalent among children of school age and least prevalent among adults. However, all members of a family may become infected, and the incidence of infection is often high among children in institutions and areas where crowded conditions exist. It has been estimated that infection rates in the United States may be as high as 20% of the general population.[4] This is an optionally reported disease in the United States, however in 1972, fifty-three cases were reported in three states. No statistics are available for Canada.

The most characteristic symptom of enterobiasis is itching about the anogenital region. The itching may lead to restlessness and loss of sleep at night, and such children may be irritable, refuse food, and lose weight. Occasional nausea and vomiting may occur. In female children and women the worms may crawl into the vulva, vagina, or urethra causing infection, and severe pruritus and irritation may result from scratching.

Diagnosis of enterobiasis is made by microscopic examination for the presence of eggs. A cellulose tape slide is applied to the skin about the anal folds, and the eggs are removed from the slide by a solvent (toluol). It is often necessary to make several slides on successive nights before specific diagnosis can be made. Occasionally worms may be observed by directing a bright light on the anal opening, or a small low enema of tap water or saline solution may wash the worms out where they may be seen.

Treatment may be with either of two therapeutic agents found to be effective for the infection—pyrvinium pamoate and piperazine. After the administration of pyrvinium pamoate, stools will be red. After a lapse of one week the treatment may be repeated. A soothing antipruritic ointment may be prescribed to relieve the irritation about the genital area. The patient should be reexamined in three months to determine if reinfection has occurred.[7]

Concomitant with treatment of the patient all members of the family or other exposed persons should be examined and treated if infected. If cure is to be achieved, a strict hygienic program must be adhered to. Recommendations include keeping the fingers out of and away from the mouth, keeping fingernails short, thorough handwashing following use of the toilet, and daily bathing with warm water and soap or a shower if possible. All sleeping garments, underwear, towels, and the like should be boiled daily and all contaminated objects washed with soap and water.

TRICHINOSIS

Trichinosis is caused by a nematode called *Trichinella spiralis*. The infection occurs in man and a large number of mammals. The source of human infection is the consumption of animal meat, principally pork and pork products, that are infected with *T. spiralis*. After the infected meat is digested in the stomach the released larvae pass into the intestine, where maturation of the adult worm occurs. The female, which becomes embedded in the wall of the intestine, releases from 1000 to 1500 larvae, which penetrate the intestinal mucosa and eventually enter the blood stream, being carried over the body in the general circulation. The larvae have an affinity for skeletal muscle tissue, which they penetrate; they grow rapidly and become encysted, and calcification of the larval cyst may occur. Muscles most commonly affected are the greater pectoral, parts of the deltoid, gastrocnemius, and biceps. Muscles of the tongue, larynx, diaphragm, neck, and thorax may also be affected.[13]

The source of the disease in man is the ingestion of insufficiently cooked pork and pork products such as sausage. The disease in hogs may result from ingestion of infected rodents such as rats; however, raw or uncooked garbage is considered the principal source of infection. The feeding of uncooked garbage in the large hog-raising centers of the United States and Canada has been greatly reduced during the past ten years. Most outbreaks of trichinosis at the present time are traced to home-grown and processed pork products that do not come under meat inspection regulations.[14] Although many rural families process pork for their own consumption, some states or counties prohibit the sale of such meat.

Trichinosis is considered a worldwide problem; however, distribution varies. The incidence is low in France, Canada, South America, and Mexico, but it remains a public health problem in the United States. The exact incidence of the disease in the United States is unknown, since not all cases are reported or are clinically recognized. Top reports that about 450 cases are reported each year.[13]

All ages and races and both sexes are susceptible to the infection, which may occur at any time of the year.

The first symptoms of trichinosis occur from two to twenty-eight days after ingestion of infected pork, with an average of about nine days.

The disease is characterized by several stages incident to the development of worms, their migration through the body, and their encystment. In the first stage, during which the larvae are being released in the stomach and the adult worms are maturing and releasing embryonated larvae, gastrointestinal symptoms predominate. There is abdominal pain, nausea, vomiting, anorexia, and diarrhea. The second, or migratory stage is acute, with severe muscle pain, fever from 101° to 104° F., edema such as puffiness around the eyes, headache, and various cutaneous manifestations that include urticaria, pruritus, tingling of the skin, and increased perspiration. One of the cardinal signs is eosinophilia. The leukocyte count may reach 20,000 to 30,000 per cubic millimeter of blood, of which 10% to 70% may be eosinophils.[10] Central nervous system symptoms may occur that mimic any of numerous conditions such as acute psychosis, tumors of the brain or spinal cord, paresis, polyneuritis, and paraplegia. The reason for the severe nervous system symptoms is not clear, but during necropsy, larvae have been found in the brain.[6] The third stage occurs when the larvae reach the muscle tissue and become encysted, the disease gradually becoming chronic with muscular rheumatic-like pains.

Clinical diagnosis of trichinosis is probably impossible. The three signs that may lead to suspected disease are muscle pain, edema, and eosinophilia, which together with a history of eating inadequately cooked pork provide the best evidence of trichinosis. Biopsy of muscle tissue and identification of the larvae in the muscle may confirm the diagnosis. In some situations it may be possible to isolate the larvae in infected pork. Laboratory methods of diagnosis are not sufficiently specific to permit reliable diagnosis. However, an intradermal skin test using an antigen consisting of an extract from dried ground trichinae may show a positive immunologic response in the presence of infection. Since cross-reactions occur as a result of other helminth infections, the test is considered to have limited value as a diagnostic tool.[10] A number of serologic tests have been used with varying degrees of success. Precipitin tests have been widely used, and the complement-fixation test is used by a number of laboratories and some believe it to be superior to the precipitin test. Recently a fluorescent antibody test has been shown to provide good results.[10]

There is no therapeutic agent specific for trichinosis. A number of drugs, including steroids, have been used. If diagnosis could be made before the larvae become embedded in the intestinal mucosa, anthelmintic agents and repeated doses of saline cathartics might remove some adult worms and reduce the number of larvae that reach the general circulation. However, the disease has usually progressed too far for such treatment to be of any value by the time the individual reaches the physician. At present the therapeutic agent being used is a broad-spectrum anthelmintic, thiabendazole. The drug is highly toxic, and most patients will experience nausea, vomiting, cutaneous rash, and central nervous system symptoms. Although the drug results in general improvement of the patient, there is insufficient evidence at present to determine if it destroys the larvae in the muscles.[7]

Other treatment may include bed rest during the acute stage of the disease, analgesics to relieve muscle pain, antihistamines to relieve the allergic manifestations of the infection, and sodium restriction with a high protein diet.

Mortality rates from trichinosis vary between 5% and 10%, and morbidity rates are about 16%. Patients who succumb to the disease usually do so between four and six weeks after onset of the disease.

PREVENTION OF HELMINTH INFECTIONS

Preventing helminth infections requires a broad program of public education and the adoption and enforcement of regulations to prevent the conditions incident to the existence and spread of helminths.

One of the most important factors in prevention is the sanitary disposal of human excreta. In rural areas proper construction of pit privies to prevent the dissemination of helminth ova and larvae is an indispensable necessity. Regulations to prevent the pollution of streams and lakes with human excreta should be adopted. Persons in underdeveloped countries who are required to enter polluted water should be taught to wear protective clothing or when possible, to use repellents. All persons in areas where hookworm is endemic should avoid going barefooted.

Public education in the necessity of thorough cooking of pork is important if trichinosis is to be prevented. Regulations should be established to prevent the feeding of uncooked garbage to hogs and to prevent sale or interstate movement of infected animals.

World eradication of helminth infections requires international as well as personal cooperation and understanding of the problem. There is need for the development of screening technics by which large numbers of persons can be examined and research in the development of simple effective therapy.

REFERENCES

1. Bergersen, Betty S.: Pharmacology in nursing, ed. 12, St. Louis, 1973, The C. V. Mosby Co.
2. Beye, Henry, Brooks, Charles, and Guinn, Elizabeth: Protozoan and helminthic infections among migratory agricultural workers, Am. J. Public Health **51**:1862-1871, Dec., 1961.
3. Cheng, Thomas C.: The biology of animal parasites, Philadelphia, 1964, W. B. Saunders Co.
4. Gordon, John E., editor: Control of communicable diseases in man, ed. 10, New York, 1965, American Public Health Assn., Inc.
5. Jung, Rodney C.: The management of intestinal parasitic infections, J. Pediatr. **53**:89-98, July, 1958.
6. Kennedy, F. Bryan, and Rege, Vishram B.: Trichinosis, Arch. Int. Med. **117**:108-112, Jan., 1966.
7. Modell, Walter, editor: Drugs of choice 1974-1975, St. Louis, 1974, The C. V. Mosby Co.
8. Pinworms, Health Information Series no. 51, Public Health Service Publication no. 108, Washington, D. C., 1966, U. S. Government Printing Office.
9. Report of WHO Expert Committee on Helminthiases, Soil-transmitted hel-

minths, Technical Report Series no. 277, Geneva, 1964, World Health Organization.

10. Samter, Max, editor: Immunological diseases, Boston, 1965, Little, Brown & Co.
11. Smith, Alice Lorraine: Carter's principles of microbiology, ed. 4, St. Louis, 1961, The C. V. Mosby Co.
12. Stoll, Norman R.: On endemic hookworm; where do we stand today? Experimental Parasitology **12**:241-252, April, 1962.
13. Top, Franklin H., and Wehrle, Paul F.: Communicable and infectious diseases, ed. 7, St. Louis, 1972, The C. V. Mosby Co.
14. Zimmerman, W. J., and Brandly, Paul J.: The current status of trichiniasis in the United States swine, Public Health Reports **80**:1061-1066, Dec., 1965.

GLOSSARY

aerobe an organism that lives only in the presence of free oxygen.

affinity mutual attraction to each other.

alopecia syphilitica the loss of hair resulting from syphilis.

anaerobe an organism that lives only in complete or nearly complete absence of oxygen.

anaphylactoid reaction an unusual and severe systemic reaction to a foreign protein or other substance to which the individual is hypersensitive.

antibody specifically adapted serum globulin with the capacity to react to or neutralize an antigen.

antigen any substance, usually protein or protein-polysaccharide, capable of stimulating antibody production.

antiserum a serum containing antibodies.

anxiety a feeling of being worried, concerned, or apprehensive.

apyrexia absence of fever.

arthropod a member of the group of vectors having paired legs and a hard segmented exoskeleton that is capable of transmitting disease.

Asiatic cholera an infectious disease caused by *Vibrio cholerae* contained in bowel discharges of infected persons and transmitted through drinking water.

attenuated diluted or rendered inactive.

autarcesis the normal activity of body cells to resist infection.

autoinoculation inoculation of new sites on one's body from an original lesion.

autopsy the postmortem examination of a body.

azotemia the presence of urea or other nitrogenous products in the blood.

bacteriophage a bacterial virus used in typing *Staphylococcus aureus.*

black vomit character of vomitus of persons infected with yellow fever, considered to be of diagnostic significance.

bubo swollen lymph gland in the groin, axilla, or neck seen in bubonic plague.

capsule a slime layer surrounding a microorganism.

caseation a cheeselike necrosis composed of lipoid material of a tubercle.

centripetal moving toward the center.

cercaria the final free-swimming larval stage of various trematodes.

chancre initial lesion of primary syphilis occurring at the site of inoculation.

cholera infantum noncontagious infantile diarrhea.

cholera morbus acute gastroenteritis, which is frequently confused with Asiatic cholera during epidemics.

coccidioidoma a coin-type pulmonary lesion occurring in pneumonitis accompanying coccidioidomycosis.

concurrent disinfection the destruction of pathogenic organisms as soon as possible after they leave the body.

condyloma latum a moist wartlike lesion occurring about the anogenital area in secondary syphilis.

conidium an asexual spore that splits off from the top of the conidiophore from the vegetative body of a fungus.

consent medical use means agreement for any medical or surgical treatment deemed necessary by the physician.

cross-infection a second communicable disease superimposed on a patient already suffering from a communicable disease.

desquamation peeling of the skin.

diphtheroids nonpathogenic organisms resembling the diphtheria bacillus.

disseminate to spread throughout a wide area.

distemper term commonly applied to a number of diseases during the early colonial period.

divalent having two strains of the infectious agent or a valence of two.

ecchymosis a form of macula appearing in large irregularly formed hemorrhagic areas of the skin.

ecology the relationship of biologic organisms to their environment.

embryo an early developmental stage of an animal within the egg.

enanthem eruptions of mucous membrane —Koplik's spots.

encystment enclosure within a capsule or sac.

endemic when disease is restricted to a given area and may be recurring but does not spread to other regions.

endogenous developing from within the body.

enterotoxin a toxin that affects the cells of the intestinal mucosa.

enzootic a disease present at all times in an animal community, but resulting in low morbidity.

eosinophilia the presence of an abnormally large number of eosinophils in the blood.

epidemic a disease that affects many people in an area and tends to spread rapidly.

epidermophytosis infection by fungi of the genus *Epidermophyton.*

epizootic a disease that affects a large number of animals of the same kind at the same time.

equine pertaining to horses.

erythema a patch of redness that may blanche on pressure.

ethnic pertaining to a group of persons with the same customs, language, national origin, religion.

exanthem the skin rash occurring in some communicable diseases.

exogenous originating outside the body.

exudate discharging material from a lesion; may be fluid or solid debris from cells.

flagellum a whiplike appendage of some bacteria that serves as an organ of locomotion.

fluoresce to produce light or to glow while being acted on by light.

fumigation the use of a gaseous substance in a closed space to kill animal forms such as insects and rodents.

haptene a particular antigen incapable of stimulating antibody production.

hematogenous spread through the bloodstream.

herbivores animals that feed primarily on grasses or plants.

herpetiform localized group of vesicles.

histoplasmin a filtrate of a culture of *Histoplasma capsulatum* that is used for skin testing in histoplasmosis.

hypoproteinemia a decrease in the amount of protein in the blood.

icteric having jaundice.

immunity possessing specific antibodies to resist infection; may be active or passive, natural or acquired.

isolation the separation of persons with communicable disease from contact with others for a specified period of time.

larva an immature stage in the life of an animal—the intermediate stage between the egg and the mature structure of the adult.

lazaretto public hospital, usually charity, for persons with communicable disease, and it may also apply to other facilities used for quarantine.

leukopenia a reduction in the number of leukocytes in the blood.

liability responsibility for any wrong act or wrongdoing.

macule a flat, circumscribed area of skin discoloration.

meningococcemia bloodstream infection caused by the meningococcus.

Metazoa a zoologic division of the animal kingdom that includes all animals except the protozoa.

migrant a person who moves from one place to another or from one region to another; frequently used to denote a person following work.

monovalent producing immunity against one strain of the infectious agent.

necropsy the postmortem examination of a body.

negligence failure to exercise the care necessary to prevent injury to another.

Negri bodies round or oval bodies found in the cytoplasm of neurons in animals with rabies.

Nematoda a class of helminths, consisting of the roundworms.

neurotropic having an affinity for and principally affecting nervous tissue.

nonofficial agency an organization that does not receive its support from public taxation.

nosocomial related to a disease occurring in the hospital.

official agency an organization or agency supported by local, state, or federal government.

pandemic an epidemic of disease that is worldwide.

papule circumscribed area of red skin varying from a few millimeters to a centimeter.

parenchyma the functional part of an organ.

pathogenesis the beginning of disease.

penicillinase an enzyme produced by certain strains of *Staphylococcus aureus.*

petechia a small hemorrhage (pin-head size) beneath the epidermis, when it occurs in large patches, it is called ecchymoses.

Peyer's patches a collection of elevated areas of lymphoid tissue on the mucosa of the small intestine forming colliculi.

plague a highly fatal disease caused by *Pasteurella pestis* and transmitted by rodents from person to person.

privacy the right of a person to withhold or refuse to allow public viewing of himself or his property.

prodromal period during which there are signs of an approaching communicable disease.

promiscuity indiscriminate sexual relations with many persons.

properdin a serum protein distinct from the serum globulins and related to nonspecific resistance.

prostitute a person who engages in sexual relations for money.

proximal nearest to the center of the body.

pyoderma neonatorum purulent skin disease of the newborn.

pustule a small circumscribed area of the skin formed when the clear vesicular fluid becomes pus.

pyrexia the elevation of body temperature above normal.

quarantine restriction of movement in or out of a place where a communicable disease exists.

resolution subsidence of inflammation and infection.

risus sardonicus spasm of facial muscles resulting in a grinning expression.

saber shin a form of periostitis causing bulging of the tibia.

segmented in zoology the division of an animal into parts.

social problem a condition or conditions regarded as undesirable or morally wrong by many persons.

society a group of persons living together under the same or similar environmental conditions.

spores bodies produced by some bacteria or fungi highly resistant to the usual methods of disinfection.

stigma a mark or characteristic that detracts from what is regarded as normal or standard.

stratification a social process that differentiates and places people into classes, high or low and superior or inferior.

S.T.S. serologic test for syphilis.

surveillance close supervision of a person, disease, or condition necessary for effective control.

susceptibility the opposite of immunity—possessing no specific antibodies to resist infection.

symbiosis the living together of dissimilar organisms with mutual advantages to each.

tenesmus painful and ineffective straining to defecate.

teratogenic tending to produce abnormal development of the fetus in utero.

terminal cleaning the ordinary cleaning of a room and its contents following recovery, transfer, or death of a person having a communicable disease.

Trematoda the class of any of the large group of flatworms.

trismus spasm of muscles of mastication resulting in the grinding of teeth.

variant one that differs in some way from others of the same kind.

vesicle sharply circumscribed collections of clear fluid in the skin; when they are larger, they are called bulbae.

vibrio the genus for microorganisms shaped like a comma or like an S, causing Asiatic cholera.

viremia the presence of viruses in the bloodstream.

viscerotome an instrument used to secure specimens of liver tissue from a corpse by a simple puncture technic.

zoonosis an infectious disease of animals that may be transmitted secondarily to man.

BIBLIOGRAPHY

BOOKS

Burt, J., and Brower, L.: Education for sexuality; concepts and programs for teaching, Philadelphia, 1970, W. B. Saunders Co.

Dubay, E. C., and Grubb, R. D.: Infection: prevention and control, St. Louis, 1973, The C. V. Mosby Co.

Elliott, H., and Ryz, K.: Venereal diseases; treatment and nursing, London, 1972, Ballière Tindall.

Fox, J. P., Hall, C. E., and Elveback, L. R.: Epidemiology; man and disease, New York, 1970, The Macmillan Co.

Frobisher, M., and Fuerst, R.: Microbiology in health and disease, Philadelphia, 1973, W. B. Saunders Co.

Goldman, R.: Principles of medical science, Toronto, 1973, McGraw-Hill Inc.

Houston, J. C., and Stockdale, M.: Principles of medicine and medical nursing, London, 1968, The English Universities Press Ltd.

Hubbard, C. W.: Family planning education: parenthood and social disease control, St. Louis, 1973, The C. V. Mosby Co.

Ingram, J. T.: The nursing care of the patient with skin disease, London, 1970, William Heinemann Ltd.

Kogan, B. A.: Health; man in a changing environment, New York, 1970, Harcourt Brace Jovanovich, Inc.

Krugman, S., and Ward, R.: Infectious diseases of children, ed. 5, St. Louis, 1973, The C. V. Mosby Co.

Latham, H. C., and Heckel, R. V.: Pediatric nursing, ed. 2, St. Louis, 1972, The C. V. Mosby Co.

Laycock, S. R.: Family living and sex education, Toronto, 1971, Mil-Mac Publications Ltd.

Marlow, D.: Textbook of pediatric nursing, Philadelphia, 1973, W. B. Saunders Co.

MacKenna, R. M. B., and Cohen, E. L.: Dermatology, London, 1970, Baillière Tindall.

National Tuberculosis and Respiratory Disease Association: Introduction to respiratory diseases, New York, 1969, The Association.

Smith, A. L.: Principles of microbiology, ed. 7, St. Louis, 1973, The C. V. Mosby Co.

Stead, W. W.: Understanding tuberculosis today; a handbook for patients, Milwaukee, 1971, Marquette University Press.

Stewart, F. S.: Bacteriology and immunology for students of medicine, London, 1971, Baillière Tindall.

United States Department of Health, Education, and Welfare: Isolation techniques for use in hospitals, Atlanta, Georgia, 1970, U. S. Department of

Health, Education, and Welfare Public Health Science Center for Disease Control.
Young, C. G., and Barger, J. D.: Introduction to medical science, ed. 2, St. Louis, 1973, The C. V. Mosby Co.

JOURNALS AND REPORTS

Ad Hoc Committee on the Treatment of Tuberculosis Patients in General Hospitals: Guidelines for the general hospital in the admission and care of tuberculosis patients, New York, 1969, National Tuberculosis and Respiratory Disease Association.
Almasy, P.: Smallpox; seek and destroy, World Health 26-29, Oct., 1971.
American Thoracic Society: Definitions and classifications of infectious reactions of the lung, New York, 1970, National Tuberculosis and Respiratory Disease Association.
Bechelli, L.: Leprosy today, World Health 10-19, Oct., 1971.
Bessudo, D., and others: Isolation of S. Typhi resistant to high concentrations of chloramphenicol, Bulletin: The Pan American Health Organization, Vol. 7, No. 3, 1973.
Committee on inquiry for smallpox outbreak: Smallpox inquiry blames systems, not individuals, Nurs. Times **70**(26): 980, June, 1974.
Egli, D.: Conquest of an epidemic, World Health 28-31, Oct., 1972.
Giesbrecht, E.: Infectious mononucleosis; the kissing disease, Canadian Nurse 37-40, Feb., 1972.
Guthe, T.: Familiarity breeds disease, World Health 30-35, Oct., 1971.
Guzman, C.: Why not outpatient rehabilitation centers for cold patients? Bulletin: Canadian Tuberculosis and Respiratory Disease Association **51**(3):2-4, Sept., 1972.
Haider, S.: Infectious diseases; Part I, Nurs. Mirror **137**(15 Suppl.): 1-5, Oct., 12, 1973.
Haider S.: Infectious diseases; Part II, Nurs. Mirror **137**(16 Suppl.): 1-8, Oct 19, 1973.
Haider, S.: Infectious diseases; Part III, Nurs. Mirror **137**(17):9-11, Oct. 26, 1973.
Haider, S.: Infectious diseases; Part IV, Nurs. Mirror **137**(18):26-27, Nov. 2, 1973.
Helming, M. G., editor: Nursing in respiratory diseases; a symposium, New York, 1968, National Tuberculosis and Respiratory Disease Association.
Henderson, D. A.: Smallpox eradication; the global strategy, World Health 8-17, Oct., 1972.
Lenczner, M. M.: Tropical and parasite diseases; new challenge to health teams, Canadian Nurse **69**:34-37, Sept., 1973.
Mirando, M., Latimer, K. P., and Brubaker, M. L.: Alternative designs and methods for V.D. control programs, Bulletin: The Pan American Health Organization **7**(3):1-8, 1973.
Newill, R.: The germs of love, Book of life, Part 42, vol. 3, London, 1969, Marshall Cavendish Ltd., pp. 1164-1167.
Noble, W. C.: Commensal bacteria of human skin, Nurs. Times **69**(40):1287-1288, Oct. 4, 1973.
NTA Ad Hoc Committee on Treatment of Tuberculosis Patients in General Hospitals: Infectiousness of tuberculosis, New York, 1967, National Tuberculosis and Respiratory Disease Association.
Palmer, P.: New approach to old pestilences, World Health 4-15, May, 1971.
Smith, A. C.: Communications and carriers, Book of life, Part 12, London, 1969, Marshall Cavendish Ltd., pp. 328-332.
Standards Committee: Canadian tuberculosis standards; for use in general and special hospitals, Ottawa, 1972, Tuberculosis and Respiratory Disease Association.
Stares, J.: Smallpox and chickenpox, Book of life, Part 94, vol. 6, London, 1970, Marshall Cavendish Ltd., pp. 2629-2632.

Thapalyal, L.: Smallpox; a grim saga, World Health 4-7, Oct., 1972.

Tigre, C. H. F., Martinez, A. V., and Fischmann, A.: Hemorrhagic smallpox caused by alastrim virus; report on a case in Rio Grande Do Sul, Brazil, Bulletin: The Pan American Health Organization **7**(3):26-28, 1973.

United States Public Health Service: Syphilis, Clinical Symposium **24**(3): 3-32, 1972.

Wellsteed, A. J.: The rubella problem, Nurs. Mirror **137**(12):34-35, Sept., 1973.

Witte, J.: A complete guide to immunization, Parents' Magazine Supplement, Nov., 1973.

World Health Organization: ABC of flu; 25 facts about influenza, Nurs. Mirror, **137**(18):39-40, Nov., 1973.

World Health Organization: Every country pays for smallpox, World Health 26-27, Oct., 1972.

World Health Organization: Facts, figures, pointers, World Health 18-19, May, 1974.

World Health Organization: Immunology, World Health 1-31, June, 1971.

World Health Organization: Ignorance and indifference; 25 facts about venereal diseases, Nurs. Mirror **138**(5):59, April, 1974.

World Health Organization: No beds for T.B.; 25 facts about tuberculosis, Nurs. Mirror **137**(16):46-47, Oct., 1973.

World Health Organization: Objective zero; 25 facts about smallpox, Nurs. Mirror **137**(13):23-24, Sept., 1973.

World Health Organization: The seventh pandemic; 25 facts about cholera, Nurs. Mirror **137**(17):26-27, Oct., 1973.

STATISTICS

Health and Welfare Division of Canada: Annual report of notifiable diseases—1972. Ottawa, 1972 Statistics Canada.

Health and Welfare Division of Canada: Notifiable diseases—weekly summary for 1974. Ottawa, 1974, Statistics Canada.

Health and Welfare Division of Canada: Selected notifiable diseases in the United States—weekly summary for 1974. Ottawa, 1974, Statistics Canada.

U. S. Department of Health, Education, and Welfare: Morbidity and mortality; annual supplement, summer 1972 and 1973, Atlanta, Georgia, 1973, Public Health Service Center for Disease Control.

APPENDIX A

Incubation periods

Disease	*Duration of incubation*
Asiatic cholera	24 hr. to 5 da.
Anthrax	2 to 4 da.; may be as long as 7 da.
Bacillary dysentery (Shigellosis)	1 to 7 da.; average of 4 da.
Blastomycosis	Unknown
Botulism (food poisoning)	Less than 24 hr.; several days after ingestion of food containing the toxin
Brucellosis (undulant fever)	5 to 30 da.
Chickenpox (varicella)	14 to 16 da.
Coccidioidomycosis (valley fever)	7 to 21 da.
Common cold	1 to 3 da.
Diarrhea, viral	3 to 5 da.
Diphtheria	2 to 6 da.; may be longer
Encephalitis	5 to 15 da.; range of 4 to 21 da.; varies as to the type
Food infection, *Salmonella*	7 to 72 hr.
Hansen's disease (leprosy, hansenosis)	Short as 5½ mo. or as long as 15 yr.; average about 5 yr.
Hepatitis	
Infectious (epidemic—virus A, catarrhal jaundice)	15 to 50 da.
Serum (virus B)	2 to 6 mo.
Herpes simplex (cold sore, fever blister)	2 to 12 da.; average of 4 da.
Herpes zoster (shingles)	4 to 24 da.; average of 4 da.
Histoplasmosis (Darling's disease)	5 to 18 da.; average of 10 da.
Infectious mononucleosis (glandular fever)	Children, less than 14 da.; adults, 33 to 49 da.; average period, 4 to 14 da.
Influenza, epidemic	24 to 72 hr.
Malaria	Varies with particular species; 12 to 14 da. or as long as 30 da.; some strains from 8 to 10 mo.
Measles (rubella, red measles)	9 to 14 da.; about 10 da. from exposure to onset of fever, and about 14 da. to appearance of rash

Continued.

Incubation periods—cont'd

Disease	*Duration of incubation*
Meningitis, bacterial	2 to 7 da.
Mumps (epidemic parotitis)	14 to 28 da.
Paratyphoid fever	1 to 10 da.
Pertussis (whooping cough)	5 to 21 da.
Plague (pasturella pestis)	
Bubonic	2 to 6 da.
Pneumonic	2 to 4 da.
Pneumococcal pneumonia, bacterial	1 to 3 da.
Poliomyelitis (infantile paralysis)	7 to 14 da.
Psittacosis (ornithosis, parrot fever)	4 to 15 da. but may vary from 5 to 28 da.; the commonest interval after exposure is 10 da.
Rabies (hydrophobia)	Dogs, 3 to 8 wk.; man, 10 da. to 2 yr. with an average of 2 to 6 wk.
Rocky Mountain spotted fever (tick fever)	2 to 12 da.; may be as long as 14 da.; average of 7 da.
Rubella (German measles)	14 to 21 da.; usually 18 da. after exposure
Scarlet fever (scarlatina) and septic sore throat	24 hr. to 10 da. but first clinical signs generally appear between 2 to 5 da.
Smallpox (variola)	7 to 16 da.; average of 12 da.
Tetanus	3 to 21 da.; average of 10 da.
Tularemia (rabbit fever)	1 to 10 da.; average of 3 da.
Typhoid fever	10 to 14 da.; may be as short as 7 da. or as long as 21 da.
Typhus fever	10 to 14 da.; variation depending on the size of the dose of the infecting organism
Venereal diseases: syphilis	10 to 90 da.; average of 3 to 4 wk.
gonorrhea	short as 2 to 10 da. or as long as 21 da.; average of 3 to 5 da.
Viral pneumonia (atypical pneumonia)	Varies widely, depending on specific virus; may be from a few days to a week or longer
Yellow fever	3 to 6 da.

APPENDIX B

Reservoirs of infection, source(s) of infection, and transmission

Disease	*Reservoir*	*Source(s)*	*Transmission*
Anthrax	Animals; soil	1. Contaminated animal hair, hides, wool, and tissue 2. Spores from contaminated soil 3. Improperly cooked meat and bones	1. Cutaneous—handling contaminated animal hair, hides, wool, or tissue 2. Pulmonary—inhaling spores from soil 3. Gastrointestinal—ingestion of contaminated or improperly cooked meat or bones 4. Commonest route—through wounds or skin abrasions
Asiatic cholera	Man	1. Feces of infectious patients 2. Convalescent carriers 3. Asymptomatic patients 4. Vomitus of infectious patients	1. Anal-oral route (feces)—poor hygiene 2. Contaminated water, milk, fruit, and vegetables
Atypical pneumonia, viral	Man	Respiratory secretions of infectious patient	1. Direct contact 2. Droplet infection 3. Indirect contact with contaminated articles
Bacillary dysentery (shigellosis)	Man	1. Feces, fingers, flies, contaminated milk, food, water, and fomites 2. Infectious patient 3. Carrier	1. Oral route—poor hygiene when in direct contact with infectious patients or articles; eating contaminated food, water, and milk 2. Direct or indirect contact with infected fomites 3. Vectors—flies 4. Contact with carriers

Continued.

Reservoirs of infection, source(s) of infection, and transmission—cont'd

Disease	*Reservoir*	*Source(s)*	*Transmission*
Bacterial pneumonia, pneumococcal	Man	Respiratory secretions of infectious patient	1. Direct contact with infectious patient 2. Direct contact with carriers 3. Indirect contact through droplets and fomites
Blastomycosis	Soil and dust	Spores of contaminated dust and soil	Not clearly understood; probably by inhalation of spores
Botulism (food poisoning)	1. Soil 2. Vegetable matter 3. Feces of domestic animals	Contaminated food	Ingestion of contaminated foods
Brucellosis (undulant fever)	Animals	1. Infected animals 2. Infected milk or milk products	1. Animals to man—not fully understood; probably through respiratory tract 2. Inoculation through cutaneous abrasions
Chickenpox (varicella)	Man	1. Discharge from skin lesions of infectious patient 2. Nose and throat secretions of infectious patients	1. Direct contact 2. Indirect contact 3. Airborne droplet infection
Cholera, Asiatic	See Asiatic cholera		
Coccidioidomycosis (valley fever)	Contaminated soil and dust	Fungus, spore laden soil and dust	Inhalation of spores
Cold sore (herpes simplex, fever blister)	Man	1. Infectious lesions of skin and mucosa of lips, mouth, and genitalia 2. Urine 3. Saliva	Close direct contact through kissing; coitus when genital lesions present
Darling's disease (histoplasmosis)	Soil, fungus	Soil contaminated with fungus produces spores	Inhaling airborne spores
Diarrhea, viral	Man	Feces of infectious patient	Not fully understood; probably through anal-oral route
Diphtheria	Man	1. Salivary and nasal discharges of infectious patient (respiratory tract infection) 2. Carriers	1. Direct or indirect contact 2. Most cases result from droplet or droplet nuclei infection from contact with a case or carrier

Disease	*Reservoir*	*Source(s)*	*Transmission*
Encephalitis	Mosquito	Animal to man (not man to man); infected mosquito	Transmitted to humans by bite of infected mosquito
Food infection, *Salmonella*	Man and animal	1. Contaminated food products 2. Human carriers	By feces of infected humans and animals
German Measles (rubella)	Man	1. Secretions from nose and throat of infectious patient; saliva 2. Urine from infectious patients	1. Direct contact 2. Airborne by droplets 3. Intimate personal contact 4. Indirect contact with fomites 5. Handling urine from infectious patients
Glandular fever (infectious mononucleosis)	Man	Saliva of infectious patient	1. Precise mode unknown 2. Direct contact; salivary interchange (kissing) 3. Eating and drinking from common utensils
Hansen's disease (leprosy, hansenosis)	Man	Lesions of skin; mucous membrane of upper respiratory tract	1. Contact with degenerative lesions of skin or mucous membrane of upper respiratory tract 2. Directly from person to person
Hepatitis, infectious and serum	Man	1. Feces (virus A) of in fectious patient 2. Blood and certain blood fractions (virus A and D)	*Infectious* 1. Person to person 2. Anal-oral route *Serum* 1. Transfusions with contaminated blood 2. Skin punctures with infected needles
Herpes zoster (shingles)	Man	Discharge from lesions of infectious patient	Appears to be the same as chickenpox and measles; method of transmission not fully understood
Hydrophobia (rabies)	Animals	Saliva of infectious animals	Bite of an infected animal where saliva may enter the wound
Influenza, epidemic	Man	Discharges from nose and throat of infectious patient	1. Not fully known 2. Probably through airborne droplet infection 3. Direct or indirect contact
Leprosy	See Hansen's disease		
Malaria	Man	Blood of infectious patient	1. Transmitted from man to mosquito (anopheles) when mosquito bites an infectious person

Continued.

Reservoirs of infection, source(s) of infection, and transmission—cont'd

Disease	*Reservoir*	*Source(s)*	*Transmission*
Malaria—cont'd			2. Bite of infected mosquito to man 3. Transmitted from man to man through blood transfusions or contaminated syringes and needles
Measles (rubeola or red)	Man	Respiratory tract secretions (nasal discharge) of infected patient	1. Direct contact 2. Airborne droplets and contaminated dust
Meningitis	Man	Nose and throat secretions; upper respiratory tract	1. Direct contact with droplet infection from nose and throat of infected person 2. Indirect contact with fomites
Mumps (parotitis)	Man	Respiratory tract secretions and urine of infectious patient	1. Direct contact 2. Droplet infection 3. Perhaps indirectly through contaminated fomites 4. Contact with urine of infectious patient
Paratyphoid fever	Man	Prepared food—meat, pies, synthetic milk, cream products, and shellfish	1. Resembles typhoid fever but much milder 2. Feces of infected patient
Parrot fever (psittacosis, ornithosis)	Birds	1. Infected birds—inoculation by bites from infected birds 2. Excreta of infected birds 3. Nose and mouth secretions of infectious patients	1. Transmission is animal to man, and man to man 2. Bites from infected birds 3. Contact of excreta from infected birds with open wounds 4. Inhalation of virus 5. Contact with nose and mouth secretions of infectious patient
Pertussis (whooping cough)	Man	Respiratory secretions of infectious patient	1. Droplet infection 2. Direct contact with infected person
Plague (Pasteurella pestis), bubonic and pneumonic	Rat flea	1. Respiratory secretions of infectious patient 2. Infected rat flea	1. Bubonic—to man by bite of rat flea; from man to man by droplet infection 2. Pneumonic—from man to man by droplet infection
Poliomyelitis (infantile paralysis)	Man	Pharyngeal and intestinal excretions of infectious patient	1. Enters through the mouth (oral contamination) 2. Direct contact 3. Droplet infection
Rabbit fever (tularemia)	Wild animals such as	1. Infected live animals 2. Infected animal tissue 3. Contaminated water	1. Animal to man (not from man to man)

Disease	*Reservoir*	*Source(s)*	*Transmission*
Rabbit fever—cont'd	rabbits, squirrels, and rodents		2. Bite of tick while handling infected animals 3. Ingestion of inadequately cooked rabbit food 4. Drinking water contaminated by rodents and other animals
Ringworm (tinea, superficial mycoses)	Fungus	Spores from fungus	Direct contact and indirect contact—through barbershops, clippers, brushes, combs, towels, swimming pools, lockers, and showers
Rocky Mountain spotted fever (tick fever)	Infected ticks	1. Infected tick 2. Tick feces 3. Tick tissue	1. Tick to man (not man to man) 2. Bite of infected tick 3. Contamination of skin with tick feces or tissue
Scarlet fever (scarlatina) and septic sore throat	Man	1. Oral and nasal secretions of patients and carriers 2. Purulent discharge from lymph nodes, ears, and other lesions	1. Direct contact 2. Indirect contact 3. Fomites 4. Droplet infection
Smallpox (variola)	Man	1. Oral and respiratory secretions of infectious patient 2. Lesions of skin and mucous membrane (pox fluid, scabs, or crusts) 3. Carriers (dead or alive)	1. Direct contact 2. Droplet infection 3. Indirect contact with contaminated fomites 4. Carried passively without causing disease by vaccinated person, patient, or even a corpse
Staphylococcus aureus infection	Man	Anterior nares, skin, and throat	1. Direct contact with infectious patient 2. Carriers 3. Dust, lint, fomites, pus
Tetanus	Soil	Intestines of certain herbivorous animals (feces)	Direct contact with open wound
Tuberculosis, pulmonary	Man and animal	Secretions from respiratory tract of infectious person	Inhaling tubercle bacilli from persons with active disease—coughing, sneezing, laughing.
Typhus fever, epidemic and murine	Louse and rat flea	1. Feces of louse 2. Infected rat flea	1. Direct contact—feces of louse enters open wound (epidemic typhus) 2. Murine typhus—bite of infected rat flea
Typhoid fever	Man	1. Feces and urine of infectious patients	Anal-oral route (bacilli must be swallowed)

Continued.

Reservoirs of infection, source(s) of infection, and transmission—cont'd

Disease	*Reservoir*	*Source(s)*	*Transmission*
Typhoid fever—cont'd		2. Feces and urine of carriers 3. Contaminated water, milk, and food products	
Venereal disease	Man	All infectious lesions	1. Intimate sexual contact including homosexual relationships; with the exception of a small number of congenital syphilis cases 2. Rare through contaminated articles 3. Blood transfusions or accidental inoculation
Yellow fever	Man and mosquito	Infected mosquito	1. Man to mosquito to man 2. Mosquito bites infected patient 3. Infected mosquito bites man

APPENDIX C

Reported cases of specified notifiable diseases per year in the United States and Canada between 1971 and 1974

Disease	*1971*	*1972*	*1973*	*1974*	*Comment*
Anthrax					
U. S.	5	2	2	‡	
Canada					
Asiatic cholera					
U. S.			1		
Canada				1	
Atypical pneumonia, viral					
U. S.*					
Canada*					
Bacillary dysentery (Shigellosis)					
U. S.	16,143	20,207	23,818	‡	
Canada	1350	1290	1912	2369	
Bacterial pneumonia, pneumococcal					
U. S.*					
Canada*					
Blastomycosis					
U. S.†	‡	45	39	‡	Reported by 11 states
Canada*					

*Not notifiable
†Optionally reported
‡Not available at writing of this book
From Statistics Canada: Annual report of notifiable diseases, Ottawa, 1972, 1973, and 1974, Health and Welfare Division, and Center for Disease Control: Morbidity and mortality; annual supplement—summary 1972 and 1973, Atlanta, Georgia. U. S. Department of Health, Education and Welfare.

Continued.

Reported cases of specified notifiable diseases per year in the United States and Canada between 1971 and 1974—cont'd

Disease	*1971*	*1972*	*1973*	*1974*	*Comment*
Botulism (food poisoning)					
U. S.	25	22	34	25	
Canada	10	9	7	9	
Brucellosis (undulant fever)					
U. S.	183	196	202	181	
Canada	8	16	7	24	
Chickenpox (varicella)					
U. S.	‡	164,114	182,927	‡	
Canada*					
Coccidioidomycosis (valley fever)					
U. S.†	‡	951	436	‡	1972—Reported by 13 states 1973—Reported by 12 states
Canada*					
Cold sore (herpes simplex, fever blister)					
U. S.†					
Canada*					
Darling's disease (histoplasmosis)					
U. S.†	‡	226	284	‡	1972—Reported by 16 states 1973—Reported by 22 states
Canada*					
Diarrhea, viral					
U. S.†					
Canada*					
Diphtheria					
U. S.	215	152	282	240	
Canada	75	69	169	174	
Encephalitis					
U. S.	1580	1524	1509	‡	
Canada		8	‡	‡	
Food Infection *Salmonella*					
U. S.	21,928	22,151	23,818	21,450	
Canada	1729	796	849	255	
German measles (Rubella)					
U. S.	45,086	25,507	27,804	11,654	
Canada	12,567	2808	3296	7705	

Disease	*1971*	*1972*	*1973*	*1974*	*Comment*
Glandular fever (infectious mononucleosis)					
U. S.†	‡	14,178	12,833	‡	1972—Reported by 35 states 1973—Reported by 32 states
Canada*					
Hansen's disease (leprosy or Hansenosis)					
U. S.	131	130	146	151	
Canada	9	10	15	11	
Hepatitis					
Infectious					
U. S.	59,606	54,074	50,749	47,908	
Canada	8682	7344	6664	5316	
Serum					
U. S.	9556	9402	8451	9574	
Canada	102	467	541	328	
Herpes Zoster (shingles)					
U. S.†					
Canada*					
Hydrophobia (rabies)					
U. S.	1	2	1		
Canada					
Influenza epidemic					
U. S.†					
Canada*					
Malaria					
U. S.	2375	742	237	255	
Canada	7	7	24	36	
Measles (Rubeola or red)					
U. S.	75,290	32,275	26,690	21,726	
Canada	7454	3136	10,840	11,932	
Meningitis					
U. S.	5176	4634	2510	1297	
Canada	209	361	436	352	
Mumps (parotitis)					
U. S.	124,939	74,215	69,612	54,895	
Canada*					
Ornithosis (parrot fever, psittacosis)					
U. S.	32	52	33	22	
Canada	3	6	2		

Continued.

Reported cases of specified notifiable diseases per year in the United States and Canada between 1971 and 1974—cont'd

Disease	*1971*	*1972*	*1973*	*1974*	*Comment*
Paratyphoid fever					
U. S.*					
Canada	24	53	46	69	
Pertussis (whooping cough)					
U. S.	3036	3287	1759	1689	
Canada	3002	1297	969	1555	
Plague (pasteurellis pestis)					
U. S.	2	1	2		
Canada					
Poliomyelitis (infantile paralysis)					
U. S.	21	31	8	5	
Canada	1	2	5	3	
Rabbit fever (tularemia)					
U. S.	187	152	171	135	
Canada	1		1	7	
Ringworm (tinea, superficial mycoses)					
U. S.†	‡	1226	953	‡	1972—Reported by 18 states 1973—Reported by 14 states
Canada	103	16	43	7	
Rocky Mountain spotted fever (tick fever)					
U. S.	432	523	668	765	
Canada		1			
Rubella syndrome, congenital					
U. S.	68	42	31	47	
Canada*					
Scarlet fever and septic sore throat					
U. S.†	‡	421,517	474,212	‡	
Canada	10,814	12,224	15,694	20,114	
Smallpox (variola)					
U. S.					
Canada					
Staphylococcus aureus					
U. S.†	‡	724	574	‡	1972—Reported by 4 states 1973—Reported by 5 states
Canada*					

Disease	*1971*	*1972*	*1973*	*1974*	*Comment*
Tetanus					
U. S.	116	128	101	93	
Canada	6	3	3	6	
Tuberculosis, pulmonary					
U. S.	35,217	39,932	31,015	‡	
Canada	3943	3909	1875	‡	
Typhus fever (epidemic and murine)					
U. S.	23	18	32	‡	
Canada					
Typhoid fever					
U. S.	407	398	680	414	
Canada	99	108	101	116	
Venereal diseases					
Syphilis					
U. S.	95,997	91,149	87,469	24,080	
Canada	2489	3064	3764	3658	
Congenital syphilis					
U. S.	2052	1758	1527	‡	
Canada*		41			
Gonorrhea					
U. S.	670,268	767,215	842,621	882,590	
Canada	34,405	41,467	45,266	46,760	
Yellow fever					
U. S.					
Canada					

INDEX

D